PREVENTING PROSTATE CANCER
Screening versus Chemoprevention

CANCER SURVEYS

Advances and Prospects in Clinical, Epidemiological and Laboratory Oncology

Published for the

Imperial Cancer Research Fund

PREVENTING PROSTATE CANCER
Screening versus Chemoprevention
Pros and Cons Based on New Views of Its Biology, Early Events and Clinical Behaviour

Guest Editors
R T D Oliver
A Belldegrun
P F M Wrigley

COLD SPRING HARBOR LABORATORY PRESS 1995

CANCER SURVEYS
Preventing Prostate Cancer: Screening versus Chemoprevention
Volume 23

Published by Cold Spring Harbor Laboratory Press
Printed in the United States of America
ISBN 0-87969-466-1
ISSN 0261-2429

Cover and book design by Leon Bolognese & Associates, Inc.

All Cold Spring Harbor Laboratory Press publications may be ordered directly from Cold Spring Harbor Laboratory Press, 10 Skyline Drive, Plainview, New York 11803-9729. Phone: Continental US & Canada 1-800-843-4388; all other locations (516) 349-1930. FAX: (516) 349-1946.

Contents

Preface

The Prostate Cancer Charitable Trust was formed to foster discussion and the exchange of ideas between clinicians and other research workers. The trustees felt that prostate cancer had not received the same attention as many other cancers. Only now is interest awakening in the common disease.

Mr Clive Bourne conceived the idea to set up a series of meetings and publications after the manner of the Helen Harris Trust in Ovarian Cancer. This book is the result of the first of the meetings about prostate cancer held in Cambridge in April 1994.

For those of us who were there it was a lively occasion in a town with a great tradition of debate and new thought. Useful contacts were made between people in different fields from across the globe. This book is the result of those encounters.

We particularly thank Mrs Shirley Claff for her organizing skills, Sir Walter Bodmer for his help in facilitating this meeting and Dr Eric Sidebottom for his hard work in organizing the meeting with Mrs Claff. We also thank Zeneca for their support of this meeting and the Trust.

P F M Wrigley

Introduction

R T D OLIVER[1] • A BELLDEGRUN[2] • P F M WRIGLEY[3]

[1]*Royal London Hospital Medical College, 1 Turner Street, London E1 2A;*[2]*UCLA Division of Urology, Department of Surgery, UCLA School of Medicine, Los Angeles, CA;*[3]*134 Harley Street, London W1A 1AH*

INTRODUCTION

With bowel and lung cancer declining in young men because of increased consumption of dietary fibre and a reduction in smoking, prostate cancer is becoming the most significant malignant cause of death in terms of rate of increase and numbers after lung cancer. However, most patients present after age 70 and most men have some evidence of "latent" malignant cells in the prostate after death from other causes at the age of 80. It has been estimated that four of five patients treated by radical surgery in the USA would not have died of their disease, even if they had not been operated on. This has been a major factor in the scepticism about radical treatment of such patients. However, the death rate is increasing, and under the age of 65 just over 1000 men a year are dying in the UK. Overall in 1992, prostate cancer was responsible for 72 000 lost years of life compared with 226 000 from breast cancer and 35 000 from cancer of the cervix.

This publication, arising out of a meeting organized by the Prostate Cancer Charitable Trust, sets out to refocus attention on the biology of prostate cancer and its treatment. The relative merits of screening versus chemoprevention as long term strategies for reducing deaths was the primary concern of the meeting and particular attention has been paid to the following areas.

WHEN ARE ATYPICAL PROSTATIC CELLS MALIGNANT?

With increasing numbers of markers of malignancy, such as androgen receptor loss, basic fibroblast growth factor, collagenase, mutated oncogenes and de-

Cancer Surveys Volume 23: *Preventing Prostate Cancer: Screening versus Chemoprevention*

leted suppresser genes, pathologists have better tools to differentiate "latent" and clinically significant malignancy. Chapters by Bostwick, Isaacs *et al,* Chung and Wilding develop this theme.

EPIDEMIOLOGY

Genetic Defects and the Possibilities of Gene Therapy

Although familial cancers are relatively rare, it is increasingly recognized that discovery of the genes involved in the rare familial cases helps in understanding how to look for those genes that are damaged in tumours arising in patients without a family history. Until recently, prostate cancer was not recognized as one of the tumours with a genetic component. There are now several reports showing that this has been due to a failure of data collection because the age of those men who have prostate cancer leads to poor recall of family history. Research is continuing to determine if it is possible to identify target genes whose defects could be corrected by gene therapy, and these efforts are reviewed in the chapters by Isaacs *et al,* Chung and Taneja *et al.*

Diet, Exercise, Smoking and Other Stress Related Factors in Preventing the Occurrence and Progression of Prostate Cancer

It is now accepted that a substantial proportion of patients with prostate cancer can have long periods of stable disease without tumour progression. Given the undesirable effects of hormone and surgical treatment, there could be considerable benefit from identifying self help factors in patients with slow growing tumours. There is mounting evidence that increasing vitamin A levels, regular exercise, stopping smoking even in non-smoking related cancers and stress relief programmes can slow the progression of some cancers. As yet, these issues have not been fully explored in prostate cancer, although the chapters by Key, Sitas and Cuzick review the limited data on these and other epidemiological aspects of the disease.

Virology and Geographical Epidemiology

The limited mainly negative literature on the HPV related virology of prostate cancer is reviewed by Cuzick. The parallel escalation of cervical and prostate cancer in Africa, particularly in the setting of the HIV epidemic, provides added interest in exploring the virology of prostate cancer in younger patients in different geographical settings with a high (such as Africa) and low (such as Israel) incidence of cervical cancer. Reports from high and low incidence areas of the world, reviewing these issues, are included in the chapters by Sitas, DeAntoni, Oishi *et al,* Kehinde, Brenner *et al* and Newling.

CLINICAL TRIALS

Two extremes of view exist with regard to clinical trials, that of the therapeutic nihilist whose aim is to postpone treatment as long as possible and that of the active interventionist. In both metastatic disease, covered in the chapters by Smith, Kirk, Oliver and Gallagher, Kehinde *et al,* Rosen and Belldegrun, and primary disease, covered in the chapters by Parkes, Adolfsson, Labrie *et al* and Schmid, this debate is pursued, and in the chapters by Oliver, Blandy and deKernion *et al*, a new agenda for the next decade is defined.

Pathology, Molecular Biology and Epidemiology of Prostate Cancer

The Pathology of Incidental Carcinoma

DAVID G BOSTWICK
Department of Pathology, Mayo Clinic, Rochester, MN 55905

INTRODUCTION

Prostate cancer is the most common cancer among men in the USA and second only to lung cancer as a cause of cancer death. It is estimated that 38 000 men died of prostate cancer in 1994 and 200 000 new cases were diagnosed (Boring *et al,* 1994). Although the majority of prostatic cancers grow relatively slowly and never become clinically manifest, the clinical course is often unpredictable in its speed of progression, perhaps because of the marked heterogeneity of histological grade and other factors that influence tumour growth. Despite an autopsy prevalence of up to 80% by age 80 years, the clinical incidence is much lower, indicating that most men die with prostate cancer rather than of prostate cancer. Little is known about the causes of prostate cancer despite the high incidence and prevalence (Morra and Das, 1993). The prevalence of incidental cancer is similar in different geographic and ethnic groups, despite wide variation in clinical incidence (Morra and Das, 1993).

Different regions of the prostate are sampled by transurethral resection (TURP) and needle biopsy (McNeal *et al,* 1988a), and specimens consist of tissue from the transition zone, urethra, periurethral area, bladder neck and anterior fibromuscular stroma. The resection does not usually include tissue from the central or peripheral zones, and not all of the transition zone is removed (Epstein *et al,* 1988; McNeal *et al,* 1988a,b; Greene *et al,* 1991a,b). Most needle biopsy specimens consist of tissue from the peripheral zone, seldom including the central or transition zones.

Well differentiated cancer found incidentally at TURP usually arises in the transition zone (McNeal *et al,* 1988a). These tumours are frequently small and

TABLE 1. Comparison of staging systems for prostate cancer

Pathological stage	American	TNM[a,b]
Non-palpable cancer		
≤5% of TURP tissue[c]	A_1	T_{1a}
>5% of TURP tissue[c]	A_2	T_{1b}
Cancer detected by biopsy (eg elevated PSA)	B_0	T_{1c}
Palpable or visible cancer clinically confined within the capsule		
≤Half of one lobe	B_1	T_{2a}
>Half of one lobe, but not both sides	B_1	T_{2b}
Both lobes	B_2	T_{2c}
Cancer with local extracapsular extension		
Unilateral	C_1	T_{3a}
Bilateral	C_1	T_{3b}
Seminal vesicle invasion	C_2	T_{3c}
Invasion of bladder neck, rectum or external sphincter	C_2	T_{4a}
Invasion of levator muscle or pelvic wall	C_2	T_{4b}
Metastatic cancer		
Single regional lymph node ≤2 cm in greater dimension	D_1	N_1[d]
Single regional lymph node 2–5 cm, or multiple regional lymph nodes ≤5 cm	D_1	N_2
Single regional lymph node >5 cm	D_1	N_3
Distant metastasis	D_2	M_1
Non-regional lymph node(s)	D_2	M_{1a}
Bone(s)	D_2	M_{1b}
Other sites	D_2	M_{1c}

[a] N_0 or N_xM_0 for T_1-T_4

[b] Stage groupings for TNM staging systems (G = grade on 1–4 scale):

Stage 0	T_{1a}	N_0	M_0	G_1
Stage I	T_{1a}	N_0	M_0	$G_{2,3,4}$
	T_{1b}	N_0	M_0	Any G
	T_{1c}	N_0	M_0	Any G
	T_1	N_0	M_0	Any G
Stage II	T_2	N_0	M_0	Any G
Stage III	T_3	N_0	M_0	Any G
Stage IV	T_4	N_0	M_0	Any G
	Any T	$N_{1,2,3}$	M_0	Any G
	Any T	Any N	M_1	Any G

[c] Different definitions exist for substaging A_1 and A_2 cancers

[d] N_x: regional lymph nodes not assessable; M_x: distant metastasis not assessable

may be completely resected by TURP. Poorly differentiated cancer in TURP chips usually represents part of a larger tumour that has invaded the transition zone from the peripheral zone. This chapter describes the pathology of incidental prostate cancer and its role in predicting outcome of patients with stage T_1 carcinoma.

DETECTION OF INCIDENTAL CARCINOMA

Clinical Detection and Staging

Current staging of early prostate cancer stratifies patients according to the method of tumour detection, separating non-palpable "incidental" cancers detected during TURP for clinically benign prostatic hyperplasia (American [Jewett-Whitmore] A; TNM T_1) from palpable cancers detected by digital rectal examination (American [Jewett-Whitmore] B; TNM T_2) (Table 1) (Shroder *et al,* 1992; Bostwick *et al,* 1994). The term "latent" is inaccurate because it describes cancer of low malignant potential, and "occult" describes metastatic cancer with unknown site of primary. About 10% of TURP specimens are incidentally found to contain carcinoma.

Current staging systems are based in part on a poor prognostic factor (method of cancer detection) that has little biological significance and utilizes digital rectal examination, a method with low sensitivity, low specificity and low positive predictive value (Friedman *et al,* 1991). Patients are separated into stages that have considerable overlap in natural history and are treated similarly. Attempts to correct these failings by separating cancer into two distinct groups according to the number of tumour foci present on TURP (T_{1a}: three or fewer foci; T_{1b}: more than three foci) have created a subset of low stage incidental cancer (T_{1b}), which frequently has a greater tumour burden and is clinically more aggressive than higher stage palpable cancer (T_{2a}). Paulson (1989) concluded that "Stage A (T_{1a}) disease is merely an artifact of detection and that patient management should be a function of identified disease (volume) and projected duration of risk". The 1992 revision of the TNM system created a new category (T_{1c}), defined as tumour identified by needle biopsy following elevated serum prostate specific antigen (PSA) level (Shroder, 1992). Recent studies indicate that this new stage identifies a heterogeneous population of patients and therefore fails to assist in stratification of patients for therapy (Table 2) (Oesterling *et al,* 1993; Epstein *et al,* 1994).

Clinical understaging of incidental carcinoma can be a significant problem. The sensitivity of TURP in detecting stage A carcinoma is only 28%; among patients with stage A_1 carcinoma, between 40% and 92% will have residual carcinoma and about 26% will be upstaged (Epstein *et al,* 1988; Greene *et al,* 1991a,b). Even in those with substantial residual tumour, the location of the tumour in the peripheral and apical regions of the prostate often makes it inaccessible to TURP. The aggregate results challenge the usefulness of examining TURP specimens to stage prostatic carcinoma; nevertheless, at present, there is no reasonable alternative method for staging incidental carcinoma.

Pathological Staging

Numerous methods have been developed to measure tumour volume in incidental prostate cancer, including TURP chip counting, estimation of the area ratio on the chips, estimation of the volume, comparison of the ratio of benign to malignant chips, comparison of the ratio of malignant chips to total chips using a volume-base "grid" method, and cancer foci counting (Table 3) (Bostwick and Choi, 1992). The "eyeball" estimate of tumour volume correlates well with morphometrically determined measures, and the predictive

TABLE 2. Pathological characteristics of prostate cancer clinical stage T1c, T2a and T2b[a]

Variable	Stage T_{1c}	Stages T_{2a} and T_{2b}
Tumour volume[b] (cm^3)	6.4 (range: 0.03–56)	5.2 (range: 0.01–98)
Maximum diameter[b] (cm)	2.1 (range: 0.1–5.0)	2.0 (range: 0.3–6.8)
Focality		
Unifocal	152 (73%)	162 (78%)
Multifocal	56 (27%)	46 (22%)
Gleason score		
2–4	48 (23%)	42 (20%)
5–6	124 (60%)	128 (62%)
7–10	36 (17%)	38 (18%)
DNA ploidy		
Diploid	153 (74%)	153 (74%)
Tetraploid	27 (13%)	30 (14%)
Aneuploid	11 (5%)	9 (4%)
Not interpretable	17 (8%)	16 (8%)
Pathological stage		
Organ confined	110 (53%)	115 (55%)
Capsular perforation	74 (35%)	75 (36%)
Seminal vesicle invasion	18 (9%)	14 (7%)
Pelvic lymph node involvement	6 (3%)	4 (2%)
Surgical margins		
Negative	138 (66%)	156 (75%)
Microscopic involvement	66 (32%)	51 (24.5%)
Macroscopic involvement	4 (2%)	1 (0.5%)
Prostate gland size[b] (cm^3)	57 (range: 20–290)	47 (range: 20–110)
Predominant tumour location		
Peripheral zone	179 (86%)	199 (96%)
Transition and/or central zone	19 (9%)	6 (3%)

[a]From Oesterling *et al* (1993) with permission from WB Saunders Company
[b]Mean value

power is similar to that of other methods of tumour quantitation. In addition, the percent tumour is slightly more predictive of tumour progression than absolute tumour volume for stage T_1 and T_2 cancers. The TNM staging system recommends the area ratio estimation method, using 5% or less of the specimen area as the cutpoint for identification of aggressive cancer.

The optimal number of TURP chips to submit for histological evaluation remains controversial, with some experts advocating complete submission even with large specimens that would require many tissue cassettes (Eble and Tejada, 1986; Murphy *et al,* 1986; Vollmer, 1986; Rohr, 1987). The Cancer Committee of the College of American Pathologists recommends a minimum of six cassettes for the first 30 g of tissue and one cassette for every 10 g thereafter (Henson *et al,* 1994).

TABLE 3. Methods of defining prostate cancer substages A_1 and A_2

Method	Description	Advantages	Disadvantages
TURP chip counting	Stage A_1: Fewer than 3 chips involved Stage A_2: More than 3 involved	Simple to use, popular	Few supporting studies for 3 chip threshold, cannot apply to enucleation specimens
Area ratio estimation	Stage A_1: 5% or less of specimen area	Simple to use, strong empirical support, used in 1992 revision of TNM system	Incompatible with current concepts of cancer risk factors, supporting studies only from one institution (Johns Hopkins)
Volume estimate	Stage A_1: 1 cm^3 or less Stage A_2: Greater than 1 cm^3 cancer volume	Theoretically sound, modest empirical support	Requires measurement and calculation, based on volume
TURP chip ratio	Ratio of benign to malignant chips in TURP specimens	Simple to use, low interobserver variability, correlates with prognosis	Does not lend itself to two tier A_1–A_2 substaging, cannot apply to enucleation specimens
TURP chip grid ratio	Ratio of malignant to total "grids" in TURP specimens	Simple to use, slightly better than area ratio estimation method	Requires grid or ruler, recently introduced, does not lend itself to two tier A_1–A_2 substaging
Cancer foci counting	Stage A_1 (T_{1a}): 3 or fewer microscopic foci Stage A_2 (T_{1b}): More than 3 foci of cancer	Simple to use, used in TNM system (until 1992)	"Foci" not defined, same problems as area ratio estimation method, addition of grade to T_{1a} and T_{1b} to obtain final stage in TNM system is awkward (T_{1a} and low grade = stage 0, T_{1a} and higher grade = stage I, T_{1b} with any grade is stage II)

PATHOLOGY OF INCIDENTAL CARCINOMA

Transition zone origin accounts for about 24% of all prostate cancers, but 78% of stage T_1 cancers originate in this zone, including 75% of stage T_{1a} and 79% of stage T_{1b} cancers (Table 4) (Greene *et al,* 1991a; Bostwick *et al,* 1992). The high percentage of incidental cancer in the transition zone is probably due to selective sampling by TURP, and up to 30% of stage T_1 tumours could theoretically be removed completely by TURP (Epstein *et al,* 1988; McNeal *et al,* 1988b; Greene *et al,* 1991a,b; Bostwick *et al,* 1992). The majority of transi-

TABLE 4. Prostatic carcinoma: comparison based on anatomical site of origin[a,b]

Variable	Transition zone cancer	Peripheral zone cancer
Incidence		
Stage A_1	75%	–
Stage A_2	79%	–
All stage A	78%	–
All stages	24%	70%
Origin		
In or near BPH	Yes	No
Near apex	Yes	Yes
Detection rate by TURP	78%	–
Pathological features		
Tumour volume	Usually small	Small to large
Tumour pattern	Alveolar-medullary	Tubular-scirrhous
Tumour grade (Gleason)	Usually 1 or 2	Usually 2, 3 or 4
Clear cell pattern	Most cases	Rare
Stromal fibrosis	Uncommon	Common
Associated putative pre-malignant changes	AAH or PIN	PIN
Aneuploidy	6%	31%
Clinical behaviour		
Extracapsular extension	11%	44%
Site of extracapsular extension	Anterolateral and apical	Lateral
Average tumour size with extracapsular extension	4.98 cm^3	3.86 cm^3
Risk of seminal vesicle invasion	0%	19%
Risk of lymph node metastases	Low	High

[a]Central zone cancers (5–10% of total) were excluded
[b]From Bostwick *et al* (1992) with permission from JB Lippincott Company

tion zone cancers arise in foci adjacent to benign prostatic hyperplasia (BPH), with about a third arising within BPH nodules; most are multifocal.

Transition zone cancer appears to be morphologically and biologically distinct from cancer arising in the peripheral zone (Epstein *et al,* 1988; McNeal *et al,* 1988b; Greene *et al,* 1991a,b; Bostwick *et al,* 1992). It tends to be better differentiated and accounts for the majority of Gleason primary grade 1 and 2 cancers (Fig. 1). Tumour volume tends to be smaller than that of tumours arising in the peripheral zone, although frequent exceptions are noted. Furthermore, most transition zone cancers display a distinctive columnar clear cell pattern, which is infrequently observed in peripheral zone cancers; there is also decreased stromal fibrosis.

The confinement of transition zone cancer to the site of origin may account in part for the favourable prognosis of clinical stage T_1 cancer. The transition zone boundary acts as a relative barrier to tumour extension, and malignant glands frequently fan out along this boundary before invasion into the peripheral and central zones. Transition zone tumours preferentially

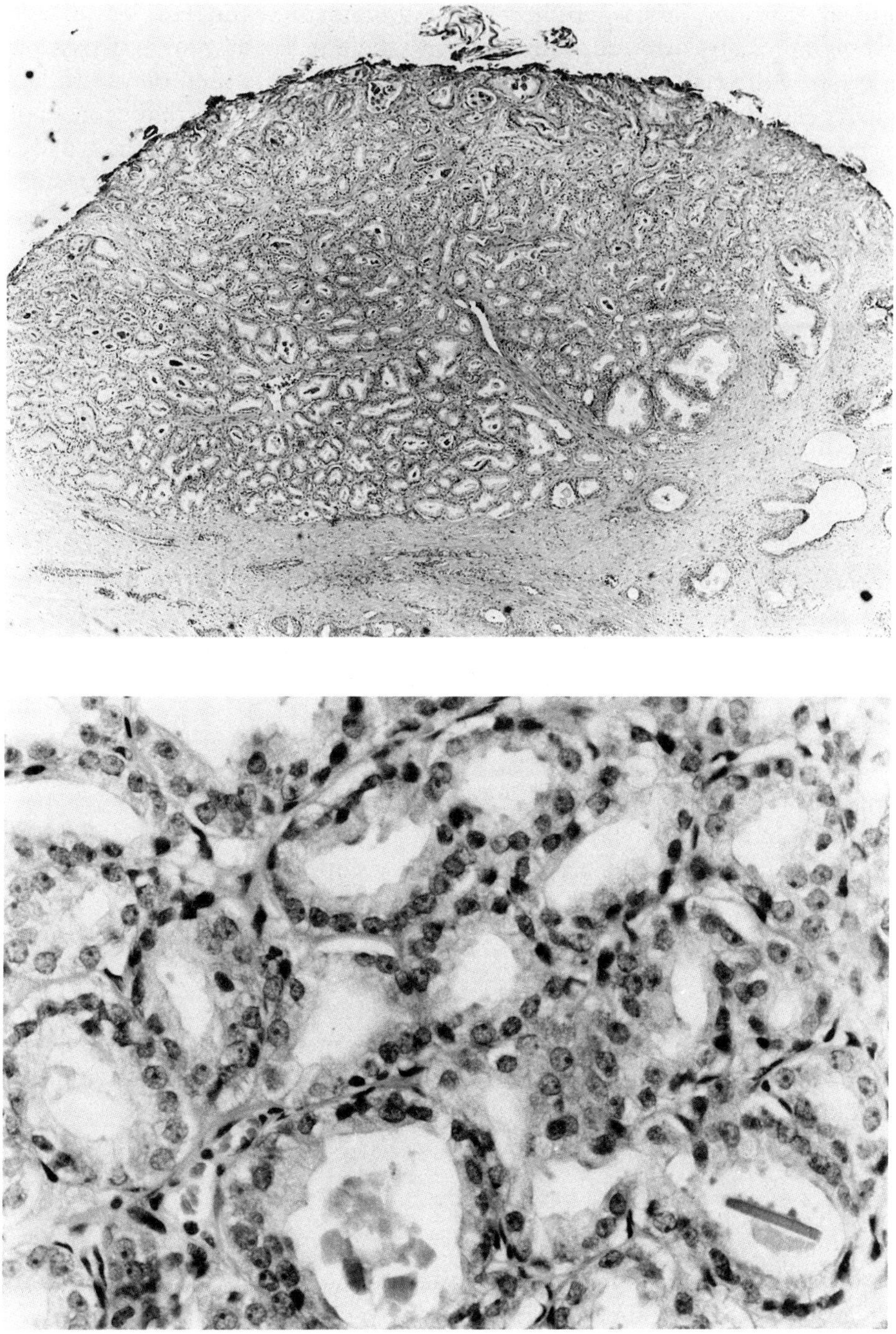

Fig. 1. Well differentiated adenocarcinoma (Gleason 1+1) arising in the transition zone in a TURP specimen. (A) At low magnification, the tumour is circumscribed, contains uniform glands and may be mistaken for benign prostatic hyperplasia. In B, the neoplastic glands display features of malignancy, including nucleomegaly, nucleolomegaly and rare luminal crystalloids (bottom right)

cluster at the apex, as do peripheral zone tumours, but they are less likely to show extraprostatic extension. Invasion into the anterior fibromuscular stroma can occur with small volume tumours, but perforation is seen only with large tumours (Bostwick, 1994). Twenty-five percent of transition zone cancers display capsular perforation or anterior fibromuscular stromal invasion, usually in the anterolateral and apical directions, where the distance from the capsule is short. The risk of spread to the seminal vesicles and regional lymph nodes is significantly less than with peripheral zone cancer.

Association between Incidental Carcinoma and Benign Prostatic Hyperplasia

There are a number of similarities between BPH and cancer (Bostwick *et al*, 1992). Both display a parallel increase in prevalence with age according to autopsy studies, although clinical cancer lags by 15–20 years. Both require androgens for growth and development, and both may respond to androgen deprivation treatment. Most cancers arise in prostates with concomitant BPH, and cancer is found incidentally in a significant number (10%) of transurethral prostatectomy specimens. Benign prostatic hyperplasia may be related to prostate cancer arising in the transition zone, perhaps in association with certain forms of hyperplasia, but BPH is neither a premalignant lesion nor a precursor of carcinoma.

Association between Incidental Carcinoma and Putative Premalignant Lesions

Two potential morphological precursors of adenocarcinoma have recently been identified, referred to as prostatic intraepithelial neoplasia (PIN) and atypical adenomatous hyperplasia (AAH) (Bostwick and Srigley, 1990). These lesions display some of the features of carcinoma, but PIN lacks stromal invasiveness and AAH lacks significant cytological atypia. High grade PIN is commonly found in association with invasive cancer in the peripheral zone, and the high predictive value of this lesion suggests that further search for carcinoma be made in cases in which high grade PIN is found on biopsy. Atypical adenomatous hyperplasia is also found in association with carcinoma but not as commonly as PIN.

Foci of AAH are usually found in the periurethral area and transition zone, occurring in 20% of prostates with BPH (Bostwick DG and Qian J, unpublished). PIN is present in the transition zone in 2–8% of TURP specimens and up to 37% of radical prostatectomies (Qian *et al*, in press).

Numerous studies suggest that AAH is a precursor of transition zone carcinoma, although no direct evidence has been found (Bostwick *et al*, 1993). Firstly, AAH shares many of the features of well differentiated adenocarcinoma, including cytological abnormalities (enlarged nucleoli) and architectural abnormalities (glandular proliferation and discontinuity of the basal cell

TABLE 5. Long term follow-up of patients with untreated clinical stage T1a (A1) adenocarcinoma of prostate

Reference	Method of defining stage T_{1a} (A_1)	Mean age in years (range)	Mean follow-up in years (range)	Progression (%)	Mean time to progression in years (range)
Thompson and Zeidman (1989)	Cancer foci counting	NA	7.5% (1–20)	3/37 (8%)	8.7 (2–19)
Zhang *et al* (1991)	Area ratio estimation	NA	8.2 (5–23)	12/132 (10%)	7 (0.5–20)
Lowe and Listrom (1988)	Area ratio estimation	NA (46–99)	NA	12/80 (15%)	13.5 (1–26.5)
Orestano (1991)	Cancer foci counting	72 (59–87)	9	11/30 (37%)	7
Epstein *et al* (1986)	Area ratio estimation	65 (50–87)	10 (8–18)	8/50 (16%)	7 (3.5–8)
Blute *et al* (1986)	Volume estimation	55 (48–59)	12.2 (10–25)	4/15 (27%)	10.2 (9–19)

NA: Data not given

layer). Secondly, the age of peak incidence of AAH precedes that of carcinoma by 5–15 years. Thirdly, AAH is increased in frequency in the presence of carcinoma, suggesting that this lesion has some predictive value for malignancy. Finally, the frequency of cell proliferation is higher in AAH than in normal prostate, similar to that of well differentiated adenocarcinoma. Most authors consider AAH to be a marker for the development of adenocarcinoma and suggest that the association of AAH with carcinoma is an epiphenomenon.

CLINICAL SIGNIFICANCE AND TREATMENT OF INCIDENTAL CARCINOMA

The clinical significance of incidental carcinoma remains controversial. Recent studies indicate an increasing long term risk for developing clinical carcinoma, progression and death in patients with stage A_1 tumours (Table 5) (Blute *et al,* 1986; Epstein *et al,* 1986; Lowe and Listrom, 1988; Thompson and Zeidman, 1989; Orestano, 1991; Zhang *et al,* 1991). Epstein *et al* (1986) reported a series of 94 men with untreated stage A_1 carcinoma identified by TURP; in patients followed for more than 8 years, 16% developed progression, with a mean time to progression of 7 years. Blute *et al* (1986) found progression in 27% of 15 patients under 60 years of age with stage A_1 carcinoma followed for 10 years or more. These two studies and others indicate that patients with stage T_{1a} prostate cancer are at risk for tumour progression.

Clinical progression is more likely with stage T_{1b} than with stage T_{1a} cancer. Residual carcinoma is usually found in prostatectomy specimens from patients with stage T_{1b} carcinoma, with capsular perforation in up to 19% of cases. Most urologists treat stage T_{1b} cancer aggressively, particularly when it is detected in younger patients (Scardino *et al*, 1992; Matzkin *et al*, 1994).

The single most significant question in treating "incidental" adenocarcinoma is how to separate tumours that will progress from those which will not progress during the expected lifetime of the patient. Important prognostic factors include the patient's age, tumour location (peripheral zone v. transition zone), tumour grade, tumour volume and serum PSA level and morphometric factors such as nuclear roundness. Studies directed at early detection allow discovery of increasingly smaller cancers (Mettlin *et al*, 1991). However, in the zeal to detect cancer in an organ confined ("curable") stage, early detection efforts may uncover a large number of innocuous tumours that would probably not be otherwise clinically detected during the patient's lifetime. Efforts should thus be directed at defining the natural history of individual tumours.

It is difficult to compare precisely the efficacy of different treatments and outcomes in prostate cancer because of the significant clinical staging error, the paucity of rigorous prospective and randomized clinical trials and the lengthy follow up needed to obtain results with a relatively slow growing tumour such as prostate cancer. The 10 year cancer specific survival for all stages of cancer is about 51%, with an estimated "cure" rate of 32% (Scardino *et al*, 1992). Clinically localized cancer has the most favourable outcome. Long term progression for untreated stage T_{1a} cancer varies from 8% to 37%, with the risk of progression increasing with additional years of follow-up; survival at 10 years is 95%, similar to the age specific survival, prompting the suggestion that treatment for this stage may be unnecessary. Larger organ confined cancers (T_{1b} and T_2) and those with local extraprostatic extension (T_3 and T_4) show progressively lower survival and "cure" rates, and the worst outcomes are observed with cancers metastatic to regional lymph nodes ($T_{1\text{-}4}N + M_0$; 40% survival at 10 years) and distant organs (M+; 10% survival).

SUMMARY

"Incidental" cancer refers to predominantly well differentiated cancer that arises in the transition zone and is found by chance in TURP chips. These tumours are frequently small and may be completely resected by TURP, although a significant number have an additional tumour that is unreachable with a resectoscope. These tumours often co-exist with benign prostatic hyperplasia. Putative precursors of incidental carcinoma include high grade PIN and AAH, and these lesions are frequently found in the transition zone in prostatectomies for cancer. The single most significant question in treating incidental adenocarcinoma is how to separate tumours that will progress from those that will not progress during the expected lifetime of the patient. The 1992 revision of the TNM staging system separated non-aggressive (T_{1a}) and aggressive (T_{1b}) incidental cancer according to the number of foci of cancer, using more than three foci as the cutpoint to identify more aggressive cancer.

However, 8–37% of patients with T_1 a cancer will develop cancer progression within 10 years if untreated, with the risk of progression increasing with additional years of follow-up. Important prognostic factors include the patient's age, tumour location (peripheral zone v. transition zone), tumour grade, tumour volume, serum PSA concentrations and morphometric factors such as nuclear roundness. Studies directed at early detection allow discovery of increasingly smaller cancers.

References

Blute ML, Zincke H and Farrow GM (1986) Long-term followup of young patients with stage A adenocarcinoma of the prostate. *Journal of Urology* **136** 840–843

Boring CC, Squires TS, Tong T and Montgomery S (1994) Cancer statistics, 1994. *CA-A Cancer Journal for Clinicians* **44** 7–26

Bostwick DG (1994) The significance of tumor volume in prostate cancer. *Urology Annual* **8** 1–21

Bostwick DG and Choi C (1992) Prognostic factors in early prostate cancer. *Urology Annual* **6** 63–101

Bostwick DG and Srigley J (1990) Premalignant lesions, In: Bostwick DG (ed). *Pathology of the Prostate,* pp 37–59, Churchill Livingstone, New York

Bostwick DG, Cooner WH, Denis L, Jones GW, Scardino PT and Murphy GP (1992) The association of benign prostatic hyperplasia and cancer of the prostate. *Cancer* **70 (Supplement)** 291–301

Bostwick DG, Srigley J, Grignon D *et al* (1993) Atypical adenomatous hyperplasia of the prostate: morphologic criteria for its distinction from well-differentiated carcinoma. *Human Pathology* **24** 819–832

Bostwick DG, Myers RP and Oesterling JE (1994a) The staging of prostate cancer. *Seminars in Surgical Oncology* **10** 60–73

Eble JN and Tejada E (1986) Cost implications of sampling strategies for prostatic transurethral resection specimens: analysis of 549 cases. *American Journal of Clinical Pathology* **85** 382–383

Epstein JI, Paull G, Eggleston JC and Walsh PC (1986) Prognosis of untreated stage A1 prostatic carcinoma: a study of 94 cases with extended followup. *Journal of Urology* **13** 837–839

Epstein JI, Oesterling JE and Walsh PC (1988) The volume and anatomical location of residual tumor in radical prostatectomy specimens removed for stage A1 prostate cancer. *Journal of Urology* **139** 975–979

Epstein JI, Walsh PC, Carmichael M and Brendler CB (1994) Pathologic and clinical findings to predict tumor extent of nonpalpable (stage T1c) prostate cancer. *Journal of the American Medical Association* **271** 368–374

Friedman GD, Hiatt RA, Quesenberry CP and Selby JV (1991) Case-control study of screening for prostate cancer by digital rectal examinations. *Lancet* **337** 1526–1530

Greene DR, Egawa S, Neerhut G *et al* (1991a) The distribution of residual cancer in radical prostatectomy specimens in stage A prostate cancer. *Journal of Urology* **145** 324–329

Greene DR, Wheeler TM, Egawa S, Dunn JK and Scardino PT (1991b) A comparison of the morphological features of cancer arising in the transition zone and in the peripheral zone of the prostate. *Journal of Urology* **146** 1069–1076

Henson DE, Hutter RVP and Farrow GM (1994) Practice protocol for the examination of specimens removed from patients with carcinoma of the prostate gland. *Archives of Pathology and Laboratory Medicine* **118** 779–784

Lowe BA and Listrom MB (1988) Incidental carcinoma of the prostate: an analysis of the predictors of progression. *Journal of Urology* **140** 1340–1344

McNeal JE, Price H, Redwine EA and Stamey TA (1988a) Stage A versus stage B adenocarcinoma of the prostate: morphologic comparison and biologic significance. *Journal of Urology* **139** 61–68

McNeal JE, Redwine EA, Freiha FS and Stamey TA (1988b) Zonal distribution of prostatic adenocarcinoma: correlation with histologic pattern and direction of spread. *American Journal of Surgical Pathology* **12** 897–906

Matzkin H, Patel JP, Altwein JE and Soloway MS (1994) Stage T1A carcinoma of prostate. *Urology* **43** 11–21

Mettlin C, Lee F, Drago J and Murphy G (1991) The American Cancer Society National Prostate Cancer Detection Project: findings on the detection of early prostate cancer in 2425 men. *Cancer* **67** 2949–2958

Morra MN and Das S (1993) Prostate cancer: epidemiology and etiology, In: Das S and Crawford ED (eds). *Cancer of the Prostate,* pp 1–12, Marcel Dekker, New York

Murphy WM, Dean PJ, Brasfield JA *et al* (1986) Incidental carcinoma of the prostate: how much sampling is adequate? *American Journal of Surgical Pathology* **10** 170–176

Oesterling JE, Suman VJ, Zincke H and Bostwick DG (1993) PSA-detected (clinical stage T1c or B0) prostate cancer. *Urologic Clinics of North America* **20** 687–694

Orestano F (1991) Problems of wait-and-see policy in incidental carcinoma of the prostate, In: Altwein JE, Faul P and Schneider W (eds). *Incidental Carcinoma of the Prostate,* pp 163–166, Springer Verlag, Berlin

Paulson DF (1989) Stage A prostatic adenocarcinoma: an artifact of detection. *World Journal of Urology* **7** 34–37

Qian J, Wollan P and Bostwick DG The extent and multicentricity of high grade prostatic intraepithelial neoplasia in clinically localized prostatic adenocarcinoma. *Human Pathology* (in press)

Rohr LR (1987) Incidental adenocarcinoma in transurethral resection of the prostate: partial versus complete microscopic examination. *American Journal of Surgical Pathology* **11** 53–58

Scardino PT, Weaver R and Hudson MA (1992) Early detection of prostate cancer. *Human Pathology* **23** 211–222

Shroder FH, Hermanek P, Denis L *et al* (1992) The TNM classification of prostate carcinoma. *Prostate* **4 (Supplement)** 129–138

Thompson IM and Zeidman EJ (1989) Extended followup of stage A1 carcinoma of the prostate. *Urology* **33** 455–458

Vollmer RT (1986) Prostate cancer and chip specimens: complete versus partial sampling. *Human Pathology* **17** 285–290

Zhang G, Wasserman NF, Sidi AM, Reinberg Y and Reddy PK (1991) Long-term follow-up results after expectant management of stage A1 prostatic cancer. *Journal of Urology* **146** 99–103

The author is responsible for the accuracy of the references.

Molecular Biology of Prostate Cancer Progression

W B ISAACS • G S BOVA • R A MORTON
M J G BUSSEMAKERS • J D BROOKS• C M EWING
Research Laboratories of the Brady Urological Institute, Johns Hopkins Medical Institutions, Baltimore, Maryland 21205

INTRODUCTION

The growth pattern of the prostate gland is somewhat unique. It is probably the only organ that continues to grow throughout life, such that the size of a prostate gland from a 65 year old man will, on average, be two- to threefold larger than that of a 20 year old man. In fact, it has been calculated that throughout the adult years, the prostate grows continuously at a rate of between 0.4 and 1.6 g per year (Berry *et al,* 1984). The factors responsible for this characteristic growth pattern are essentially unknown. Whereas most of this age related increase in prostatic mass is due to frequent hyperplasia of the periurethral or transition zone of the prostate, lesions that are histologically identifiable as prostate cancer can be found with a frequency of similar magnitude. Although, fortunately, few of these latter lesions progress to clinical disease, these features of the natural history of the prostate emphasize the tremendous predilection of the prostate to undergo abnormal growth. (However, if abnormal means unusual, it is not an appropriate modifier.) Understanding this characteristic of the prostate in molecular terms is an important goal in the study of the molecular biology of the prostate.

With respect to prostate cancer, a particularly important question from a clinical point of view is what are the molecular events responsible for the prog-

Cancer Surveys Volume 23: *Preventing Prostate Cancer: Screening versus Chemoprevention*

ression of prostate cancer, or why and how does prostate cancer evolve from an indolent to a life threatening disease? Furthermore, is this evolution inevitable or are some prostate cancers destined not to progress to life threatening disease, or clinically detectable disease, regardless of the time frame? We have undertaken a study of prostate cancer DNA as a starting point to identify and characterize genetic changes that may answer these questions.

THE SEARCH FOR CANCER GENES

The molecular biology of human cancer has seen enormous progress in the last decade. This has been the result of both technical and conceptual advances, reinforcing certain concepts in carcinogenesis and providing the basis for the formulation of many more. For example, the concept of clonality as a fundamental aspect of cancer biology has been abundantly demonstrated, although the mechanisms that drive expansion and selection of clonal cell populations are less well defined. This is particularly important in prostate cancer, where recent evidence suggests that multiple clonal populations may arise. Perhaps the most striking example of progress in molecular oncology is the identification and characterization of cancer susceptibility genes, which has provided the foundation for understanding the relationship between inherited and sporadic forms of common human cancers (see below).

This laboratory has focused on the identification and characterization of consistent genetic alterations in human prostate cancer. Although we have concentrated primarily on somatic alterations associated with prostate cancer, we have initiated linkage studies in families in which prostate cancer occurs to characterize hereditary forms of this common disease. It is expected that these efforts will provide markers capable of identifying individuals at high risk of developing prostate cancer, and which may be of prognostic value in evaluating the aggressiveness of the disease once diagnosed.

As the quest to define "cancer genes" in prostate and other forms of cancer continues, it has become apparent that the definitions of oncogenes and tumour suppressor genes have become somewhat blurred, particularly in the case of tumour suppressor genes that can act essentially as dominantly acting oncogenes when mutated (eg *TP53*). Furthermore, a new category of genes needs to be included in this group, the genes involved in DNA repair. The recent finding of mutations of a DNA repair enzyme gene, the *hMSH2* gene, in the germ line of patients with hereditary non-polyposis colon cancer (Leach *et al*, 1993) and that tumours from such individuals have literally thousands of somatic mutations, has verified a hypothesis that was espoused by several researchers almost 20 years ago (Loeb *et al*, 1974; Nowell, 1976) that a mutator phenotype could play a critical part in human carcinogenesis. That fidelity of DNA replication and repair should play such a prominent part in human carcinogenesis is not surprising but has been overshadowed by the search for oncogenes and tumour suppressor genes, as these are most likely the critical growth regulatory targets of mutational events. This apparent neglect of the role of DNA repair in carcinogenesis is in large part due to the operational methodologies used to search for cancer genes. In the DNA transfection approaches used so commonly in the early 1980s to identify dominantly acting oncogenes and the allelic loss strategies used subsequently to locate tumour suppressor genes, genes coding for DNA repair enzymes would not be detected. A possible exception to this is the identification of the *TP53* gene as a tumour suppressor gene, in that a primary function of this gene is to inhibit cell cycle progression in response to DNA damage (Kastan *et al,* 1991). In any case, new methodologies, or more likely adaptation of existing methodologies to search for alterations in DNA repair processes, will undoubtedly become a major area of activity in oncological research. At the same time, the overall contribution of inherited or acquired abnormalities in a cell's ability to repair DNA to carcinogenesis of the prostate and other organs should become apparent.

Recently, we examined prostate cancer DNA for the presence of replication errors similar to those seen in hereditary non-polyposis colon cancer. Although the frequency is low, certain prostate cancers do show the replication error or RER phenotype as defined by Aaltonen *et al* (1993). Analysis of microsatellite repeats has shown instability in both primary cancers and at least one prostate cancer cell line (Bussemakers *et al,* 1994). A particularly intriguing aspect of this instability in colon cancer is that it is much more common in hereditary cancers (ie hereditary non-polyposis colorectal cancer) than sporadic ones. It will be of great interest to analyse tumours from men with hereditary form(s) of prostate cancer for this type of genetic instability.

STUDY POPULATION

The study of prostate cancer DNA and the changes therein obviously necessitates the availability of such DNA. Our primary source of tissue for research is from men who are undergoing radical prostatectomy for treatment of clinically localized prostate cancer. From these cases, we obtain seminal vesicle tissue and benign prostatic tissue as well as tumour tissue. Freezing in liquid nitrogen and maintenance of such specimens at $-70^{o}C$ allow for the efficient extraction of DNA, RNA and protein for analysis. We have begun to take more advantage of archival paraffin embedded samples from which nucleic acids can be obtained, but with considerably less yield and size. Bova *et al* (1993a) have described the technique that we use to obtain and process adequate tissue for analysis and not compromise any aspect of the pathological evaluation.

As mentioned above, by far the largest number of specimens analysed have been clinically localized tumours. Although these samples are invaluable because of the numbers available, and their representation of prostate cancer at defined stage, they need to be complemented with tumours from either end of the spectrum (ie very early lesions [stage A, prostatic intraepithelial neoplasia] and tissue from men with widely disseminated disease) if a true picture of the natural history of this disease is to emerge. Indeed, analysis of such samples are needed if we are to understand the molecular events involved in the transition of incidental prostate cancer to clinical prostate cancer, as well as the genetic alterations associated with progression of localized cancer to lethal, metastatic disease. The ability of polymerase chain reaction (PCR) to analyse very small prostatic lesions (Wolman *et al,* 1992, Macoska *et al,* 1993) and a greater effort to obtain tissue from men with advanced disease should provide the keys to these questions.

Ras IN PROSTATE CANCER

The Ha-*ras* gene has the distinction of being the first gene found to be mutated in a human cancer cell (Reddy *et al,* 1982). On the basis of evidence suggesting a potentially important role for activated *ras* genes in prostate cancer (Peehl *et al,* 1987; Treiger and Isaacs, 1988; Thompson *et al,* 1989), we examined prostate cancers for the presence of *ras* gene mutations using differential oligodeoxy-nucleotide hybridization of DNA amplified using the PCR (Carter *et al,* 1990a). Overall, with our subsequent studies, we have assayed 51 samples of prostate cancer, including both acinar and ductal carcinomas, primary tumours and metastatic deposits and prostate cancer cell lines. Only two mutations have been detected: an A to G transition causing a glutamate to arginine substitution at codon 61 of the Ha-*ras* gene in a primary prostatic duct adenocarcinoma and a G to T transversion causing a glycine to valine substitution at codon 12 of the Ha-*ras* gene in a prostate cell line (TSU-Pr1) derived from a lymph node metastasis. Two subsequent reports have found similar low frequencies of *ras* gene mutations in prostate cancer (Gumerlock *et al,* 1991; Moul *et al,* 1992). When these three independent studies were combined, a total of three *ras* gene mutations (all in Ha-*ras*) were found in 94 samples assayed, for an overall frequency of less than 4%. These results, all obtained in American patients, demonstrate that activation of *ras* oncogenes via point mutation is not a common event in either the initiation or progression of prostatic neoplasia. In contrast to these studies, however, two reports have appeared which suggest that *ras* gene mutations *do* occur at significant frequencies (~25%) in prostate cancer, both in latent carcinoma (Konishi *et al,* 1992) and in clinical disease (Anwar *et al,* 1992). In both studies, prostate tissue from Japanese men was examined, raising the intriguing possibility that significant differences may exist in the genetic events associated with prostate cancer in American men versus Japanese men (wherein the latter has an incidence rate about fivefold less for clinical disease). Curiously, in latent prostate carcinoma, the mutations were found in the Ki-*ras* gene, whereas in the clinical cancers, mutations were found predominantly in the Ha-*ras* gene and were associated with late stage. In fact, the same Ha-*ras* mutation, an A→T transversion at codon 61, accounted for each mutation found in this gene. These results suggest that Ki-*ras* mutations do not appear to be associated with progression of latent lesions to clinical disease, and in fact may be associated with lack of progression. A clearer picture of this may emerge with additional, confirmatory studies.

In addition, in the study by Anwar *et al* (1992), human papillomavirus (HPV) DNA was detected in more than 40% of the prostate cancer samples analysed. The presence of HPV DNA in prostate cancer from North American men is controversial, but the most recent evidence suggests that this family of viruses is not commonly found in prostate cancer, at least not at levels comparable to those found in cervical cancer, where a definite aetiological link has been established.

LOSS OF HETEROZYGOSITY STUDIES

We have carried out loss of heterozygosity (LOH) studies to search for sites of consistent chromosomal deletion, possibly uncovering the location of tumour suppressor genes that become inactivated in prostatic carcinogenesis. Cytogenetic analyses of prostate cancer have not revealed consistent chromosomal deletions (see Brothman *et al,* 1990; Lundgren *et al,* 1992; Sandberg, 1992), which might provide information on the location of such genes. An early study by Atkin and Baker (1985), however, showed that four of four patients with late stage prostate carcinomas showed chromosome 10q deletions and three of four showed chromosome 7q deletions. Since that time, alterations of the long arm of chromosome 10, although by no means ubiquitous, have been the most consistently observed karyotypic abnormality in prostate cancer.

To pursue these observations at a molecular level, we studied allelic loss in prostate cancer using polymorphic DNA probes for chromosomes 10q and 7q as well as probes for chromosomes containing documented and putative tumour suppressor genes (3p, 9q, 11p, 13q, 17p, 18q). We examined specimens from 28 primary prostate cancers, most of which were localized stage B lesions, measuring <2 cm in diameter. Briefly, we found that the majority (61%) of the tumours showed allelic loss on at least one of the chromosomes examined (Carter *et al,* 1990b). The regions most frequently deleted are found on the long arms of chromosomes 10 and 16. These results suggested that clonal populations of cells with gross chromosomal deletions are common in prostate cancer specimens, even at a relatively early stage. This contrasts with most cytogenetic analyses that reveal primarily normal diploid karyotypes (see above references), suggesting that perhaps, in culture, prostate cancer cells, or least those with chromosomal deletions, are at a growth *dis*advantage.

In addition to our study, Kunimi *et al* (1991) examined ten primary tumour specimens, as well as eight metastatic lesions, for allelic loss on every non-acrocentric autosomal chromosomal arm. Interestingly, chromosomes 10 and 16, along with chromosome 8, most frequently showed allelic loss in this study.

Taken together, these results provide evidence for the specificity of allelic loss on chromosomes 8, 10 and 16 in prostate cancer.

Critical deletion mapping studies performed by Bergerheim *et al* (1991) demonstrated that chromosome 8 LOH in prostate cancer was restricted to the short arm. To refine this observation further, we recently completed a deletion mapping study of this chromosome in over 50 samples of prostate cancer. Similar to that found by Bergerheim *et al* (1991), we found high rates of loss of alleles on chromosome 8p in these samples (Bova *et al,* 1993b). In fact, we found a locus at chromosome 8p22 (MSR) that is deleted in almost 70% of the prostate cancers examined, and in one case, a homozygous deletion at this locus was observed. A chromosome 8p deletion map defines the smallest region of overlap to a 14 cM interval between D8S163 and LPL, flanking the MSR locus. These data strongly suggest the presence of a tumour suppressor gene in this region. Evidence for increased copy number of sequences on the long arm of chromosome 8 was found in 5 of 32 (16%) tumours, suggesting the presence of an activated oncogene on this chromosome as well. Interestingly, the short arm of chromosome 8 shows frequent LOH in a variety of common human tumours including colorectal and lung cancer (Vogelstein *et al,* 1989; Emi *et al,* 1992). Whether the same gene is the target of these LOH events in prostate, colorectal and lung cancer is unclear, but it is interesting to speculate that a gene that is inactivated in a large fraction of human cancers may reside in this region of the genome. In any case, the identification of the chromosome 8p gene(s) involved in prostate carcinogenesis should provide insight into this process.

To confirm and extend the results of our initial study of LOH on chromosome 16q in prostate cancer, we examined this chromosomal arm in 52 additional samples of prostate cancer (47 primary, 5 metastases) using five different polymorphic probes for this region. Overall, of 39 tumours for which the markers were informative, 14 showed loss of alleles on chromosome 16q. This fraction (36%) is slightly higher than our previous quantitation of this event (30%) in a smaller number of tumours. Interestingly, whereas 11 of 34 (32%) primary tumours had chromosome 16q deletions, 3 of 5 (60%) metastatic tumours showed deletions on this arm, suggesting a possible role for inactivation of gene(s) in this region in tumour metastasis.

E-CADHERIN/α CATENIN IN PROSTATE CANCER

Our finding of allelic loss on chromosome 16q led to an examination of putative candidate genes in this region. The *E-cadherin* gene, mapped to chromosome 16q22.1 (Natt *et al,* 1989), is of particular interest. The product of this gene, originally termed uvomorulin by Peyrieras *et al* (1983), Arc-1 by Berhrens *et al* (1985) and E-cadherin (reviewed in Takeichi, 1991), had been shown to play a critical part in embryogenesis and organogenesis by mediating epithelial cell-cell recognition and adhesion processes. Indeed, the appearance of E-cadherin protein on the surface of cells of the early mouse embryo was shown to be required for normal development. The cadherin family of proteins has now been determined to be quite large, with expression in numerous cell types. The role of E-cadherin in maintaining various aspects of cell differentiation led investigators to examine E-cadherin in adenocarcinoma cells. It was found that E-cadherin protein levels were frequently reduced or absent in cancer cell lines, and such lines were often more fibroblastic in morphology and invasive in experimental assays (Frixen *et al,* 1991; Sommers *et al,* 1991). Vleminckx *et al* (1991) demonstrated that experimental inactivation of E-cadherin with either antibodies or anti-sense RNA resulted in the acquisition of invasive potential and that transfection of invasive adenocarcinoma cells with *E-cadherin* cDNA rendered the expressing cells non-invasive.

The first studies to examine E-cadherin in prostate cancer were carried out by Bussemakers *et al* (1992) in the Dunning rat model where a strong correlation between the lack of E-cadherin and metastatic and/or invasive potential was found. This correlation was strengthened by the direct observation of the progression of a non-invasive E-cadherin positive tumour to an E-cadherin negative highly metastatic tumour. To extend these observations to human prostate cancer, in collaboration with J Schalken's laboratory in Nijmegen, we examined a series of more than 90 samples of prostate cancer for E-cadherin protein levels by immunohistochemistry (Umbas *et al,* 1992). Whereas all benign samples stained uniformly, with strong intensity at cell-cell borders, approximately one-half of the tumours examined showed reduced or absent E-cadherin protein staining. When compared with Gleason grade, there was a strong association between high grade and aberrant E-cadherin staining. In fact, no tumours with a grade of 9 and 10 had normal staining, whereas all tumours with a Gleason score of less than 6 had normal staining patterns. A subsequent study of the potential prognostic significance of E-cadherin staining shows that, indeed, aberrant E-cadherin staining is a powerful predictor of poor outcome, in terms of both disease progression and overall survival (Umbas *et al,* 1994).

To extend our understanding of the role of E-cadherin mediated cell-cell adhesion in prostate cancer, we examined the synthesis and organization of this protein and its associated proteins in prostate cancer cell lines (Morton *et al,* 1993b). Using immunoprecipitation experiments, we found that cultured normal prostatic epithelial cells make abundant E-cadherin, which can be observed to form complexes with a series of cytoplasmic proteins termed catenins, α and β. These proteins, in particular α catenin, are thought to link E-cadherin to the microfilament cytoskeleton, and the interaction of E-cadherin with these proteins has been shown to be required for induction of cell-cell adhesion (Ozawa *et al,* 1989). In cultured prostatic cancer cell lines, E-cadherin levels are frequently reduced or absent, as in surgical specimens of prostate cancer. Furthermore, this study provided the unexpected finding that the levels of the E-cadherin associated protein, α catenin, are also frequently reduced in prostate cancer cells. Loss of this protein in the PC-3 prostate cancer cells is associated with their decreased ability to aggregate when compared to cells expressing normal levels of E-cadherin and α catenin. Thus, the E-cadherin mediated pathway of cell-cell adhesion may become inactivated in a variety of ways. The lack of α catenin expression in PC-3 cells is due to a homozygous deletion within the α catenin gene (Morton *et al,* 1993b). We have recently mapped the α catenin gene to chromosome 5q22 (McPherson *et al,* 1994), and preliminary results suggest that LOH in this region occurs in approximately 25% of prostate cancers analysed.

MICROCELL TRANSFER STUDIES

As a functional test for the presence of genes on various chromosomes that are capable of suppressing tumour growth, we have used the microcell transfer technique to insert a normal copy of a given chromosome into prostate cancer cell lines. We have successfully transferred chromosomes 5, 8, 10, 11 and 17 into a number of prostate cancer cell lines, including TSU-Pr1, DU145 and PC-3. The presence of transferred chromosomes has been confirmed by in situ hybridization with centromeric probes and Southern and microsatellite repeat analysis with polymorphic markers that can discriminate endogenous from exogenous chromosomes. The most striking results are observed after reintroduction of a normal copy of chromosome 5 into PC-3 cells (Isaacs WB, Ewing CM and Morton RA, unpublished). Not only do the cells undergo a dramatic change in morphology to form tightly packed, more epithelioid colonies in vitro, but also the tumorigenicity of the cells is essentially abolished when they are placed in nude mice. These alterations in growth characteristics are accompanied by dramatic alterations in the organization of the actin based cytoskeleton. Importantly, this reversion to a more normal phenotype is correlated with the re-expression of α catenin with restoration of E-cadherin mediated cell-cell adhesion.

In experiments with chromosome 10, in the TSU-Pr1 cells, in vivo growth suppression is seen following microcell transfer, but only in clones of cancer cells that have taken up two or more copies of chromosome 10. The growth suppression is not observed in vitro and is not complete in vivo, but rather is manifest as an increase in lag time before tumours appear. Experiments with the PC-3 have been more dramatic in that, following microcell transfer and selection of resistant clones in neomycin, two types of colonies appear. The most numerous are small colonies in which cells undergo only a limited number of divisions and subsequently appear to senesce. Less frequently, colonies of rapidly growing cells form; these cells are fully tumorigenic when injected into nude mice. Experiments with chromosome 17 show a definite tumour suppressive activity (Bova *et al,* 1993c), which, curiously, appears to be independent of restoration of *TP53* function (see below). No consistent suppression of tumour formation has yet been observed upon transfer of either chromosomes 8 or 11 into prostate cancer cells.

TP53 AND *RB*

In addition to detection of allelic loss on chromosomes 10q and 16q, approximately one fifth of the prostatic tumours analysed in our initial study were deleted at chromosomes 17p, 18q and 13q. These regions harbour the tumour suppressor genes *TP53, DCC* and *RB,* respectively. Thus, the possibility exists that inactivation of these genes plays a part in at least a subset of prostatic neoplasms. The importance of *RB* gene inactivation in prostate cancer has been suggested by the studies of Bookstein *et al* (1990a,b). To examine the *RB* gene more closely, we studied additional tumours for allelic loss of the *RB* gene using a PCR based detection of a VNTR in intron 20 of the gene. Of 41 informative tumours, 11 (27%) demonstrated allelic loss of one copy of the *RB* gene (Brooks *et al,* in press), suggesting that inactivation of the *RB* gene may be important in a significant subset of prostatic adenocarcinomas.

With regard to the *TP53* gene, we have found that three of five prostate cancer cell lines (TSUPr-1, PC-3 and DU145) contain mutations in the coding sequence of the *TP53* gene and that the growth of these lines can be suppressed by the introduction of a wild type copy of this gene (Isaacs *et al,* 1991). Studies by others have revealed that the frequency of mutations in primary prostate cancer is low (10–15%) in comparison to many other common cancers (Visakorpi *et al,* 1992; Bookstein *et al,* 1993), whereas preliminary evidence from a number of laboratories suggests that bone metastases of prostate cancer may frequently show mutant *TP53*. These results suggest that *TP53* mutations are late events in the progression of prostate cancer

To pursue this, we analysed 71 primary prostate cancers for allelic loss of chromosome 17p and the *TP53* gene. Of the 56 informative tumours, 11 (20%) demonstrated allelic loss. Furthermore, allelic loss was directly correlated with increasing Gleason grade and appeared to be correlated with disease stage. Curiously, however, sequence analysis of the remaining allele in the 11 primary tumours with LOH on chromosome 17p reveals a lack of mutations in exons 5–8 of the remaining *TP53* allele, suggesting the existence of a different gene that may be the target of these LOH events. A closer examination of the roles of this gene in prostatic cancer is warranted, particularly with respect to progression of this disease.

DNA METHYLATION

In addition to deletions, mutations and chromosomal translocations, alterations in DNA methylation can affect gene expression. Hypermethylation of CpG islands (areas of the genome that are rich in the sequence CpG, associated with the 5′ regulatory regions of genes) has been associated with gene inactivation. We examined the methylation status of a highly polymorphic locus, D17S5, located at chromosome 17p13.3 with the probe YNZ22.1. This locus lies within a cluster of NotI restriction sites (GC\GGCCGC), a finding consistent with the presence of a CpG island. Previous studies by Makos *et al* (1992) have observed hypermethylation at this locus in both colon and lung cancer. Furthermore, deletions of the D17S5 locus at 17p13.3 have been identified in some breast cancers when other commonly deleted areas of 17p, including the *TP53* gene at 17p13.1, are retained (Sato *et al,* 1990). In prostate cancer, probing NotI digested DNA with the probe YNZ22.1, we found hypermethylation at this site in 14 of 15 tumours and 4 of 5 prostate cancer cell lines (Morton *et al,* 1993a). These findings further suggest that there may be a tumour suppressor gene on chromosome 17p, separate from *TP53,* that has a role in prostate carcinogenesis and is frequently inactivated via hypermethylation. Further studies such as identification of the affected gene will be necessary to clarify the role of this methylation process in the development of prostate cancer.

HEREDITARY PROSTATE CANCER

Finally, Carter *et al* (1992, 1993) have recently shown in a study of familial aggregation of prostate cancer that this clustering can be best explained by the mendelian inheritance of a rare autosomal dominant allele that predisposes men to develop this disease. From the study population examined, it was estimated that the gene responsible for this predisposition accounts for approximately 9% of the total number of cases of prostate cancer and 45% of the cases observed in men under 55 years of age. In collaboration with Drs Patrick Walsh, Terri Beaty, Roy Levitt and Deborah Meyers at our institution, we are initiating efforts to map this gene by linkage studies. Analysis of candidate regions, including BRCA1, FCC and chromosome 8p22 are under way. Although prostate cancer poses some unique obstacles to such an analysis, it is expected that such studies will provide critical information on the genetic mechanisms of hereditary prostate cancer and also on the more common sporadic disease.

SUMMARY

A number of genetic changes have been documented in prostate cancer, ranging from allelic loss to point mutations and changes in DNA methylation patterns (summarized in Fig. 1). The most consistent changes seen are those of allelic loss events, with the majority of tumours examined showing loss of alleles from at least one chromosomal arm. The short arm of chromosome 8, followed by the long arm of chromosome 16, seem to be the most frequent regions of loss, suggesting the presence of novel tumour suppressor genes. Deletions of one copy of the *RB* and *TP53* genes are less frequent as are mutations of the *TP53* gene, and accumulating evidence suggests the presence of an additional tumour suppressor gene on chromosome 17p, which is frequently inactivated in prostate cancer. Alterations in the E-cadherin/α catenin mediated cell-cell adhesion mechanism appear to be present in almost half of all prostate cancers and may be critical to the acquisition of metastatic potential

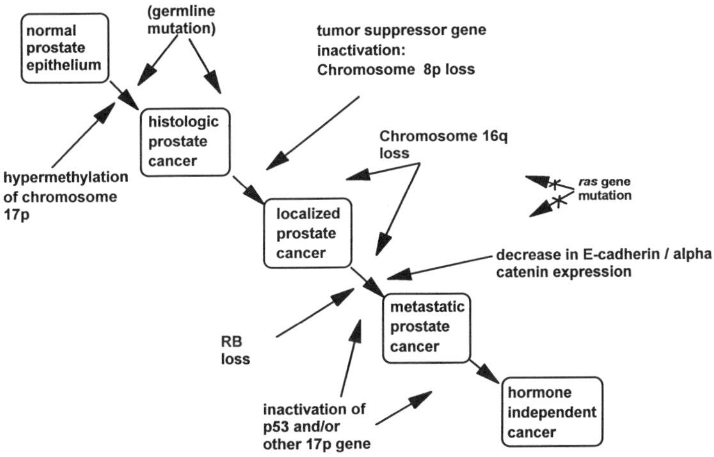

Fig. 1. Summary of genetic alterations in the progression of prostate cancer

of aggressive prostate cancers. Finally, altered DNA methylation patterns have been found in the majority of prostate cancers examined, suggesting widespread alterations in methylation modulated gene expression. The presence of multiple changes in these tumours is consistent with the multistep nature of the transformation process. Finally, efforts to identify prostate cancer susceptibility loci are under way, which may elucidate critical early events in prostatic carcinogenesis.

Acknowledgements

This work was supported by the United States Public Health Service (CA-55231, CA-58236).

References

Aaltonen LA, Peltomaki P, Leach FS *et al* (1993) Clues to the pathogenesis of familial colorectal cancer. *Science* **260** 812–816

Anwar K, Nakakuki K, Shiraishi T, Naiki H, Yatani R and Inuzuka M (1992) Presence of *ras* oncogene mutations and human papilloma virus DNA in human prostate carcinoma. *Cancer Research* **52** 5991

Atkin NB and Baker MC (1985) Chromosome study of five cancers of the prostate. *Human Genetics* **70** 359

Behrens J, Birchmeier W, Goodman SL and Imhof BA (1985) Dissociation of Madin-Darby canine kidney epithelial cells by the monoclonal antibody anti-Arc1: mechanistic aspects and identification of the antigen as a component related to uvomorulin. *Journal Cell Biology* **101** 1307–1315

Bergerheim US, Kunimi K, Collins VP and Ekman P (1991) Deletion mapping of chromosomes 8, 10, and 16 in human prostate carcinoma. *Genes, Chromosomes & Cancer* **3** 215

Berry SJ, Coffey DS, Walsh PC and Ewing LL (1984) The development of human benign prostatic hyperplasia with age. *Journal of Urology* **132** 474–479

Bookstein R, Shew J, Chen P, Scully P and Lee W-H (1990a) Suppression of tumorigenicity of

human prostate carcinoma cells by replacing a mutated *Rb* gene. *Science* **247** 712
Bookstein R, Rio P, Madreperla S, Hong F, Allred C, Grizzle W and Lee W-H (1990b) Promoter deletion and loss of retinoblastoma gene expression in human prostate carcinoma. *Proceedings of the National Academy of Sciences of the USA* **87** 7762–7767
Bookstein R, MacGrogan D, Milsenbeck SG, Sharkey F and Allred D (1993) *p53* is mutated in a subset of advanced-stage prostate cancer. *Cancer Research* **53** 3369–3373
Bova GS, Fox WM and Epstein JI (1993a) Methods of radical prostatectomy specimen processing: a novel technique for harvesting fresh prostate cancer tissue and review of processing techniques. *Modern Pathology* **6** 201–207
Bova GS, Carter BS, Bussemakers MJG *et al* (1993b) Homozygous deletion and frequent allelic loss of chromosome 8p22 loci in human prostate cancer. *Cancer Research* **53** 3869–3873
Bova GS, Robinson JC and Isaacs WB (1993c) Chromosome 17 suppresses tumorigenicity of a human prostate cancer cell line. *Proceedings of the American Association for Cancer Research* **34** 540
Brooks JD, Bova GS and Isaacs WB Allelic loss of the retinoblastoma gene in primary human prostatic adenocarcinoma. *Prostate* (in press)
Brothman A, Peehl D, Patel A and McNeal J (1990) Frequency and pattern of karyotypic abnormalities in human prostate cancer. *Cancer Research* **50** 3795
Bussemakers MJG, Van Moorselaar RJA, Giroldi LA *et al* (1992) Decreased expression of E-cadherin in the progression of rat prostatic cancer. *Cancer Research* **52** 2916–2922
Bussemakers MJG, Bova GS, Schoeberg MP, Hakimi JM, Barrack ER and Isaacs WB (1994) Microsatellite instability in human prostate cancer. *Journal of Urology* **151** 468A [Abstract]
Carter BS, Epstein JI and Isaacs WB (1990a) *Ras* gene mutations in human prostate cancer. *Cancer Research* **50** 6830
Carter BS, Ewing CM, Ward SW *et al* (1990b) Allelic loss of chromosomes 16q and 10q in human prostate cancer. *Proceedings of the National Academy of Sciences of the USA* **87** 8751
Carter BS, Beaty TH, Steinberg GD, Childs B and Walsh PC (1992) Mendelian inheritance of familial prostate cancer. *Proceedings of the National Academy of Sciences of the USA* **89** 3367
Carter BS, Bova GS, Beaty TH *et al* (1993) Hereditary prostate cancer: epidemiology and clinical features. *Journal of Urology* **150** 797
Emi M, Fujiwara Y, Nakajima T *et al* (1992) Frequent loss of heterozygosity for loci on chromosome 8p in hepatocellular carcinoma, colorectal cancer, and lung cancer. *Cancer Research* **52** 5368
Frixen UH, Behrens J, Sachs M *et al* (1991) E-cadherin-mediated cell-cell adhesion prevents invasiveness of human carcinoma cells. *Journal of Cell Biology* **113** 173
Gumerlock PH, Poonamallee UR, Meyers FJ and de Vere White RW (1991) Activated *ras* alleles in human prostate cancer are rare. *Cancer Research* **51** 1632–1637
Isaacs WB, Carter BS and Ewing CM (1991) Wild-type *p53* suppresses growth of human prostate cancer cells containing mutant *p53* alleles. *Cancer Research* **51** 4716
Kastan MB, Onyekwere O, Sidransky D, Vogelstein B and Craig RW (1991) Participation of *p53* protein in the cellular response to DNA damage. *Cancer Research* **51** 6304–6311
Konishi N, Enomoto T, Buzard G, Oshima M, Ward JM and Rice JM (1992) K-*ras* activation and *ras* p21 expression in latent prostatic carcinoma in Japanese men. *Cancer* **69** 2293
Kunimi K, Bergerheim USR, Larsson I-L, Ekman P and Collins VP (1991) Allelotyping of human prostatic adenocarcinoma. *Genomics* **11** 530
Leach FS, Papadopoulos N, Liu B *et al* (1993) Mutations of a *mutS* homolog in hereditary nonpolyposis colorectal cancer. *Cell* **75** 1215–1225
Loeb LA, Springgate CF and Battula N (1974) Errors in DNA replication as a basis of malignant change. *Cancer Research* **34** 2311–2321
Lundgren R, Mandahl N, Heim S, Limon J, Henrikson H and Mitelman F (1992) Cytogenetic analysis of 57 primary prostatic adenocarcinomas. *Genes, Chromosomes & Cancer* **4** 16–24
Macoska JA, Micale MA, Sakr WA, Benson PD and Wolman SR (1993) Extensive genetic altera-

tions in prostate cancer revealed by dual PCR and FISH analysis. *Genes, Chromosomes & Cancer* **8** 88–97

Makos M, Nelkin BD, Lerman MI, Latif F, Zbar B and Baylin SB (1992) Distinct hypermethylation patterns occur at altered chromosome loci in human lung and colon cancer. *Proceedings of the National Academy of Sciences of the USA* **89** 1929

McPherson JD, Morton RA, Ewing CM *et al* (1994) Assignment of the human α catenin gene to chromosome 5q21-q22. *Genomics* **19** 188–190

Morton RA, Bova GS and Isaacs WB (1993a) Hypermethylation of chromosome 17p13.3 in human adenocarcinoma of the prostate. *Journal of Urology* **149** 376A [Abstract]

Morton RA, Ewing CM, Nagafuchi A, Tsukita S and Isaacs WB (1993b) Reduction of E-cadherin levels and deletion of the α catenin gene in human prostate cancer cells. *Cancer Research* **53** 3585

Moul JW, Friedrichs PA, Lance RS, Theune SM and Chung E (1992) Infrequent *ras* oncogene mutations in human prostate cancer. *Prostate* **20** 327–338

Natt E, Magenis RE, Zimmer J, Mansouri A and Scherer G (1989) Regional assignment of the human loci for uvomorulin and chymotrypsinogen B with the help of two overlapping deletions on the long arm of chromosome 16. *Cytogenetics and Cell Genetics* **50** 145

Nowell P (1976) The clonal evolution of tumor cell progression: a review. *Science* **194** 3074–3079

Ozawa M, Baribault H and Kemler R (1989) The cytoplasmic domain of the cell adhesion molecule uvomorulin associates with three independent proteins structurally related in different species. *EMBO Journal* **8** 1711–1717

Peehl DM, Wehner N and Stamey TA (1987) Activated Ki-*ras* oncogene in human prostatic adenocarcinoma. *Prostate* **10** 281

Peyrieras N, Hyafil F, Louvard D, Ploegh HL and Jacob F (1983) Uvomorulin a nonintegral membrane protein of early mouse embryo. *Proceedings of the National Academy of Sciences of the USA* **80** 6274–6277

Reddy EP, Reynolds R, Santos E and Barbacid M (1982) A point mutation is responsible for the acquisition of transforming properties of the T24 human bladder carcinoma oncogene. *Nature* **300** 149–152

Sandberg AA (1992) Chromosomal abnormalities and related events in prostate cancer. *Human Pathology* **23** 368–382

Sato T, Tanigami A, Yamakawa K *et al* (1990) Allelotype of breast cancer cumulative allele losses promote tumor progression in primary breast cancer. *Cancer Research* **50** 7184

Sommers CL, Thompson EW, Torri JA, Kemler R, Gelmann EP and Byers SW (1991) Cell adhesion molecule uvomorulin expression in human breast cancer cell lines: relationship to morphology and invasive capacities. *Cell Growth Differentiation* **2** 365–372

Takeichi M (1991) Cadherin cell adhesion receptors as a morphogenetic regulator. *Science* **251** 1451–1455

Thompson TC, Southgate J, Kitchener G and Land H (1989) Multistage carcinogenesis induced by *ras* and *myc* oncogenes in a reconstituted organ. *Cell* **56** 917

Treiger BF and Isaacs JT (1988) Expression of a transfected v-Ha-*ras* oncogene in a Dunning rat prostate adenocarcinoma and the development of high metastatic ability. *Journal of Urology* **140** 1580

Umbas R, Schalken JA, Aalders TW *et al* (1992) Expression of the cellular adhesion molecule, E-cadherin, is reduced or absent in high grade prostate cancer. *Cancer Research* **52** 5104

Umbas R, Isaacs WB, Bringuier PP *et al* (1994) Decreased E-cadherin expression is associated with poor prognosis in patients with prostate cancer. *Cancer Research* **54** 3929–3933

Visakorpi T, Kallioniemi OP, Heikkinen A, Koivula T and Isola J (1992) Small subgroup of aggressive, highly proliferative prostatic carcinomas defined by p53 accumulation. *Journal National Cancer Institute* **84** 883–887

Vleminckx K, Vakaet L, Mareel M, Fiers W and Van Roy F (1991) Genetic manipulation of E-cadherin expression by epithelial tumor cells reveals an invasion suppressor role. *Cell* **66**

107–119

Vogelstein B, Fearon ER, Kern SE *et al* (1989) Allelotype of colorectal carcinomas. *Science* **244** 207

Wolman SR, Macoska JA, Micale MA and Sakr WA (1992) An approach to definition of genetic alterations in prostate cancer. *Diagnostic Molecular Pathology* **1** 192–199

The authors are responsible for the accuracy of the references.

The Role of Stromal-Epithelial Interaction in Normal and Malignant Growth

LELAND W K CHUNG

Urology Research Laboratory, University of Texas MD Anderson Cancer Center, 1515 Holcombe Boulevard, Houston, Texas 77030

INTRODUCTION

To understand and appreciate the molecular and cellular basis of prostate growth, development and neoplastic transformation, key players that affect these biological processes need to be identified and characterized. In the past decades, remarkable advances have been made in the understanding of the complexity and interplay between androgen growth factors, stromal-epithelial interaction and the temporal and spatial relationships between prostate cells and their surrounding microenvironment during the active phases of glandular growth and neoplastic progression (Chung *et al,* 1990a; Coffey, 1992). In addition, knowledge has been refined at the molecular level on the structural and nuclear organization of prostate cells, pathways of signal transduction, steroid hormone action, roles of the cell cycle and programmed cell death in prostate cell growth and neoplastic transformation, overexpression or amplification of oncogenes, loss of tumour suppressors and the possible presence of as yet unidentified gene(s) that may be associated with familial clusters of prostate cancer. These factors will contribute to our understanding of the fundamental biological processes that influence the rate of prostate cancer progression. The ultimate goal of these efforts is the translation of the enormous knowledge gained from the laboratory to the clinic for the improvement of diagnosis, prognosis and treatment of prostate diseases.

Cancer Surveys Volume 23: *Preventing Prostate Cancer: Screening versus Chemoprevention*

In this context, this chapter summarizes efforts made primarily by our laboratory in defining the molecular and cellular events associated with androgen regulation of prostate growth and neoplastic progression.

ROLES OF MESENCHYMAL CELLS IN NORMAL PROSTATE EPITHELIAL GROWTH AND ITS NEOPLASTIC TRANSFORMATION

Reciprocal cellular interaction between mesenchyme and epithelium has been demonstrated as a key determinant in the morphogenesis and cytodifferentiation of both endocrine (eg prostate and breast) and non-endocrine (eg lung, salivary gland and urinary bladder) target organs. Using a tissue recombinant technique, we and others (Cunha and Chung, 1981; Chung and Cunha, 1983; Naubauer *et al,* 1986) have shown that mesenchymal cells are probably the target cells for androgen steroids, which promote the growth and differentiation of the responding prostate epithelium. Under androgen treatment, mesenchymal cells also mediate regressive changes of the glandular epithelium in the mammary gland (Kratochwil and Schwartz, 1976). Fetal urogenital sinus mesenchyme (UGM), when implanted directly into the prostate glands of intact mice, remarkably reduces local prostate hyperplasia (Chung *et al,* 1984), suggesting that adult prostate remains responsive to growth induction when placed in contact with competent inductive fetal tissues. These results also illustrate that cellular interaction is a continuing process, even in the adult gland, that could contribute to the pathology of the prostate gland. This observation is supported by clinical evidence that human benign prostatic hyperplasia (BPH) may result from reactivation of the embryonic growth inductive potential in the adult prostate gland (McNeal, 1990). In addition to promoting growth, fetal UGM also induces prostate cancer differentiation (Chung *et al,* 1990b; Hayashi *et al,* 1990). Some hormone responsive (Chung *et al,* 1990b; Hayashi *et al,* 1990), but not hormone unresponsive (Chung *et al,* 1990b), rat prostate tumours are induced by UGM to redifferentiate to form normal ductal acinar architecture and assume secretory functions.

Because of the requirement of mesenchymal and epithelial cells to establish an intercellular communication network before committing to certain morphogenetic and differentiation programs, we have developed a cell-cell, rather than tissue-tissue, recombination model in which the roles of specific mesenchymal cell types and their specificities in the induction of human prostate epithelial tumour growth in vivo can be defined. Results of our study clearly demonstrate that prostate and bone, but not lung, kidney or 3T3, fibroblasts confer androgen induced growth responsiveness to a human prostate cancer epithelial cell line (LNCaP) (Gleave *et al,* 1991). We also found that rat UGM (rUGM) cells confer androgen induced growth responsiveness to both androgen receptor positive and receptor negative prostate and non-prostate epithelial cells in vivo (Fig. 1). Rat UGM cells, when co-

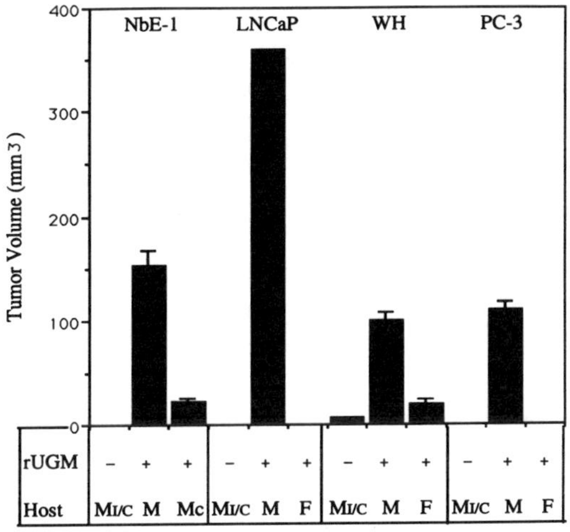

Fig. 1. Rat urogenital sinus mesenchymal cells (rUGM) conferred androgen induced growth responses to both prostate (eg normal rat prostate epithelial cells [NbE-1]; see Chung *et al,* 1989), androgen receptor positive human prostate cancer epithelial cell line, LNCaP (see Horoszewicz *et al,* 1983 and androgen receptor negative human prostate cancer epithelial cell line, PC-3, (see Kaighn *et al,* 1979) and non-prostate epithelial cell line (eg human urinary bladder cell line WH derived from a bladder transition cell carcinoma (Zhau *et al,* 1994). All epithelial cell growth in vivo in the male hosts was accelerated by co-inoculation with rUGM cells. The tumours formed were predominantly human and were found to stain positively with cytokeratin antibody (Zhau *et al,* 1994). MI/c intact or castrated males; M and F = male or female hosts, respectively; Mc = castrated male hosts

inoculated with the target epithelial cells in male hosts, elicited enhanced growth responsiveness in the resulting chimaeric tumours, which in most cases consisted primarily of epithelial cells. These results suggest that the possible production of soluble growth factors and/or extracellular matrix molecules by fetal rUGM cells might account for the stimulation of local growth of chimaeric tumours in vivo (Gleave *et al,* 1992a; Chung, 1993). Alternatively, reciprocal interactions between rUGM and target epithelial cells, mediated by soluble growth factors and/or extracellular matrices, might be the local signalling that contributes to chimaeric tumour growth (Chung *et al,* 1991a).

Another important characteristic of selected mesenchymal cells (eg osteoblasts) is that they induce LNCaP to progress from androgen dependent to androgen independent and from androgen independent to metastatic. The lack of an androgen microenvironment appears to facilitate the emergence of androgen independent and metastatic phenotypes. Figure 2 presents a scheme of the derivation of tumour cells from hosts harbouring solid LNCaP tumours. As can been seen, when the LNCaP tumours were maintained and passaged twice with human bone stromal cells (MS cell line) in castrated hosts, the resulting tumour cells (C4-2 subline) acquired androgen independence and osseous metastatic potential; neither of these behavioural phenotypes was found in the parent LNCaP cell line (Wu *et al,* 1994; Thalmann *et al,* 1994). This is a novel finding that has important biological implications. Firstly, the

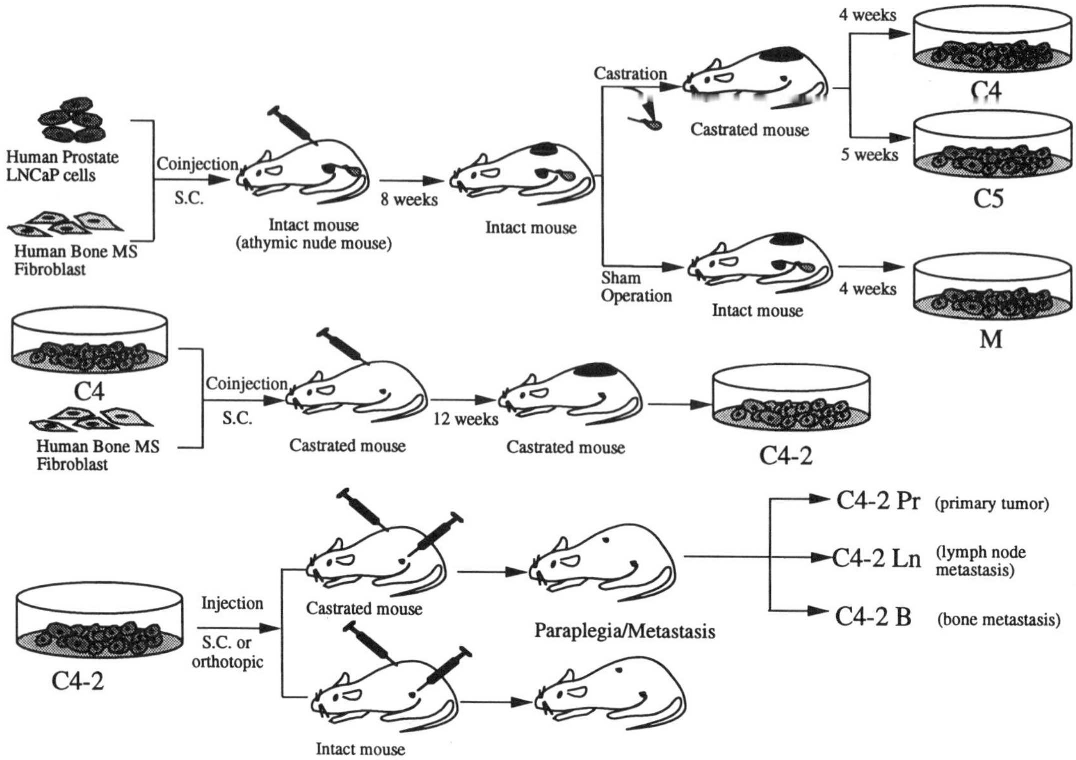

Fig. 2. Generation of androgen independent (eg C4, C5, C4-2) and metastatic (eg C4-2) human prostate cancer cell lines. The basis of this scheme relies upon the positive interaction between human prostate epithelial (LNCaP) and human bone stromal (MS) cell lines in vivo in castrated hosts to create a condition that may "select" or facilitate "adaptation" and hence the emergence of more aggressive androgen independent and metastatic human prostate cancer cells. This is the first time that androgen independent and metastatic human prostate cancer cell lines were generated

fact that stromal cells exhibited specificity in promoting prostate cancer progression from androgen dependent (eg LNCaP cells) to androgen independent (eg C4, C5 and C4-2 sublines) and further to metastatic (eg C4-2 subline) in a castrated host indicates that the host microenvironment promotes prostate tumour progression. Secondly, in the stromal microenvironment surrounding the tumour cells, which may promote the acquisition of androgen independent and invasive properties by the tumour cells, a large number of cell types are known to exist, including fibroblasts, smooth muscle cells, epithelial cells, neuroendocrine cells, macrophages, lymphocytes and other cell types associated with inflammatory responses. Our results showed that a spindle shaped cell (ie a fibroblast) that stained negatively with cytokeratin and desmin antibodies but positively with the vimentin antibody is the primary cell type that induces reciprocal cellular interaction with tumour cells in vivo; after cellular interaction with fibroblasts, androgen independent and metastatic prostate cancer epithelial cells emerged. Thirdly, an androgen deficient microenvironment may select for or allow the inductive events to occur more frequently, resulting in the emergence of more aggressive and metastatic prostate epithelial cell clones. Androgenic steroids both induce and suppress gene expression by prostate epithelial cells. It can be hypothesized that in the absence of androgen, certain clusters of genes may no longer be suppressed, and this could set off a chain of events that may link to the emergence of androgen independent and metastatic cell clones. Finally, our results suggest that both the soluble and matrix associated factors produced by the organ specific fibroblasts are of particular importance and can function as paracrine, autocrine or neuroendocrine mediators to induce prostate cancer progression.

EVIDENCE FOR PERMANENT BEHAVIOURAL AND CYTOGENETIC ALTERATIONS OF PROSTATE EPITHELIAL CELLS FOLLOWING CELLULAR INTERACTIONS WITH COMPETENT INDUCTIVE STROMAL CELLS IN VIVO

LNCaP cells were obtained from the lymph nodes of a patient with androgen independent and metastatic prostate cancer (Horoszewicz *et al,* 1983). LNCaP cells were demonstrated initially to be tumorigenic, androgen dependent and non-metastatic, but after repeated cell culture, the cell line lost its tumorigenicity. In athymic nude mice, however, tumorigenicity of LNCaP cells can be "recreated" by interaction either with organ specific fibroblasts (Gleave *et al,* 1991) or with reconstituted basement membrane (Matrigel) (Pretlow *et al,* 1991) or by injecting the cells orthotopically, presumably creating a condition of interacting with host fibroblasts (Gleave *et al,* 1992b; Stephenson *et al,* 1992). This is the only human prostate cancer cell line that grows readily in vitro, responds to androgen and synthesizes and secretes a clinically useful human prostate cancer marker, prostate specific antigen (PSA). Although the biology of LNCaP cells appears to be complex, the "evolution" of this cell line in vivo, which results in the acquisition of tumorigenic, androgen independent and metastatic phenotypes, is predictable and non-random. Using bone fibroblasts as inducers, our laboratory has cloned several LNCaP sublines that exhibit diverse tumorigenic, androgen dependent and metastatic behaviours (Thalmann *et al,* 1994; Wu *et al,* 1994). We consider these behavioural changes of LNCaP cells in vivo to be the consequence of "progression" resulting from cellular interaction with fibroblasts in an androgen deficient microenvironment. Mechanistically, how do organ specific fibroblasts "instruct" LNCaP cells to progress from non-tumorigenic to tumorigenic status and from androgen dependent to androgen independent and osseous metastatic phenotypes? It is unlikely that "clonal expansion" or "clonal evolution" alone can account for these experimental observations, because the acquisition of the androgen independent and metastatic phenotypes is rapid (~4 weeks) and massive cell death is absent. A more likely explanation for the alterations of the behavioural traits of the LNCaP cells could be "adap-

TABLE 1. Distinction between "clonal expansion" and "genomic adaptation" mechanisms for acquisition of tumour cell heterogeneity

Parameter	Clonal expansion	Genomic adaptation
Cell proliferation	Required	Not required
Cell death	Required	Not required
Rate of occurrence	Affected by the rate of cell growth and death	Affected by neither cell proliferation nor cell death
Genotype of subclones	Must pre-exist	Acquired, but can pre-exist

tive mutation" (Foster, 1993), in which both the dividing and non-dividing cells may undergo a "non-random genomic adaptation", so that certain favoured genotypes and phenotypes are selected and evolve under the influence of the host microenvironment. This hypothesis expanded from the current concept that genomic changes occur not only in cells that undergo mitosis, but also in cells that do not enter or complete their proliferative cell cycles (see Foster, 1993). Table 1 lists the differences between clonal expansion and "genomic adaptation" as the potential mechanisms explaining the evolution of tumour cells that leads to the acquisition of tumour cell heterogeneity.

IDENTIFICATION OF SOLUBLE MEDIATORS AND EXTRACELLULAR MATRICES THAT SERVE AS SIGNAL MOLECULES IN STROMAL-EPITHELIAL INTERACTION

We have focused on the characterizations of soluble growth factors produced by a human bone osteoblast cell line, MS, that is capable of stimulating prostate tumour growth in vivo and anchorage independent growth of prostate epithelial cells in vitro. MS1, a heparin Sepharose affinity column bound fraction, eluted by 1 mol/l NaCl, was shown to possess growth stimulating activity (Chung *et al,* 1992). We have fractionated this material further with high performance liquid chromatography and polyacrylamide gel electrophoresis. Results show that a high molecular mass (apparently >200 kDa) protein is active in stimulating prostate tumour cell anchorage independent growth (Li W and Chung LWK, unpublished).

Another approach is to use a polyclonal antibody prepared against the biologically active growth factor fraction MS1, obtained from the heparin affinity column, as a reagent to screen against a cDNA library prepared from a human MS bone stromal cell line. Screening this cDNA library MS1 antibody has resulted in the detection of several positive clones. We have isolated and characterized one of such clone, termed BPGF1 (bone-prostate growth factor 1). BPGF1 is a 3.2 kb novel paracrine growth factor cDNA with an estimated molecular mass of 59 kDa expressed in *Escherichia coli*. The cDNA reading frame of this gene is 1.6 kb. Northern blot hybridization has revealed two BPGF1 transcripts of 3.3 kb and 2.5 kb. The transcripts were detected in bone

TABLE 2. Expression of BPGF1 mRNA in various human and rodent cell lines and tissues

Human	BPGF1	Rodent	BPGF1
MS (bone osteosarcoma)	+++++	NbE-1 (normal prostate epithelial cell line)	–
BS (normal bone stroma)	++++	rUGM (normal rat UGM cell line)	–
TZ (prostate transition zone)	++	NIH3T3	–
PZ (prostate peripheral zone)	+		
LNCaP (AR+ prostate cancer)	+/–		
PC-3 (AR– prostate cancer)	+/–		
WH (urinary bladder)	+/–		
HeLa (cervical cancer cells)	–		
Brain tissue	–		
CEM (leukaemic cells)	–		
H3229 (lung cancer cells)	–		
MCF-7 (breast cancer cells	–		
CAPAN-1 (pancreatic cells)	–		
CRL1502 (skin fibroblasts)	–		
HT144 (melanoma cells)	–		
UPS7 (ovarian cells	–		
SMS (colon cells)	–		
KS-1 (kidney cells)	–		

and prostate fibroblasts but not in the cell extracts of a host of other human and rodent cells and tissues (Table 2). BPGF1 cDNA, when expressed in COS cells, stimulates prostate cancer epithelial cell growth (Fig. 3). These results support the hypothesis that certain novel and organ specific paracrine mesenchymal factors stimulate prostate cancer epithelial growth in vivo.

CLINICAL IMPLICATIONS OF STROMAL-EPITHELIAL INTERACTION IN PROSTATE GROWTH AND DISEASE PROGRESSION

We have demonstrated that stroma can confer androgen sensitivity to target epithelial cells. We have demonstrated that organ specific fibroblasts may be required to accelerate prostate epithelial cell growth and induce the progression of prostate tumours from androgen dependent to androgen independent and metastatic states in vivo. The underlying mechanism of this interaction can be promoted by soluble and matrix associated factors (Gleave *et al,* 1992b).

To eliminate or slow down the progression of prostate tumours from androgen dependent to androgen independent, we propose that the stromal microenvironment surrounding the tumour epithelium be considered as a therapeutic target for future chemotherapy. By modifying the host microenvironment and the stromal milieu, we may expect tumour regression or a

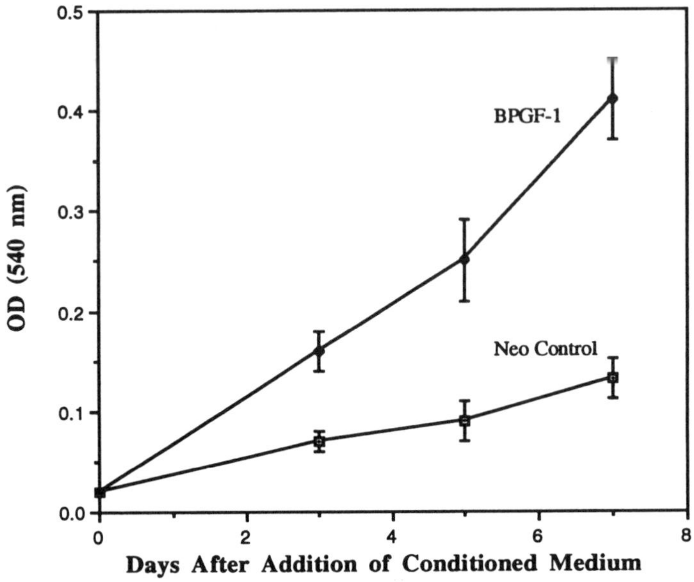

Fig. 3. BPGF1 protein expression in COS cells induced anchorage independent growth of NbE-1 cells. Control medium obtained from neo-expression vector failed to induce NbE-1 cell growth

slowing of growth. This approach will expand our current armamentarium of chemotherapeutic agents into a new era of therapy. Identification of active growth factor, growth factor receptor pathways and extracellular matrix molecules, using model systems such as ours, may assist the design of potential therapeutic agents.

Another potential use of this model is the elucidation of biomarkers that may be associated with various stages of prostate cancer progression and could be used to predict cancer progression. This approach is particularly relevant since it has been suggested, the basis of epidemiological surveys, that the rates of progression of latent to clinical cancer in different populations may be vastly different (Carter and Coffey, 1990; Carter *et al,* 1990). By using the current model system, we hope to uncover the factors that may contribute either positively or negatively to prostate cancer progression. This model may assist the future development of rational therapy for either the prevention or the inhibition of prostate cancer growth, progression and metastasis.

SUMMARY

Stromal-epithelial interaction has a fundamental role in determining normal prostate development. Aberrant interaction between stroma and epithelium in the prostate is thought to contribute to neoplastic progression. Using a cell-cell interaction model, we observed that an inductive fibroblast cell line derived from fetal urogenital sinuses can confer growth responsiveness to androgen in both prostate and non-prostate epithelial cells in vivo. This concept was applied to test whether inductive stromal cells from bone or prostate alter cancer growth and metastasis. We observed that when a non-tumorigenic stromal cell line derived from a human osteosarcoma interacted with a non-tumorigenic androgen dependent prostate cancer cell line (LNCaP) in vivo, there was a marked alteration of both genotypes and phenotypes of the subsequently derived LNCaP sublines. One such subline, C4-2, acquired androgen independence as well as osseous-metastatic potential. These results support the concept that "genomic adaptation" is the most likely mechanism to explain the phenomenon of prostate cancer cell lines being permanently altered as a result of stromal-epithelial interaction in vivo. The establishment and further refinement of this cell-cell interaction model will allow us to define the roles of growth factors, growth factor receptors and extracellular matrices in prostate carcinogenesis. This approach could lead to the development of new therapeutic modalities that influence the rate of human prostate cancer progression.

Acknowledgements

This work was supported in part by National Institutes of Health Public Health Service grant CA-56307.

References

Carter BS, Pianatadosi S and Issacs JT (1990) Clinical evidence for the implications of multistep development of prostate cancer. *Journal of Urology* **143** 742–746

Carter HB and Coffey DS (1990) The prostate: an increasing medical problem. *Prostate* **16** 39–48

Chung LWK (1991) Fibroblasts are critical determinants in prostatic cancer growth and dissemination. *Cancer and Metastasis Review* **10** 263–274

Chung LWK (1993) Implication of stromal-epithelial interaction in human prostate cancer growth, progression and differentiation. *Seminars in Cancer Biology* **4** 183–192

Chung LWK and Cunha GR (1983) Stromal-epithelial interactions, II Regulation of prostate growth by embryonic urogenital sinus mesenchyme. *Prostate* **4** 503–511

Chung LWK, Matsuura J and Runner MN (1984) Tissue interactions and prostatic growth, I Induction of adult mouse prostatic hyperplasia by fetal urogenital sinus implants. *Biology of Reproduction* **31** 155–163

Chung LWK, Chang SM, Bell C, Zhau HE, Ro JY and von Eschenbach AC (1989) Co-inoculation of tumorigenic rat prostate mesenchymal cells with non-tumorigenic epithelial cells results in the development of carcinosarcoma in syngeneic and athymic animals. *International Journal of Cancer* **43** 1179–1187

Chung LWK, Camps JL and von Eschenbach AC (1990a) Cancer biology, In: Chisholm GD and Fair W (eds). *Scientific Foundations of Urology*, pp 459–474, Year Book Medical Publishers Inc, Chicago

Chung LWK, Zhau HE and Ro JY (1990b) Morphologic and biochemical alterations in rat prostatic tumors induced by fetal urogenital sinus mesenchyme. *The Prostate* **17** 165–174

Chung LWK, Gleave ME, Hsieh J-T, Hong S-J and Zhau HE (1991a) Reciprocal mesenchymal-epithelial interaction affecting prostate tumour growth and hormonal responsiveness. *Cancer Surveys* **11** 91–121

Chung LWK, Hong SJ, Zhau HE *et al* (1991b) Fibroblast-mediated human epithelial tumor growth and hormonal responsiveness in vivo, In: Karr JP, Coffey DS, Smith RG and Tindall

DJ (eds). *Molecular and Cellular Biology of Cancer,* pp 91–102, Penum Press, New York and London

Chung LWK, Li W, Gleave M *et al* (1992) Human prostate cancer model roles of growth factors and extracellular matrices. *Journal of Cellular Biochemistry* **16H** 99–105

Coffey DS (1992) The molecular biology, endocrinology and physiology of prostate and seminal vesicles, In: Walsh PC, Retiki AB, Stamey TA and Vaughan ED Jr (eds). *Campbell's Urology,* 6th Edition, Vol I, pp 221–251, AB Saunders Company, Philadelphia

Cunha GR and Chung LWK (1981) Stromal-epithelial interaction, I Induction of prostatic phenotype in urothelium of testicular feminized (TFm/y) mice. *Journal of Steroid Biochemistry* **14** 1317–1321

Foster PL (1993) Adaptive mutation: the uses of adversity. *Annual Review of Microbiology* **47** 467–504

Gleave ME, Hsieh JT, Gao C, Chung LWK and von Eschenbach AC (1991) Acceleration of human prostate cancer growth in vivo by prostate and bone fibroblasts. *Cancer Research* **51** 3753–3761

Gleave ME, Hsieh JT, von Eschenbach AC and Chung LWK (1992a) Prostate and bone fibroblasts induce human prostate cancer growth in vivo: implications for bidirectional stromal-epithelial interaction in prostate carcinoma growth and metastasis. *Journal of Urology* **147** 1151–1159

Gleave ME, Hsieh JT, Wu HC, von Eschenbach AC and Chung LWK (1992b) Serum prostate specific antigen levels in mice bearing human prostate LNCaP tumors are determined by tumor volume and endocrine and growth factors. *Cancer Research* **52** 1598–1605

Hayashi N, Cunha GR and Wong YC (1990) Influence of male genital tract mesenchymes on differentiation of Dunning prostatic adenocarcinoma. *Cancer Research* **50** 4747–4754

Horoszewicz JS, Leong SS, Kavinski E *et al* (1983) LNCaP model of human prostatic carcinoma. *Cancer Research* **43** 1809–1818

Kaighn MD, Narayan KS, Ohnuki Y, Lechner JF and Jones LW (1979) Establishment and characterization of a human prostate cell line (PC-3). *Investigative Urology* **17** 16–23

Kratochwil K and Schwartz P (1976) Tissue interaction in androgen response of embryonic mammary rudiment of mouse: identification of target for testosterone. *Proceedings of the National Academy of Sciences of the USA* **73** 4041–4044

McNeal J (1990) Pathology of benign prostatic hyperplasia: insight into etiology. *Urologic Clinic of North America* **17** 477–486

Naubauer BL, Best KL, Hoover DM, Slisz ML, vanFrank RM and Goode RL (1986) Mesenchymal-epithelial interactions as factors influencing male accessory sex organ growth in the rate. *Federation Proceedings* **45** 2618–2626

Pretlow TG, Delmoro CM, Dilley GG, Spadafora CG and Pretlow TP (1991) Transplantation of human prostatic carcinoma into nude mice in Matrigel. *Cancer Research* **51** 3814–3817

Stephenson RA, Dinney CPN, Gohji K, Ordonez NG, Killion JJ and Fidler IJ (1992) Metastatic model for human prostate cancer using orthotopic implantation in nude mice. *Journal of the National Cancer Institute* **84** 951–957

Thalmann GN, Anezinis PE, Chang SM *et al* (1994) Androgen-independent cancer progression and bone metastasis in the LNCaP model of human prostate cancer. *Cancer Research* **54** 2577–2581

Wu HS, Hsieh JT, Gleave ME, Brown NM, Pathak S and Chung LWK (1994) Derivation of androgen-independent human LNCaP prostatic cancer cell sublines: role of bone stromal cells. *International Journal of Cancer* **57** 406–412

Zhau HE, Hong SJ and Chung LWK (1994) A fetal rate urogenital sinus mesenchymal cell line (rUGM): accelerated growth and conferral of androgen-induced growth responsiveness upon a human bladder cancer epithelial cell line in vivo. *International Journal of Cancer* **56** 706–714

The author is responsible for the accuracy of the references.

Endocrine Control of Prostate Cancer

G WILDING

University of Wisconsin Comprehensive Cancer Center, 600 Highland Avenue, Madison, Wisconsin 53792

INTRODUCTION

From the time of embryonic development to old age, steroid hormones strongly influence and at times control the development, growth, function and pathogenesis of the human prostate gland. Throughout a man's lifespan, the steroid hormone milieu surrounding his prostate gland changes and so does the biology of the gland. Although androgens are clearly the most influential hormones, others such as oestrogens, retinoids and vitamin D compounds might also have a part to play. The effects of these hormones are transmitted via their receptors which act as transcription factors. With the cloning of the receptor genes, the search for receptor mutations as a cause for various abnormal phenotypes has begun. Since the ligand-receptor complex serves as part of a transcription activating complex, the products of the genes activated serve as the ultimate mediators of the steroid hormone induced cellular phenotypes. This chapter reviews the role of steroid hormones in prostate biology, focusing on the influence of androgens on pathological processes.

Approximately 200 000 new cases of prostate cancer will be diagnosed annually in the USA. Prostate cancer is the most common malignancy in American men in both incidence and prevalence (Catalona and Scott, 1986; Scardino, 1989; Dhom, 1991; Boring *et al,* 1994), and black men in the USA have the highest incidence of prostate cancer in the world (Mettlin and Natarajan, 1983). Prostate cancer accounts for more than 38 000 deaths each year in the USA and is second only to lung cancer as a cause of cancer deaths in American men (Feldman *et al,* 1986).

A number of epidemiological observations of prostate cancer in various populations suggest a vital role for steroid hormones in prostate carcinogenesis. Firstly, prostate cancer does not occur in eunuchs; an intact hormonal

Cancer Surveys Volume 23: *Preventing Prostate Cancer: Screening versus Chemoprevention*

milieu seems to be important for the development of prostate cancer. Secondly, the incidence of microscopic, latent prostate cancer shows a very close correlation with increasing age regardless of the population examined. This suggests a fundamental change with aging in all men that permits the transformation of prostate epithelial cells in a large proportion of those men. Other changes that occur with advancing age include a decline in serum testosterone levels and an increase in the incidence of benign prostatic hyperplasia. Neither of these changes seems to be causally related to the prostate carcinogenesis. Thirdly, there is large variation in the incidence of clinical prostate cancer among populations around the world despite a similar incidence of latent cancer among those populations. For example, men in Japan and Taiwan have one of the lowest rates of clinical prostate cancer in the world, whereas Japanese men living in the continental USA show an incidence of clinical prostate cancer approaching the much higher rate seen in caucasian men in the USA. The incidence of clinical prostate cancer in Japanese men residing in Hawaii is intermediate between the rates for the USA and Asian countries. The proportion of latent cancers in Japan showing invasive characteristics is rising, although the overall incidence of latent cancer has not changed. This might predict a rise in clinical prostate câncer in the future in this population (Yatani *et al*, 1988). Similarly, although black men in the USA and Nigerian black men show a similar incidence of latent cancer, black men in the USA have the highest rate of clinical prostate cancer in the world, significantly higher than their counterparts in Nigeria. Finally, a critical dilemma facing clinicians treating patients with prostate cancer is what to do with patients with androgen independent cancers. This dilemma results from our lack of understanding and inability to control the growth of hormone independent prostate cancer cells. When first diagnosed, more than 75% of men with metastatic disease have tumours that are at least in part dependent on and responsive to androgens. However, virtually all such patients inevitably develop hormone independent disease. Because androgen withdrawal constitutes the only effective form of systemic therapy for metastatic prostate cancer at this time, the appearance of androgen independent clones of tumour cells heralds the end of our ability effectively to control the course of a patient's disease (Labrie *et al*, 1986; Isaacs and Kyprianou, 1987).

The mechanisms by which prostate epithelial cells are commonly transformed with increasing age and exposure to androgens to microscopic cancer, then to clinical cancer and, ultimately, to hormone independent cancer are not understood. Neither are the underlying reasons for the wide variations in the incidence of clinical cancer with geographical changes understood. The evidence clearly points to a multistep process of carcinogenesis. One important element in the development of prostate cancer is the presence of androgens, generally over a long period of time. Surprisingly, little is known about what variation occurs in androgen receptor (*AR*) expression with aging, in men of various races, at different geographical locations or with the development of latent, clinical or hormone independent prostate cancer. In addition to a lack of information on *AR* mRNA and protein levels in these circumstances, the frequency of *AR* mutations has not been determined in these populations of men.

Likewise, although it is apparent that transforming growth factors (TGFs) A and B and other growth factors have autocrine and paracrine roles in the biology of hormone responsive tissues such as the prostate and breast (Dickson and Lippman, 1987; Wilding *et al,* 1989a,b; Thompson, 1990), little is known of their expression in prostate tissue under the conditions listed above. It has been demonstrated that the constitutive expression of *TGFA* in transgenic mice leads to hyperplasia and tumours in the mammary tissue of mice (Sandgreen *et al,* 1990) and that the expression of *TGFB* rises in prostate cancers induced by *ras/myc* transfection of prostate tissue of mice (Thompson *et al,* 1989; Thompson, 1990). The expression of these transforming factors has been shown to be regulated by oestrogens and androgens in both in vivo and in vitro settings (Kyprianou and Isaacs, 1988, 1989; Wilding *et al,* 1989b).

Prostate cancer is now first in solid tumour incidence and prevalence and second as a cause of cancer related death in American men. American black men develop prostate cancer at the highest rate in the world (Boring et al, 1994). In addition to the 200 000 men diagnosed with prostate cancer in the USA each year, benign prostatic hyperplasia affects more than two thirds of all males over the age of 50, with approximately 20–25% of these men requiring surgery for the relief of urinary obstruction (Carter and Coffey, 1990). This affliction accounts for more than 400 000 transurethral resections of the prostate each year in the USA. Clearly, diseases of the prostate have become a major health issue in terms of the number of men affected, the cost to the medical system and the morbidity inflicted.

HORMONE ACTIONS IN PROSTATE BIOLOGY

What is the role of androgens and the *AR* in prostate carcinogenesis? The answer has two dimensions: (a) the strong evidence that androgens and the *AR* have a seminal role in prostate carcinogenesis, suggesting a permissive or initiating role for androgens, and (b) the actions of the *AR* as a transcription factor regulating the expression of proto-oncogenes, TGFs and growth factor receptors in prostate epithelial cells.

Evidence exists in experimental models that androgens might act as initiators or permissive agents in prostate carcinogenesis. For example, Bosland and co-workers have demonstrated that androgens increase the incidence of *N*-methyl-nitrosourea induced prostate cancer in Noble (Nb) rats (Bosland, 1988; Bosland *et al,* 1990). Additional studies showed that testosterone treatment of rats resulted in a 10–20% incidence of prostate cancer, whereas all of the rats treated with testosterone plus oestradiol developed prostate cancer. The Nb rats were then treated with testosterone, 5-α-dihydrotestosterone (DHT) or a combination of one of these androgens plus oestradiol. In those studies, DHT did not induce any tumours, whereas testosterone induced 23%; DHT plus oestradiol induced prostatic dysplasia after 16 weeks and <50% carcinoma incidence with chronic administration. These results seem to indicate that (a) aromatization to oestradiol is critical in the induction of prostate cancer by testosterone, (b) the combination of testosterone and oestradiol is more effective in producing prostate cancers than DHT and oestradiol, suggesting that factors other than aromatization are also involved, and (c) testosterone plus oestradiol induced prostatic dysplasia, which is a reversible lesion (Bosland *et al*, 1994). Noble (1977) has also shown an increase in the incidence of prostate cancer in Nb rats through the chronic administration of testosterone and oestrogen.

Similarly, there is a vast literature delineating oestrogen induced carcinogenesis. The potential for steroid hormones, especially the oestrogens, to induce DNA damage has been reported (Henderson *et al*, 1988), but the mitogenic effects of steroid hormones might place the cells in a proliferative state thus leading to increased genetic instability or the expression of mutated genes that then could alter the cell's phenotype. Members of the steroid hormone receptor superfamily of genes act as transcription factors when complexed with their ligand regulating the expression of a large subset of genes such as oncogenes, for example, *fos*, *jun* and *myc* (Wilding *et al*, 1988; Weisaz *et al*, 1990); growth factors, for example, *TGFA* and *TGFB* (Wilding *et al*, 1989a; Jeng and Jordan, 1991); receptors, for example, epidermal growth factor receptor (*EGFR*) (Schuurmans *et al*, 1988); and other genes coding for proteins such as proteases, for example, prostate specific antigen (Clements *et al*, 1988) and tPA, which could be involved in the processes of invasion and metastasis (Dickson and Lippman, 1987). Mutation of the *AR* has been shown to inactivate the receptor (Brown *et al*, 1988) or to broaden its ability to be activated by a broad range of ligands including anti-androgens (Wilding *et al*, 1989c; Harris *et al*, 1991). Although the *AR* cannot be viewed as a proto-oncogene, the importance of its presence and its transcriptional regulation of a host of gene products that have been proved to be important in cellular transformation cannot be overlooked.

As a male accessory sex organ, both during normal development and as a mature gland, the prostate is extremely sensitive and responsive to the presence of androgenic hormones and the *AR* (Coffey, 1988). Embryologically, the *AR* mediates androgenic regulation of prostate epithelial differentiation via stromal-epithelial interactions. Using tissue recombinant studies of the urogenital sinus and its epithelial and stromal components, Cunha *et al* (1983) have shown that androgens regulate the growth, differentiation and morphogenesis of the prostate epithelium indirectly via the surrounding stroma. Analysis of the *AR* in these tissue components demonstrates that a functional *AR* in the stroma, not the epithelium, during embryogenesis is the crucial factor for normal prostate development. The manner in which the androgen stimulated stroma mediates its influence on the developing epithelium is unclear, although extracellular matrix components and soluble growth factors are potential factors. Chung and others have documented prostate stromal-epithelial interactions in vitro that lend credence to the possible indirect effects of androgens on the prostate epithelium (Chang and Chung, 1989; Kabalin *et al,* 1989).

The regulation of the adult prostate epithelium appears to be more complex, with both direct and indirect androgenic actions taking place. Again, tissue recombination studies have shed some light on the potential influence of stroma on prostate cancer growth. Studies using fetal and neonatal urogenital mesenchymes in combination with the transplantable Dunning rat prostate adenocarcinoma have shown that the cancer cells can be induced to undergo coordinated growth and differentiation in the presence of specific mesenchymes (Hayashi *et al,* 1990). Thompson *et al* (1989), using *ras* and *myc* infected components in a mouse recombinant model, have shown that *ras/myc* infected epithelium combined with uninfected stroma produces benign hyperplasia. However, *ras/myc* infected stroma combined with *ras/myc* infected epithelium results in poorly differentiated adenocarcinoma (Thompson *et al,* 1989). These authors' studies demonstrate that normal mesenchyme is non-permissive for high frequency conversion to malignancy and suggest that *ras/myc* infected urogenital sinus mesenchyme lacks the potential to inhibit malignant conversion of epithelium and/or promotes the conversion process (Thompson, 1990). Of interest, combinations of *ras/myc* infected mesenchyme and uninfected epithelium showed elevated levels of *TGFB*. In castrated animals with *ras/myc* induced tumours, *TGFB1*, *TGFB3* and tPA were all elevated two- to fourfold compared to non-castrated animals. These results indicate that the *ras/myc* induced carcinomas responded to androgen deprivation by upregulating genes that are involved in cell growth and differentiation. In addition, mesenchyme derived *TGFB* might play an important part in the conversion of premalignant epithelium to malignant carcinomas (Egawa *et al,* 1991; Ripoll *et al,* 1991). In other words, mesenchymal mediators that normally control discrete steps of development might, under the right circumstances, promote a malignant phenotype in transformed epithelial cells. Similar paracrine activities may also underlie malignant progression of prostate cancer in humans.

HORMONES IN PROSTATE CARCINOGENESIS

If androgens and mediation of their action through the *AR* are important in maintaining a normal, functioning prostate gland through adulthood, what are the data on the variations in androgen or *AR* levels with age and are there correlative changes with the development of pathological states in the gland? Firstly, it is generally agreed that there is a progressive impairment of Leydig cell function with advancing age (Nahoui and Roger, 1990). This impairment consists of a diminished capacity of Leydig cells to synthesize and secrete androgens (Serio *et al,* 1979; Takahashi *et al,* 1983; Hammar, 1985) as well as a decline in their responsiveness to human chorionic gonadotrophin (HCG) (Longcope, 1970). Although studies measuring plasma testosterone in a variety of assays have been inconsistent in documenting a decline in plasma testosterone with age, the sum of free plus albumin bound T, called non-sex hormone binding globulin (non-SHBG) or bioavailable T, has been demonstrated to be the best index for evaluating androgen activity (Cumming and Wall, 1985). In addition, it has been shown to decrease in elderly men in comparison with young men (Bartsch, 1980; Nankin and Caulkins, 1986; Tenover *et al*, 1987).

In general, although some data suggest a higher risk of prostate cancer in men with elevated testosterone levels (Hsing and Comstock, 1989), other matched control studies have not confirmed this finding (Hill *et al*, 1980). Higher testosterone levels have been associated with a Western versus a vegetarian diet (Hill *et al*, 1979). Finally, although higher DHT levels in prostate cancer tissue have correlated with a higher rate of hormone response (Geller *et al*, 1984), no conclusive correlation can be made pertaining to DHT levels and the development of prostate cancer. For example, a recent prospective epidemiological study linked high plasma androgen levels with the development of prostate cancer when an increased androstenedione level was associated with a greater risk of later developing prostate cancer in a cohort followed up for 14 years (Barrett-Connor *et al*, 1990). On the other hand, Nomura *et al* (1988) prospectively obtained serum samples from 6860 men in Hawaii. After a surveillance period of 14 years, sera from 98 incident cases of prostate cancer and 98 matched controls were assayed for testosterone, DHT, oestrone, oestradiol and SHBG. Although there was a suggestion that DHT levels were lower in the patients with prostate cancer, no strongly significant association could be made between hormone levels and prostate cancer. Others have suggested the possibility that 5-α-reductase activity in converting testosterone to DHT might be important. They note that Japanese and Chinese men have among the lowest rates of prostate cancer in the world. Both of these populations have been shown to have reduced 5-α-reductase activity relative to American blacks and whites (Lookinbill *et al*, 1991; Ross *et al*, 1992). These data have contributed to the basis for a large prevention trial with 18 000 patients of the 5-α-reductase inhibitor finasteride. In summary, although there are data suggesting that alterations in androgen levels are associated with the development of prostate cancer, consistency is a major problem in the data and no clear conclusions can be drawn. The question thus arises of whether variation in *AR* expression occurs during prostate carcinogenesis.

In men with prostate cancer, a broad range of testosterone levels are found. Retrospective analysis from one study showed that the higher the pretreatment plasma level, the greater the survival rate in patients with metastatic prostate cancer receiving primary hormone therapy (Hickey *et al*, 1988). Conversely, low testosterone levels at the time of diagnosis have been shown to carry a poor prognosis (Ishikawa *et al*, 1989). Chodak *et al* (1991) assessed the independent prognostic factors affecting survival in 240 men undergoing treatment for metastatic prostate cancer as part of a randomized clinical trial comparing a gonadotrophin releasing hormone analogue with castration. In a multivariate analysis, one of the most highly significant predictors was the serum testosterone level in addition to bone pain, performance status and serum alkaline phosphatase levels. Patients with all four factors favourable for survival had a 2 year survival rate of 84% compared with a rate of only 8% for patients with none of the four factors favourable for survival. A separate analysis of serum testosterone levels revealed that the higher the pretreatment serum testosterone level, the greater the survival rate. Compared with patients with serum testosterone levels of less than 6.9 nmol/l, significant differences in survival were observed for patients with levels of 10.4–13.9, 13.9–17.3 and over 17.3 nmol/l.

The mainstay of hormone therapy for metastatic prostate cancer is bilateral orchidectomy. Proved by Huggins in the 1940s to be an effective palliative therapy, this remains the "gold standard" against which other hormone therapies are compared. Orchidectomy removes the primary source of testosterone in men, the testicles. There exists a viewpoint that even after hormone failure, a patient should be maintained in an orchidectomized state. The rationale for this approach is that although a patient's tumour may no longer be dependent for growth on testosterone, it still may be responsive to testosterone stimulation.

Additive steroid therapy has also been used in the treatment of metastatic prostate cancer. Diethylstilbestrol (DES) and other oestrogens have been extensively studied. One of the primary conclusions of the Veterans Administration Cooperative Urologic Research Group (Byar, 1973) was that DES 1–5 mg/day was as effective as orchidectomy at palliating the symptoms of metastatic prostate cancer. Although 1 mg/day was as effective as 5 mg/day and less toxic, 1 mg/day does not achieve a drop in testosterone levels as low as those achieved with orchidectomy. Because of the availability of less toxic, although much more expensive, non-surgical hormone therapies, such as gonadotrophin releasing hormone (GnRH) agonists, the use of this form of additive steroid therapy has declined in recent years. Another additive therapy that has been used less often than oestrogens is megestrol acetate, a progestogen. Both of these additive therapies decrease serum testosterone levels by disrupting the hypothalamic–pituitary–gonadal axis by decreasing gonadotrophin release from the pituitary.

Although the testes produce over 90% of the circulating androgens in men, the adrenal glands make and secrete weak androgens that can be converted in one or two enzymatic steps to testosterone. Therefore, the concept of combining a GnRH agonist or orchidectomy with an anti-androgen was developed in an attempt to achieve maximal androgen blockade. One of the larger randomized studies of this concept compared the use of a GnRH analogue with or without the anti-androgen flutamide in men with metastatic prostate cancer (Crawford *et al*, 1989). The patients receiving the combined therapy had a longer progression free survival (16.5 v. 13.9 months) and an increase in the median length of survival (35.6 v. 28.3 months) compared with the patients receiving GnRH analogue alone. Most striking was the improved survival of the 41 patients with minimal metastatic disease who were treated with the combination therapy. If confirmed in subsequent studies, this would support earlier intervention with hormone therapy in patients with metastatic prostate cancer. Of interest, the patients receiving the combination therapy showed the greatest improvement in symptoms during the first 12 weeks of therapy, which suggests amelioration of possible GnRH induced flare effects during this period.

Primary hormone therapy ultimately fails in all patients as hormone independent disease emerges. Secondary attempts at hormone manipulation yield palliative results, generally subjective in nature, in approximately 20% of the patients and are of short duration. Secondary hormone therapies are usually aimed at reducing or blocking adrenal androgens. Most recently, withdrawal responses to the discontinuation of flutamide have been noted (Scher and Kelly, 1993).

ANDROGEN RECEPTORS IN PROSTATE CANCER

What is known about *AR* expression and protein levels in the aging process and in prostate carcinogenesis? Until recently, the assessment of *AR* levels and localization in prostate tissues and cancers have been hampered by technical difficulties. Assays on homogenized tissues do not address heterogeneity issues. The condition of the tissue—fresh, frozen, cauterized, etc—has led to variable results. Attempts to separate cellular compartments can lead to mechanical damage of cells and a shift of the receptor between the cytoplasm and nucleus of cells. With the cloning of the human *AR* gene and the development of monoclonal antibodies against the receptor, the issues of heterogeneity, intracellular distribution, transcriptional versus translational control, mutational frequency and structure-activity relationships can be addressed. Summarized below are the studies performed during the period since *AR* cDNA and monoclonal antibody reagents have become available.

The human *AR* gene is a nuclear hormone receptor. The receptor contains highly conserved regions analogous to the hormone binding and DNA binding domains of other steroid receptors such as progesterone, mineralocorticoid, glucocorticoid, oestrogen and vitamin D. These receptors comprise a superfamily of ligand modulated transcription factors that regulate homoeostasis, reproduction, development and differentiation. The cDNA sequence of the *AR* was initially reported in 1988 by several groups, including C Chang (Chang *et al,* 1988a,b; Lubahn *et al,* 1988a; Faber *et al,* 1989; Tilley *et al,* 1989). The coding region of the human *AR* encompasses approximately 3580 nucleotides from which the deduced 919 aminoacids predict a protein of 99 kDa (Lubahn *et al,* 1988b; Tan *et al,* 1988). Northern blot analysis surprisingly has shown hybridization of cDNA clones to mRNA species of 9.6 and 7 kb (Lubahn *et al,*

1988b; Chang *et al,* 1989a; Takeda *et al,* 1991). Immunohistochemical analyses of human prostate tissue sections have localized the AR protein predominantly in the nuclei of glandular epithelial cells using polyclonal antibodies or monoclonal antibodies (Lubahn *et al,* 1988b; Chang *et al,* 1989a,b; Takeda *et al,* 1991). The *AR* gene has been localized to the X chromosome between the centromere and q13.

With the development of reagents such as cDNAs and antibodies against the human *AR,* studies have begun to emerge that characterize the expression of the *AR* in human prostate tissue. Initial reports have confirmed localization of the *AR* predominantly to the nucleus of prostate epithelial cells in normal, benign hyperplastic and cancerous prostate and other tissues (Lubahn *et al,* 1988b; Takeda *et al,* 1989; Takeda and Chang, 1991). As noted above, a major limitation of previous studies using homogenized tissue was that the *AR* content was an average of all the cells in the homogenized specimen. Sadi *et al* (1991) recently tried to overcome this problem by performing an immunohistochemical analysis of the *AR* in 17 patients with prostate cancer. Needle biopsy specimens were used to determine the extent of *AR* expression in prostate cancer specimens. They found that prostate cancer contains *AR* positive and *AR* negative malignant cells before androgen withdrawal therapy, but the percentage of *AR* positive cells did not predict the time to tumour progression after androgen withdrawal therapy.

Similarly, van Aubel *et al* (1988) examined the nuclear *AR* content by a binding assay of nuclear extracts of 42 patients treated with orchidectomy and followed up for a minimum of 30 months. No relationship was found between nuclear *AR* content and the time to progression after orchidectomy in these patients. In a refinement of their earlier study, Sadi and Barrack (1993) used computer assisted image analysis to evaluate the immunohistochemical staining intensity of 200 nuclei from each of 17 stage D2 patients obtained before hormone therapy was instituted. Their analysis showed that the *AR* concentration per cell was significantly more heterogeneous in poor responders, which possibly reflected greater genetic instability in tumours that have progressed further towards androgen independence.

Other small studies have reached a variety of conclusions. Brolin *et al* (1992a,b) examined tissue from six patients with benign hyperplasia and from 24 patients with prostate cancer with fine needle aspirates. *AR* immunostaining was found in the majority of benign and malignant cells with no obvious relation in the intensity of staining between benign and malignant cells. The relative number of androgen receptor positive cells was highest in smears from poorly differentiated cancers. Van der Kwast *et al* (1991) found that in 13 of 17 tumours from patients who had failed hormone therapy, more than 80% of tumour cells stained positive for *AR*. Miyamoto *et al* (1993) found greater heterogeneity of *AR* staining in cancer tissue but also thought cancer tissue stained less intensely than normal tissue.

A larger study provided additional insight into this problem (Chodak *et al,* 1992). To facilitate an understanding of how androgens participate in the genesis of benign hyperplasia and carcinoma in humans, *AR* was assayed in the stroma and epithelium of human prostate tissue from 57 patients. Immunohistochemical staining of human *AR* was performed on 106 sections of normal, hyperplastic and cancerous prostate tissue. To determine the variability of *AR* staining, sections taken from different portions of the gland were studied. Frozen tissue sections were incubated with monoclonal *AR* antibodies and staining was completed by indirect avidin-biotin peroxidase methods. Antibody staining was found mainly in the nucleus of prostate epithelial cells, although some stromal cells also showed positive staining. Unlike normal prostate, there was a heterogeneous distribution of *AR* in benign prostatic hyperplasia and prostate cancer. The *AR* content in well differentiated adenocarcinoma epithelium was significantly higher compared to moderately ($p<0.05$) and poorly ($p<0.05$) differentiated carcinomas. Regardless of the origin of stromal tissue, some staining was observed. In each specimen studied, *AR* staining was consistent both qualitatively and quantitatively for each pathological component throughout the specimen. These data confirm that AR is a nuclear receptor protein. Furthermore, it shows the ability of monoclonal antibodies to reveal cellular/subcellular distribution of AR and demonstrates a correlation between the degree of tumour differentiation and AR content in epithelial but not stromal cells. These studies might help us to understand variable tumour response to hormonal therapy.

The mechanism by which androgen binding activates the AR and results in the regulation of expression of a specific subset of genes has not been determined. Models have been proposed, involving the C-terminal region, which attempt to link the events of ligand binding, dimerization and hormone relieved transcriptional inactivation (Forman and Samuel, 1990). Since the nuclear matrix is known to bind androgen receptors in a tissue and steroid specific manner, Getzenberg and Coffey (1990) have proposed that the tissue specificity of the nuclear matrix arranges the DNA in a unique conformation, which may be involved in the specific interaction of transcription factors with DNA sequences, resulting in tissue specific patterns of protein expression. Expression of AR is regulated by many factors including androgens and growth factors such as epidermal growth factor (Mizokami *et al,* 1992).

Detection of abnormal *AR* genes in patients with testicular feminization (Tfm) was evaluated using polymerase chain reaction technology. We were able directly to sequence the abnormal *AR* gene from patients with Tfm. Total RNA from genital skin fibroblast lines of patients was isolated by the guanidinium thiocyanate method. The first and second strand cDNAs were synthesized and the hormone binding domain of these double-stranded cDNAs were then amplified for 30 cycles. The amplified DNAs were sequenced directly. One patient was found to have a deletion of the *AR* gene from exon 1 to exon 7 (Trifio *et al,* 1989), and the other patient was found to have a mutation (Trp-717 to stop codon) in exon 7 that abolished most of the *AR* binding domain (Sai *et al,* 1990).

Wilding *et al* (1989c) conducted studies on the androgen responsive human prostate cancer cell line LNCaP to determine the direct effects of a variety of androgens, anti-androgens and other steroid hormones on hormone responsive prostate cancer cells in vitro. These cells contain approximately 30 000 high affinity androgen binding sites per cell. In the absence of any androgenic stimulation, the cells were shown to be stimulated by three different anti-androgens. These cells were subsequently shown to have a point mutation in the hormone binding region of their *AR* by Harris *et al* (1991). The data noted above verify and confirm that androgen sensitivity can be lost or altered both through subtle changes such as point mutations or by deletions of significant portions of the *AR* gene.

In recent years, data have begun to accumulate on the frequency and nature of *AR* mutations in prostate cancer. Unfortunately, virtually all of the studies were small, and they used different techniques; prostate tissues were used from multiple stages and prior treatment varied. As a result, the findings were not conclusive. In summary, the findings were as follows: Gaddipati *et al* (1994) analysed prostate tissue specimens derived from transurethral resections in patients with metastatic prostate cancer for genetic alterations in the hormone binding domain of the *AR* gene. Direct sequencing of the polymerase chain reaction derived DNAs of 6 of 24 specimens revealed a codon 877 mutation (ACT→GCT, Thr→Ala) in the hormone binding domain of the *AR* gene. This is the same mutation found in the *AR* LNCaP cells, which are stimulated by anti-androgens. This specific *AR* mutation might represent the molecular basis for flutamide withdrawal responses seen in some patients. Although all of the specimens in this study were derived from patients with stage C or D disease, prior treatment status and response to treatment were not discussed. Other studies have shown this or other mutations. For example, a study of 26 early stage B prostate cancers showed a codon 730 *AR* mutation in one specimen (Newmark, 1992). Examination of the *AR* gene in advanced prostate cancers revealed mutations in codons 701 and 877 in one of eight specimens (Suzucki *et al,* 1993), in codons 340 and 798 in two of ten specimens (Castagnaro *et al,* 1993) and in codon 715 in one of seven specimens (Cullig *et al,* 1993a,b). Not all studies have found point mutations. Sharief *et al* (1994) found no mutations in specimens from the primary tumours of 20 patients. de Vere White *et al* (1994) found none, but they did see *AR* gene expression in 13 of 19 (685) samples from patients after adequate hormone therapy.

Schoenberg *et al* (1994) have examined another aspect of the *AR* gene structure that might lead to abnormal behaviour of the *AR* in prostate cancer. The *AR* gene contains a CAG microsatellite, a homopolymeric trinucleotide repeat sequence that codes for a glutamine report that varies in length in the population (13–30 CAGs). Since trinucleotide repeat instability has been associated with several neurological diseases and colon cancer, these authors screened 40 human prostate cancers for expansion or deletions of the *AR* CAG microsatellite. In one patient, non-malignant tissue contained 24 CAGs, whereas the tumour contained one fragment with 24 CAGs, presumably from normal cells, and a second fragment with 18 CAGs, possibly a mutant derived from the cancer cells. This patient had had a flutamide withdrawal response.

Yuan *et al* (1993) introduced a full length *AR* gene cDNA driven by an SV40 promoter into the *AR* negative PC-3 cells to determine whether androgen sensitivity could be restored in these cells. *AR* was expressed and showed high affinity binding characteristics. However, in cells expressing the transfected *AR*, androgens decreased the proliferation rate and induced a more differentiated phenotype.

From these data, it seems apparent that (a) *AR* mutations do not occur at a high frequency in prostate cancer at various clinical stages. (b) When mutations are present, they tend to be point mutations. (c) Codon 877 mutations have been observed in clinical specimens and a cell line. This mutation might account for the aberrant response of the LNCaP cell line to flutamide, and it could provide insight into the flutamide withdrawal responses seen in some patients after flutamide is discontinued in the face of progressive disease. (d) *AR* continues to be expressed in patients with prostate cancer even after adequate hormone therapy. This could explain why patients with hormone refractory prostate cancer will show growth stimulation of their cancer if given androgens, but their cancer is no longer dependent on androgens to maintain a level of cancer growth or progression.

PEPTIDE GROWTH FACTORS AND OTHER STEROIDS IN PROSTATE CANCER

The androgen/*AR* complex, acting as a transcription factor, mediates its effects on a cell through transcriptional control of a specific subset of genes. The influence of the activated androgen receptor on the growth of human prostate cancer and its relationship to the surrounding stroma are controlled by complex mechanisms that are incompletely understood. Clearly, a wide range of peptide growth factors play crucial parts in these processes (Thompson, 1990). I have chosen to focus on one of these factors, *TGFB* and its related family members (Keski-Oja *et al*, 1988), because of its wide spectrum of biological effects, its influence on the transcription of a variety of oncogene products such as *myc*, *jun* and *fos* (Keski-Oja *et al*, 1988; Li *et al*, 1988; Moses *et al*, 1990), its potential interaction with suppressor genes such as retinoblastoma (*RB*) (Pietenpol *et al*, 1990a,b) and its link with androgens, not only through androgen mediated control of its transcription (Kyprianou and Isaacs, 1988), but also through its role in the androgen controlled process of apoptosis (Kyprianou and Isaacs, 1989).

In terms of growth, *TGFB* inhibits the growth of prostate cancer cells in a cytostatic fashion while stimulating the growth of critical stromal cells, such as fibroblasts (Wilding, 1991). Since the inhibitory effects of *TGFB* on prostate cancer cells appear to diminish as the process of transformation progresses towards less differentiated states, the net effect on prostate tumour growth may be positive. Recent evidence suggests that at least the inhibitory effects of *TGFB* on growth might be mediated through the RB tumour suppressor gene product and the proto-oncogene c-*myc* (Pietenpol *et al,* 1990a,b). Beyond its direct growth effects, *TGFB* also alters the response of prostate cancer cells to positive mitogenic factors, such as members of the epidermal and fibroblast growth factor families (McKeehan and Adams, 1988), suggesting that growth control is in fact a delicate balance between positive and negative influences. Non-mitogenic responses to *TGFB* by prostate cancer cells, the immune system, the stroma and the vascular system provide evidence that *TGFB* might also be important in the processes of carcinogenesis, tumour establishment and metastasis (Keski-Oja *et al,* 1988). In addition, *TGFB* appears to influence metabolic pathways important to drug metabolism and steroidogenesis (Chapekar *et al,* 1990; Rainey *et al,* 1990). Limited evidence suggests that in vivo, *TGFB* can alter the growth and differentiation of some tumour types but appears to be very toxic when administered in high doses. A better understanding of the response of prostate cancer cells to members of the *TGFB* family may open new avenues of treating and controlling this disease.

Members of the retinoic acid family might represent an opportunity to use steroid hormones to modulate growth factor expression in prostate cancer (Sporn and Roberts, 1991). For example, it has been shown that retinoic acid is a potent inducer of *TGFB2* in mouse keratinocytes, both in vitro and in vivo, but has minimal effects on *TGFB1* mRNA levels (Glick *et al,* 1989). The association between treatment with retinoic acid and the state of phosphorylation of RB protein during induction of differentiation of leukaemia cells has been reported by Mihara *et al* (1989). In addition, as noted above, *TGFB* might exert its growth inhibitory effects through a pathway involving RB. These observations suggest that retinoids might have a role in disrupting prostate carcinogenesis in humans.

Retinoids have also been noted to regulate the proliferation and differentiation of prostate cancer cells (Fong *et al,* 1993; Peehl *et al,* 1993). This regulation has led others to explore retinoids as possible preventive agents for prostate cancer. Using the Lobund-Wistar rat, Pollard *et al* (1991) recently demonstrated the prevention of primary prostate cancer using *N*-(4-hydroxyphenyl) retinamide (4HPR). In this model, 88% of rats inoculated with *N*-methyl-nitrosourea (NMU) at 3 months of age and then chronically treated with testosterone propionate (TP) developed prostate carcinomas, and 61% of the animals also developed metastases. Untreated animals spontaneously develop prostate carcinomas at a rate of 26%. When 4HPR was added to the diet of NMU/TP treated rats, the incidence of primary prostate carcinomas and metastases dropped to 21% and 16%, respectively. In addition to being a promising preventive of prostate cancer, 4HPR appears to be well tolerated. In more than 1000 women at high risk of developing breast cancer, 4HPR has been tolerated very well, with a minimum of side effects during chronic administration (200 mg/day) (Rotmensz *et al,* 1991).

Finally, note must be made of the presence of receptors for vitamin D3 in human prostate cancer cells (Miller *et al,* 1991). Not only did Miller *et al* document the presence of vitamin D3 receptors in LNCaP cells, but these cells were also stimulated to grow in the absence of androgens by vitamin D3. Petkovich *et al* (1987) have previously shown that vitamin D3 increases epidermal growth factor receptors and *TGFB* activity in bone derived cells. Likewise, Peehl *et al* (1994) have examined the effect yof 1,25-dihydroxyvitamin D3 on prostate cancer cell growth and found inhibition of cell growth. These observations raise the possibility that manipulation of vitamin D activity in prostate cancer cells might not only alter their growth, but also modulate growth factor response in these cells.

SUMMARY

Steroid hormones play an important part in prostate biology. Androgens are crucial for the normal development of the prostate gland and in maintaining its functional state in the adult. It seems that the prolonged presence of androgens might also be an important factor in the development of prostate cancer. In addition, androgens and oestrogens appear to play a part in the development of benign prostatic hypertrophy, although the exact nature of their role has not been clearly defined. Stimulation of prostate cancer growth by androgens is well established with androgen withdrawal therapy being the most effective therapy in men with prostate cancer. Additive steroid therapy of metastatic prostate cancer with oestrogens or progestogens has also proved effective. The effects of androgens on prostate cancer cell growth might be mediated through modulation of growth factor expression and alteration of growth factor receptor levels. Androgen response can be modulated by the expression of mutated oncogenes such as *ras*. Androgen independence can occur through a loss of *AR* expression or mutation of the *AR*; however, the patterns of *AR* expression in normal prostatic tissue from development to adulthood and in cancer are now just beginning to be described. Other steroids, such as the retinoids, show promise as preventive agents, possibly through the modulation of growth factors. Vitamin D compounds modulate prostate cancer cell growth, but their role in prevention and therapy is unclear.

References

Barrett-Connor E, Garland C, McPhillips JB, Khaw KT and Wingard DL (1990) A prospective, population based study of androstenedione, estrogens and prostate cancer. *Cancer Research* **50** 169–173

Bartsch W (1980) Interrelationships between sex hormone binding globulin and testosterone, 5α dihydrotestosterone and estradiol 17α in blood of normal men. *Maturitas* **2** 109–118

Boring CC, Squires TS, Tong T and Montgomery S (1994) Cancer statistics. *CA-A Cancer Journal for Clinicians* **44** 7–26

Bosland MC (1988) The etiopathogenesis of prostate cancer with special reference to environmental factors. *Advances in Cancer Research* **51** 1–106

Bosland MC, Prinsen MK, Dirksen TJM and Spit BJ (1990) Characterization of adenocarcinomas of the dorsolateral prostate induced in Wistar rats by N-methyl-N-nitrosourea 7,12-dimethyl benzanthracene and 3,2′ dimethyl-4-amino biphenyl following sequential treatment with cyproterone acetate and testosterone propionate. *Cancer Research* **50** 700–709

Bosland MC, Horton L, Dennison J, Ward L and Ritter M (1994) The role of estrogen in the induction of prostate carcinomas by androgens in rats. *Proceedings of the American Association for Cancer Research* **35** 1562

Brolin J, Lowhagen T and Skoog L (1992a) Immunocytochemical detection of the androgen receptor in fine needle aspirates from benign and malignant human prostate. *Cytopathology* **3** 351–357

Brolin J, Skoog L and Ekman P (1992b) Immunohistochemistry and biochemistry in detection of androgen, progesterone, and estrogen receptors in benign and malignant human prostatic tissue. *Prostate* **20** 281–295

Brown TR, Lubahn DB, Wilson EM, Joseph DR, French FW and Midgeon CJ (1988) Deletion of the steroid binding domain of the human androgen receptor gene in one family with complete androgen insensitivity syndrome: evidence for further genetic heterogeneity in this syndrome. *Proceedings of the National Academy of Sciences of the USA* **85** 8151–8155

Byar DP (1973) Proceedings: The Veteran's Administration Cooperative Urologic Research Group's studies of cancer of the prostate. *Cancer* **32** 1126–1130

Carter HB and Coffey DS (1990) The prostate: an increasing medical problem. *Prostate* **16** 39–48

Castagnaro M, Yandell DW, Dockhorn-Dworhiczak B, Wolfe HJ and Poremba C (1993) Human androgen receptor gene mutations and p.53 gene analysis in advanced prostate cancer. *Verhandlungen der Deutschen Gesellschaft fur Pathologie* **77** 119–123

Catalona WJ and Scott WW (1986) Carcinoma of the prostate, In: Walsh PC, Gittes RF, Perlmutter AD and Stamey TA (eds). *Campbell's Urology,* 5th ed, pp 1463-1534, Saunders Philadelphia

Chang C, Kokontis J and Liao S (1988a) Structural analysis of complementary DNA and amino acid sequences of human and rat androgen receptors. *Proceedings of the National Academy of Sciences of USA* **85** 7211–7215

Chang C, Kokontis J and Liao S (1988b) Molecular cloning of human and rat complementary DNA encoding androgen receptors. *Science* **240** 324–326

Chang C, Chodak G, Sarac E, Takeda H and Liao S (1989a) Prostate androgen receptor: immunohistochemical localization and mRNA characterization. *Steroid Biochemistry* **34** 311–313

Chang C, Whelan CT, Popovich JC, Kokontis J and Liao S (1989b) Fusion proteins containing androgen receptor sequences and their use in the production of poly- and monoclonal antiandrogen receptor antibodies. *Endocrinology* **123** 1097–1099

Chang SM and Chung LWK (1989) Interactions between prostatic fibroblast and epithelial cells in culture: role of androgen. *Endocrinology* **125** 2719–2727

Chapekar MS, Huggett AC, Chang CC, Hampton LL, Lin KH and Thorgeirsson SS (1990) Isolation and characterization of a rat liver epithelial cell line resistant to the antiproliferative effects of transforming growth factor β (Type 1). *Cancer Research* **50** 3600–3604

Chodak GW, Vogelzang NJ, Caplan RJ, Soloway M and Smith JA (1991) Independent prognostic factors in patients with metastatic (stage D2) prostate cancer. *Journal of the American Medical Association* **265** 618–621

Chodak GW, Kranc DM, Puy LA, Takeda H, Johnson K and Chang C (1992) Nuclear localization of androgen receptor in the normal, hyperplastic and neoplastic human prostate. *Journal of Urology* **147** 798–803

Clements JA, Matheson BA, Wines DR, Brady JM, McDonald RJ and Fouder JW (1988) Androgen dependence of specific kallikrein gene family members expressed in rat prostate. *Journal of Biological Chemistry* **263** 16132–16137

Coffey DS (1988) Androgen action in the sex accessary tissues, In: Knobil J and Neill J (eds).

The Physiology of Reproduction, pp 1081–1119, Raven Press, New York

Crawford ED, Eisenerger MA, McLeod DG *et al* (1989) A controlled trial of leuprolide with and without flutamide in prostatic carcinoma. *New England Journal of Medicine* **321** 419–424

Cullig Z, Klocker H, Eberle J *et al* (1993a) DNA sequence of the androgen receptor in prostatic tumor cell lines and tissue specimens assessed by means of the polymerase chain reaction. *Prostate* **22** 11–22

Cullig Z, Hobisen A, Cronauer MV *et al* (1993b) Mutant androgen receptor detected in an advanced-stage prostatic carcinoma is activated by adrenal androgens and progesterone. *Molecular Endocrinology* **7** 1541–1550

Cumming DC and Wall SR (1985) Non-sex hormone binding globulin-bound testosterone as a marker for hyperandrogenism. *Journal of Clinical Endocrinology and Metabolism* **61** 873–876

Cunha GR, Chung LWK, Shannon JM, Taquchi O and Fujii H (1983) Hormone induced morphogenesis and growth: role of mesenchymal-epithelial interactions. *Recent Progress in Hormone Research* **39** 559–598

de Vere White R, Gumerlock PH, Chamberlain SR, Lee F and Siders DB (1994) Human androgen receptor analysis in prostate cancer. *Journal of Urology* **151** 962A [Abstract]

Dhom G (1991) Epidemiology of hormone depending tumors, In: Voight KD and Knabbe C (eds). *Endocrine Dependent Tumors,* pp 1–37, Raven Press, New York

Dickson RB and Lippman ME (1987) Estrogenic regulation of growth and polypeptide growth factor secretion in human breast carcinoma. *Endocrine Review* **8** 29–43

Eqawa S, Kadmon D, Greene DR, Scardino PT and Thompson TC (1991) Adaptive changes in gene expression following androgen ablation in clonal mouse adenocarcinoma. *Journal of Urology* **145** 539

Faber PW, Kuiper GGJM, van Roij HCJ, van der Korput JAGM, Brinkman AO and Trapman J (1989) The N terminal domain of the human androgen receptor is encoded by one large exon. *Molecular and Cellular Endocrinology* **61** 257–262

Feldman AR, Kessler L, Myers MH and Naughton MD (1986) The prevalence of cancer: estimates based on the Connecticut Tumor Registry. *New England Journal of Medicine* **315** 1394–1397

Fong CJ, Sutkowski DM, Braun EJ *et al* (1993) Effect of retinoic acid on the proliferation and secretory activity of androgen responsive prostatic carcinoma cells. *Journal of Urology* **149** 1190–1194

Forman BM and Samuel HH (1990) Interactions among a subfamily of nuclear hormone receptors: the regulatory zipper model. *Molecular Endocrinology* **4** 1293–1301

Gaddipati JP, McLeod DG, Heidenberg HB *et al* (1994) Frequent detection of codon 877 mutation in the androgen receptor gene in advanced prostate cancer. *Cancer Research* **54** 2861–2864

Geller J, Albert JD, Nachtsheim DA and Loza D (1984) Tissue dihydrotestosterone levels and clinical response to hormonal therapy in patients with advanced prostate cancer. *Journal of Clinical Endocrinology and Metabolism* **58** 36–40

Getzenberg RH and Coffey DS (1990) Tissue specificity of the hormone response in sex accessary tissues is associated with nuclear matrix protein patterns. *Molecular Endocrinology* **4** 1336–1352

Glick AB, Flanders KC, Danielpour D, Yuspa H and Sporn M (1989) Retinoic acid induces transforming growth factor β2 in cultured keratinocytes and mouse epidermis. *Cell Regulation* **1** 87–97

Hammar M (1985) Impaired in vitro testicular endocrine function in elderly men. *Andrologia* **17** 444–449

Harris S, Harris MA, Rong Z *et al* (1991) Androgen regulation of HGBF I (aFGF) and characterization of the androgen receptor mRNA in the human prostate carcinoma cell line LNCaP/A-dep, In: Karr JP, Coffey DS, Smith RG and Tindall DJ (eds). *Molecular and Cel-*

lular Biology of Prostate Cancer, pp 315–330, Plenum Press, New York
Hayashi N, Cunha GR and Wong YC (1990) Influence of male genital tract mesenchyme on differentiation of Dunning prostatic adenocarcinoma. *Cancer Research* **50** 4747–4754
Henderson BE, Ross R and Bernstein L (1988) Estrogens as a cause of human cancer. *Cancer Research* **48** 246–253
Hickey D, Todd B and Soloway MS (1988) Pretreatment testosterone levels: significance in androgen deprivation therapy. *Journal of Urology* **136** 1038–1040
Hill P, Wynder E, Garbaczewski L, Garnen H and Walker ARP (1979) Diet and urinary steroids in black and white North American men and black South African men. *Cancer Research* **39** 5101–5105
Hill P, Wynder E, Garnes H and Walker A (1980) Environmental factors, hormone status and prostate cancer. *Preventive Medicine* **9** 657–666
Hsing A and Comstock G (1989) Serum hormones and risk of subsequent prostate cancer. *American Journal of Epidemiology* **130** 829
Isaacs JT and Kyprianou N (1987) Development of androgen-independent tumor cells and their implication for the treatment of prostate cancer. *Urologic Research* **15** 133–138
Ishikawa S, Soloway MS, Van Der Zwang R and Todd B (1989) Prognostic factors in survival free of progression after androgen deprivation therapy for treatment of prostate cancer. *Journal of Urology* **141** 1139–1142
Jeng MH and Jordan VC (1991) Growth stimulation and differential regulation of TGFβ1 TGFβ2 and TGFβ3 messenger RNA levels by norethindrone in MCF-7 breast cancer cells. *Molecular Endocrinolology* **5** 1120–1128
Kabalin JN, Peehl DM and Stamey TA (1989) Clonal growth of human prostate epithelial cells is stimulated by fibroblasts. *Prostate* **14** 251–263
Keski-Oja J, Postlethwaite AE and Moses HL (1988) Transforming growth factors in the regulation of malignant cell growth and invasion. *Cancer Investigation* **6** 705–724
Kyprianou N and Isaacs JT (1988) Identification of a cellular receptor for transforming growth factor β in rat ventral prostate and its regulation by androgens. *Endocrinology* **123** 2124–2131
Kyprianou N and Isaacs JT (1989) Expression of transforming growth factor beta in the rat ventral prostate during castration induced program cell death. *Molecular Endocrinology* **3** 1515–1522
Labrie F, Dupont A and Giguere M (1986) Advantages of the combination therapy in previously untreated and treated patients with advanced prostate cancer. *Journal of Steroid Biochemistry* **25** 877–883
Li L, Hu JS and Olsen EN (1990) Different members of the *jun* proto-oncogene family exhibit distinct patterns of expression in response to type β transforming growth factor. *Journal of Biological Chemistry* **265** 1556–1652
Longcope C (1973) The effect of human chorionic gonadotropin on plasma steroid levels in young and old men. *Steroids* **21** 583–592
Lookinbill DP, Demers LM and Wang C (1991) Clinical and biological parameters of androgen action in normal healthy Caucasian versus Chinese subjects. *Journal of Clinical Endocrinology and Metabolism* **72** 1242–1248
Lubahn DB, Joseph DR, Sullivan PM, Willard HF, French FS and Wilson EM (1988a) Cloning of human androgen receptor complementary DNA and localization to the X chromosome. *Science* **240** 327–330
Lubahn DB, Joseph DR, Sar M *et al* (1988b) The human androgen receptor: complementary deoxyribonucleic acid cloning, sequence analysis and gene expression in prostate. *Molecular Endocrinology* **2** 1265–1275
McKeehan WL and Adams PS (1988) Heparin binding growth factor/prostatropin attenuates inhibition of rat prostate tumor epithelial cell growth by transforming growth factor beta. *In Vitro Cellular and Developmental Biology* **24** 243–246
Mettlin C and Natarajan N (1983) Epidemiologic observations from the American College of

Surgeons survey on prostate cancer. *Prostate* **4** 323–331

Mihara K, Cao X-R, Yen A *et al* (1989) Cell cycle-dependent regulation of phosphorylation of the human retinoblastoma gene product. *Science* **246** 1300–1303

Miller GJ, Stapleton GE, Houmiel KL and Ferrara JA (1991) Specific receptors for vitamin D_3 in human prostatic carcinoma cells, In: Karr JP, Coffey DS, Smith RG and Tindall DJ (eds). *Molecular and Cellular Biology of Prostate Cancer,* pp 253–260, Plenum Press, New York

Miyamoto KK, McSherry SA, Dent GA *et al* (1993) Immunohistochemistry of the androgen receptor in human benign and malignant prostate tissue. *Journal of Urology* **149** 1015–1011q

Mizokami A, Saiga H, Matsui T, Mita T and Sugita A (1992) Regulation of androgen receptor by androgen and epidermal growth factor in a human prostatic cancer cell line LNCaP. *Endocrinologica Japonica* **39** 235–243

Moses HL, Yang EY and Pietenpol JA (1990) TGFβ stimulation and inhibition of cell proliferation: new mechanistic insights. *Cell* **63** 245–247

Nahoui K and Roger M (1990) Age-related decline of plasma bioavailable testosterone in adult men. *Journal of Steroid Biochemistry* **35** 293–299

Nankin HR and Caulkins JH (1986) Decreased bioavailable testosterone in aging normal and impotent men. *Journal of Clinical Endocrinology and Metabolism* **63** 1418–1420

Newmark JR, Hardy DO, Tonb DC *et al* (1992) Androgen receptor gene mutations in human prostate cancer. *Proceedings of the National Academy of Sciences of the USA* **89** 6314–6323

Noble K (1977) The development of prostatic adenocarcinoma in Nb rats, following prolonged sex hormone administration. *Cancer Research* **37** 1929–1933

Nomura A, Heilbrun LK, Stemmermann GN and Judd HL (1988) Prediagnostic serum hormones and the risk of prostate cancer. *Cancer Research* **48** 3515–3517

Peehl DM, Wong ST and Stamey TA (1993) Vitamin A regulates proliferation and differentiation of human prostatic epithelial cells. *Prostate* **23** 69–78

Peehl DM, Skowronski RJ, Leung GK, Wong ST, Stamey TA and Feldman D (1994) Antiproliferative effects of 1,25 dihydroxyvitamin D_3 on primary cultures of human prostatic cells. *Cancer Research* **54** 805–810

Petkovich PM, Wrang JL, Grigoriadis AE, Heersche JNM and Sodek J (1987) 1,25 dihydroxy vitamin D_3 increases epidermal growth factor receptors and transforming growth factor beta-like activity in a bone-derived cell line. *Journal of Biological Chemistry* **262** 13424–13428

Pietenpol JA, Holt JT, Stein RW and Moses HL (1990a) Transforming growth factor, suppression of *c-myc* gene transcription: role in inhibition of keratinocyte proliferation. *Proceedings of the National Academy of Sciences of the USA* **87** 3758–3762

Pietenpol JA, Stein RW, Moran E *et al* (1990b) TGFβ1 inhibition of *c-myc* transcription and growth in keratinocytes is abrogated by viral transforming proteins with pRB binding domains. *Cell* **61** 777–785

Pollard M, Luckert Ph and Sporn MB (1991) Prevention of prostate cancer in Lobund-Wistar rats by 4-hydroxyphenylretinamide. *Cancer Research* **51** 3610–3611

Rainey WE, Naville D, Saez JM *et al* (1990) Transforming growth factor β inhibits steroid 17αhydroxylase cytochrome p-450 expression in ovine adrenocortical cells. *Endocrinology* **127** 1910–1915

Ripoll E, Morz VW, Kadmon D *et al* (1991) Mesenchyme-derived factors are responsible for the conversion of oncogene-transformed epithelial cells to malignant adenocarcinomas in mouse prostate. *Journal of Urology* **145** 540

Ross RK, Bernstein L and Lobo RA (1992) Evidence for reduced 5-alpha-reductase activity in Japanese compared to US white and black males: implications for prostate cancer risk. *Lancet* **339** 887–889

Rotmensz N, DePalo G, Formell F *et al* (1991) Longterm tolerability of fenretinide (4HPR) in breast cancer patients. *European Journal of Cancer* **27** 1127–1131

Sadi MV and Barrack ER (1993) Image analysis of androgen receptor immunostaining in metastatic prostate cancer: heterogeneity as a predictor of response to hormonal therapy. *Cancer* **71** 2574–2580

Sadi MV, Walsh PC and Barrack ER (1991) Immunohistochemical study of androgen receptors in metastatic prostate cancer. *Cancer* **67** 3057–3064

Sai T, Seino S, Chang C *et al* (1990) An exonic point mutation of the androgen receptor gene in a family with complete androgen insensitivity. *American Journal of Human Genetics* **46** 1095–1100

Sandgren EP, Luettke NC, Pelmeter RD, Brinster RL and Lee DC (1990) Overexpression of TGFα in transgenic mice: induction of epithelial hyperplasia, pancreatic metaplasia and carcinoma of the prostate. *Cell* **61** 1121–1135

Scardino PT (1989) Early detection of prostate cancer. *Urology Clinics of North America* **16** 635–655

Scher HI and Kelly WK (1993) Flutamide withdrawal syndrome: its impact on clinical trials in hormone refractory prostate cancer. *Journal of Clinical Oncology* **11** 1566–1572

Schoenberg MD, Hakimi JM, Wang S *et al* (1994) Microsatellite mutation CAG (24→18) in the androgen receptor gene in human prostate cancer. *Journal of Urology* **151** 923A [Abstract]

Schuurmans ALG, Bolt J and Mulder E (1988) Androgens stimulate both growth rate and epidermal growth factor receptor activity of the human prostate tumor cell line LNCaP. *Prostate* **12** 55–64

Serio M, Gonnell P and Borelli D (1979) Human testicular secretion with increasing age. *Journal of Steroid Biochemistry* **11** 893–897

Sharief Y, Wilson E, Gumerlock P *et al* (1994) Is hormone refractory prostatic carcinoma associated with androgen receptor gene mutations or mRNA splicing errors? *Journal of Urology* **151** 566A [Abstract]

Sporn MB and Roberts AB (1991) Interactions of retinoids and transforming growth factor β in regulation of cell differentiation and proliferation. *Molecular Endocrinology* **5** 3–7

Suzucki H, Sato N, Watabe Y, Masai M, Seino S and Shimazaki J (1993) Androgen receptor gene mutations in human prostate cancer. *Journal of Steroid Biochemistry and Molecular Biology* **46** 759–765

Takahashi J, Higash Y, LaNasa JA *et al* (1983) Stimulation measurement of nine testicular steroids: evidence for reduced mitochondrial function in testis of elderly men. *Journal of Clinical Endocrinology and Metabolism* **56** 1178–1187

Takeda H and Chang C (1991) Immunocytochemical and *in situ* hybridization analysis of androgen receptor expression during the development of the mouse prostate gland. *Journal of Endocrinology* **129** 83–89

Takeda H, Chodak G, Mutchnik S, Nakamoto T and Chang C (1989) Immunohistochemical localization of androgen receptors with mono- and polyclonal antibodies to the androgen receptor. *Journal of Endocrinology* **126** 17–25

Takeda H, Nakamoto T, Kokontis J, Chodak GW and Chang C (1991) Autoregulatiuon of androgen receptor expression in rodent prostate: immunohistochemical and *in situ* hybridization analysis. *Biochemical and Biophysical Research Communications* **177** 488–496

Tan J, Joseph DR, Quarmby VE *et al* (1988) The rat androgen receptor: primary structure, autoregulation of its messenger ribonucleic acid, and immunocytochemical localization of the receptor protein. *Molecular Endocrinology* **2** 1276–1285

Tenover JS, Matsumoto AM, Plymate SR and Bremmer WJ (1987) The effects of aging in normal men on bioavailable testosterone and leutinizing hormone secretion: response to clomiphene citrate. *Journal of Clinical Endocrinology and Metabolism* **65** 118–1126

Thompson TC (1990) Growth factors and oncogenes in prostate cancer. *Cancer Cells* **2** 345–354

Thompson TC, Southgate J, Kitchner G and Land H (1989) Multistage carcinogenesis induced by *ras* and *myc* oncogenes in a reconstituted organ. *Cell* **56** 917–930

Tilley WK, Marcelli M, Wilson JD and McPhaul MJ (1989) Characterization and expression of a cDNA encoding the human androgen receptor. *Proceedings of the National Academy of*

Sciences of the USA **86** 327–331

Trifio M, Prior L, Pinsky L *et al* (1989) A single transition at an exonic CpG site apparently abolishes androgen receptor binding activity in a family with complete androgen insensitivity. *American Journal of Human Genetics* **45 (Supplement)** A225 [Abstract]

van Aubel O, Bolr-de Vries J, Blakenstein MA and Schröder FH (1988) Prediction of time to progression after orchiectomy by the nuclear androgen receptor content from multiple biopsy specimens in patients with advanced prostate cancer. *Prostate* **12** 191–198

Van Der Kwast TH, Schalken J, Ruizeveld de Winter JA *et al* (1991) Androgen receptors in endocrine therapy resistant human prostate cancer. *International Journal of Cancer* **48** 189–193

Weisz A, Cicatiello L, Persico E, Scalona M and Bresciani F (1990) Estrogen stimulates expression of *c-jun* proto-oncogene. *Molecular Endocrinology* **4** 1041–1050

Wilding G (1991) Response of prostate cancer cells to peptide growth factors: transforming growth factor beta. *Cancer Surveys* **11** 147–164

Wilding G, Lippman ME and Gelmann EP (1988) The effects of steroid hormones and peptide growth factors on *c-fos* oncogene expression in human breast cancer cells. *Cancer Research* **48** 802–805

Wilding G, Valvarius E, Knabbe C and Gelmann EP (1989a) The role of transforming growth factor alpha in human prostate cancer cell growth. *Prostate* **15** 1–12

Wilding G, Knabbe C, Zugmaier G, Flanders K and Gelmann EP (1989b) Differential effects of TGFβ on human prostate cancer cells *in vitro*. *Molecular and Cellular Endocrinology* **62** 79–87

Wilding G, Chen M and Gelmann EP (1989c) Aberrent response in vitro of hormone responsive prostate cancer cells to antiandrogens. *Prostate* **14** 103–115

Yatani R, Shiraishi T, Nakakuki K *et al* (1988) Trends in the frequency of latent prostate carcinoma in Japan from 1965-1979 to 1982-1986. *Journal of the National Cancer Institute* **80** 683–687

Yuan S, Trachtenberg J, Mills GB, Brown TJ, Xu F and Keating A (1993) Androgen-induced inhibition of cell proliferation in an androgen-insensitive prostate cancer cell line (PC-3) transfected with a human androgen receptor complementary DNA. *Cancer Research* **53** 1304–1311

The author is responsible for the accuracy of the references.

Risk Factors for Prostate Cancer

TIMOTHY KEY
Imperial Cancer Research Fund, Cancer Epidemiology Unit, Gibson Building, Radcliffe Infirmary, Oxford OX2 6HE

INTRODUCTION

The aim of this chapter is to summarize current knowledge of factors associated with the risk for prostate cancer. Following a brief discussion of the established risk factors, the possible roles of diet, smoking, sexual behaviour, sexually transmitted disease and vasectomy are assessed by a systematic review of published results. The two subsequent chapters in this book discuss the geographical epidemiology of prostate cancer and the relevance of human papillomavirus. Other aspects of the epidemiology of prostate cancer have been covered by a recent detailed review (Nomura and Kolonel, 1991).

ESTABLISHED RISK FACTORS FOR PROSTATE CANCER

There are only three well established risk factors for prostate cancer: age, family history of the disease and ethnic group/country of residence.

Men with a father or brother affected with prostate cancer have about twice the risk for developing the disease than do men without affected rela-

Cancer Surveys Volume 23: *Preventing Prostate Cancer: Screening versus Chemoprevention*

tives. The risk is higher still for men with more than one affected relative and for men with a relative who developed the disease at a young age (Carter *et al,* 1993). Carter *et al* (1992) conducted a segregation analysis and concluded that the familial clustering of prostate cancer could be explained by the autosomal dominant inheritance of a rare high risk allele giving a cumulative lifetime risk of prostate cancer of about 90% and responsible for about 10% of all prostate cancers by age 85.

Both incidence and mortality rates for prostate cancer vary widely between different populations, with very low rates in the Far East, moderate rates in southern and western Europe, and very high rates in northern Europe and the USA, with the highest rates in the world among blacks in the USA (Nomura and Kolonel, 1991). There is about a tenfold difference in mortality rates between non-white men in the USA and men in Hong Kong and Japan. Although migrant studies suggest that much of this variation is due to environmental factors rather than genetic factors (Nomura and Kolonel, 1991), some of the differences in rates between countries are due to differences in registration practices (Shimizu *et al,* 1991). The much higher rates in blacks than in whites in the USA suggest the possibility that genetic differences between populations may play a larger part in determining population rates of prostate cancer than in determining population rates of other common cancers such as breast cancer and large bowel cancer.

The risk for prostate cancer is increased by occupational exposure to certain radionuclides (Rooney *et al,* 1993). However, occupational exposure to these agents is rare and is not a major cause of prostate cancer.

SYSTEMATIC REVIEW OF DIET, SMOKING, SEXUAL BEHAVIOUR, SEXUALLY TRANSMITTED DISEASE AND VASECTOMY

Method

The approach in this review has been to select a limited number of variables and to present all the published results from different studies for each variable on the same figure. This allows the reader to see the results and the width of the confidence intervals for each study separately and to compare the results of the different studies. Summary relative risks are plotted on each figure, but these summary relative risks should be interpreted cautiously because of the different designs of the studies, the variation (for some variables) in the categories combined and the tendency of authors to present estimates of relative risk for significant results and not to present non-significant results. The summary relative risks are intended only as a guide and must not be taken as a statement of the overall effect (as they might be in an overview of clinical trials when trials have the same design and when reviewers attempt to include all published and unpublished trials).

Relevant publications were identified from previous reviews and by searching journals. Variables for review were chosen on the basis that they were related to hypotheses currently under consideration and that reasonably comparable data were available from several studies.

For each variable considered in this review, one estimate of relative risk was taken from each study. For dichotomous variables, the relative risk estimate taken was for exposed subjects compared to unexposed subjects. For continuous variables, the relative risk estimate taken was for subjects with the highest level of the variable compared to those with the lowest level. It should be noted that, because the cut off points used vary between studies, the estimates of relative risk presented for continuous variables are not strictly comparable.

In addition, the following criteria were used to choose which results to include in the figures and summary relative risks: (a) If results were given for both hospital and community controls, those for community controls were used. Results for white men were used if the men studied were from more than one ethnic group and there were few non-white men. (b) If both unadjusted and adjusted results were given, the adjusted results were used if the adjustments were judged to be appropriate. (c) Results were rounded to two decimal places. (d) Where the published relative risk was for the lowest rather than the highest level of a variable, the inverse of the lowest category and its confidence interval was used. (e) Where results for advanced prostate cancer were given as a subset of the study results (eg Giovannucci *et al,* 1993a), the results for all cases were taken if possible. (f) If foods within one class were reported separately (eg different types of meat), a summary relative risk for the individual foods was calculated. (g) The results presented for carotene are for beta-carotene where possible, otherwise for total carotene or carotene unspecified. (h) The variable meat excludes poultry unless this had already been included by the authors. (i) Smoking is classified as current or ever smokers.

The results for each variable are plotted on a logarithmic scale with the point estimate of relative risk and 95% confidence interval. At the foot of each plot, there is an estimate of the summary of the relative risks from the individual studies, calculated as the weighted average of the individual relative risks, with the weighting proportional to the inverse of the variance of each relative risk.

For some variables in some studies, the results were given in forms other than a relative risk estimate with 95% confidence interval. In these circumstances, the relative risk estimate and confidence interval were estimated using standard methods if sufficient data were given; it should be noted that these estimates are unmatched and unadjusted for other risk factors.

Some publications gave a point estimate of relative risk but no confidence interval and insufficient data to produce an estimate of the confidence interval. In these circumstances, the point estimate of relative risk has been included on the figure but such estimates do not contribute to the summary relative risk estimate.

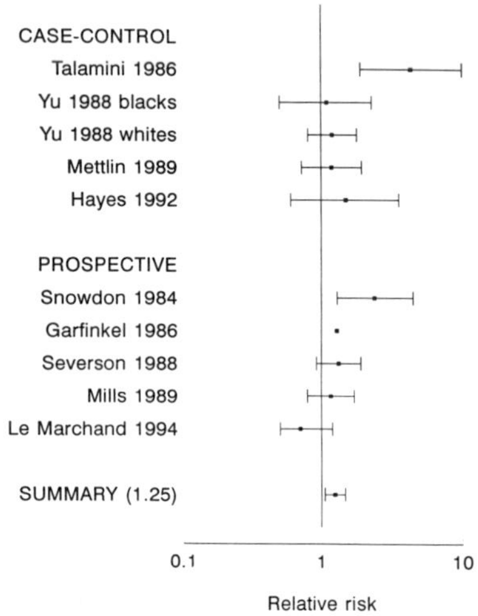

Fig. 1. Obesity and prostate cancer. Risk for highest v. lowest category

Results

Diet and related factors

Obesity is included here because it is controlled by diet and because it can be measured more accurately than food intake. Nine out of ten studies that reported relative risks for obesity noted an increase in risk with increasing obesity (measured in most studies as Quetelet's index). The summary relative risk is 1.25 for the most obese versus the least obese (Fig. 1; see Table 1 for summary of dietary risk factors).

Eleven studies reported on meat consumption and five on consumption of dairy products. Most found a higher relative risk for prostate cancer for men with the highest levels of consumption of meat or dairy products, with summary relative risks of 1.34 and 1.30, respectively (Figs. 2 and 3). Eight of ten

TABLE 1. Summary of overview of dietary risk factors for prostate cancer (see Figs. 1–8)

	Relative Risk[a]
Obesity	1.25 (1.06–1.48)
Meat consumption	1.34 (1.16–1.55)
Dairy product consumption	1.30 (1.11–1.51)
Total fat consumption	1.31 (1.10–1.54)
Animal fat consumption	1.54 (1.19–1.99)
Carrot consumption	0.66 (0.51–0.87)
Green vegetable consumption	0.93 (0.73–1.18)
Carotene consumption	0.99 (0.85–1.16)

[a]Estimate of summay relative risk for highest v. lowest category, with 95% confidence interval in brackets

studies reported a high risk with high consumption of total dietary fat (summary relative risk 1.31; Fig. 4); five of six reported a high risk with high consumption of animal fat (summary relative risk 1.54; Fig. 5). Two further studies that did not present relative risks reported a weak positive association between total fat intake and risk of prostate cancer (Heshmat *et al* 1985; Kaul *et al,* 1987).

For carrots, four of five studies reported a low risk associated with high consumption (summary relative risk 0.66; Fig. 6). No consistent pattern is evident for green vegetables (summary relative risk for high consumption 0.93; Fig. 7). Two of the earlier studies suggested that a high carotene consumption was associated with a low risk (Ross *et al,* 1987; Ohno *et al,* 1988), but most subsequent studies have not supported these findings and the summary relative risk for carotene is 0.99 (Fig. 8). Some studies have suggested that the association of carotene with risk may be different in different age groups; for example, Hsing *et al* (1990a) reported an elevated relative risk of borderline statistical significance in younger men but a strongly protective association in older men (Fig. 9). It can be seen, however, that the pattern is not consistent between studies and that the summary relative risks are very close to 1 in both younger men (summary 0.89) and older men (summary 1.04).

In addition to the studies of dietary carotene intake shown in Fig. 8, two prospective studies have reported the risk of prostate cancer in relation to serum carotene concentration (Hsing *et al,* 1990b; Knekt *et al,* 1990); the summary relative risk for these two studies is 1.66 (95% confidence interval 0.84 to 3.28). The recently published Alpha-Tocopherol, Beta Carotene Prevention Study, a randomized placebo controlled cancer prevention trial, reported 138 prostate cancers among the men who received beta carotene and 112 among those who did not (Alpha-Tocopherol, Beta Carotene Cancer Prevention Study Group, 1994). (There was, however, a deficit of prostate cancers among men who received alpha-tocopherol; 99 cases v. 151 in controls.)

Twelve studies have reported the association of alcohol intake with prostate cancer risk (Fig. 10); none of the individual studies reported a significant association, and the summary relative risk is 1.07.

Smoking

Ten of twenty studies reported an increase in risk of prostate cancer associated with cigarette smoking (Fig. 11). The summary relative risk is very close to 1 (1.16) but is statistically significant, partly because of the positive results of the very large study by Hsing *et al* (1991) and partly because some of the negative studies were not included in the summary because confidence intervals were not published.

Sexual behaviour

The summary relative risks for early first intercourse and for multiple sexual partners are both raised (1.31 and 1.24, respectively; Figs. 12 and 13; see Table 2 for summary of sexual behaviour risk factors). Much of the association

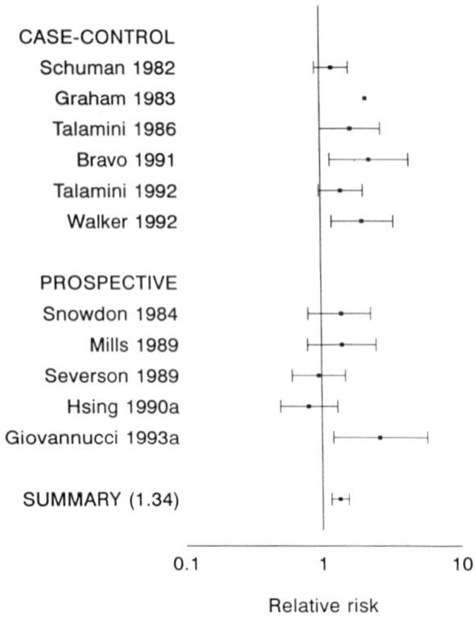

Fig. 2. Meat and prostate cancer. Risk for highest v. lowest intake group

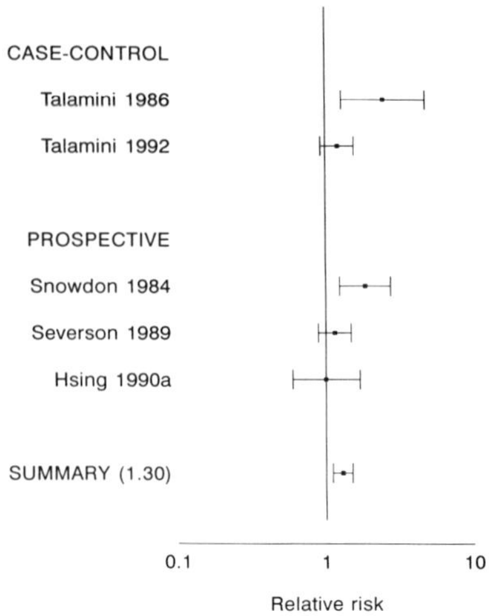

Fig. 3. Dairy products and prostate cancer. Risk for highest v. lowest intake group

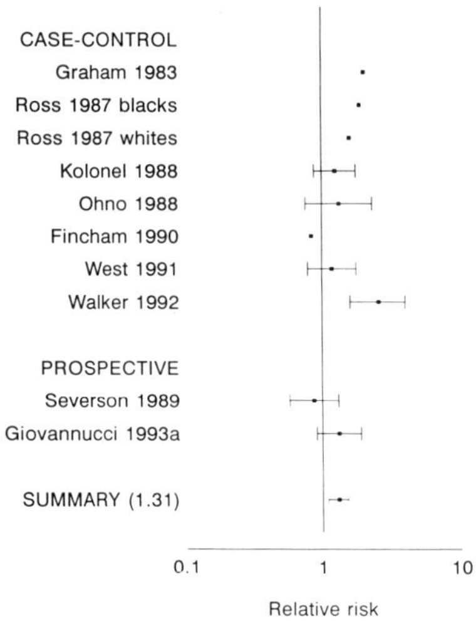

Fig. 4. Total fat consumption and prostate cancer. Risk for highest v. lowest intake group

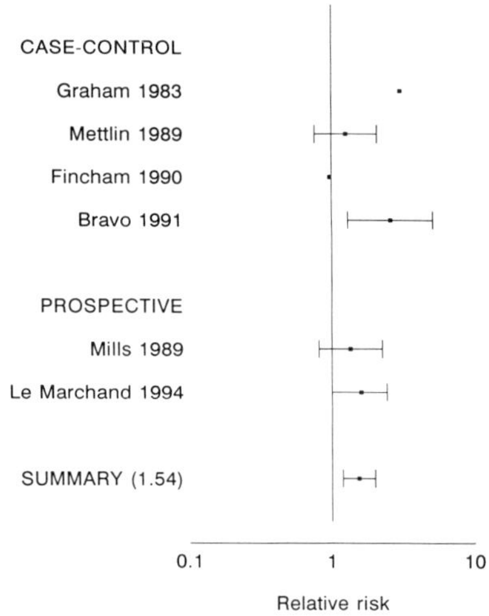

Fig. 5. Animal fat consumption and prostate cancer. Risk for highest v. lowest intake group

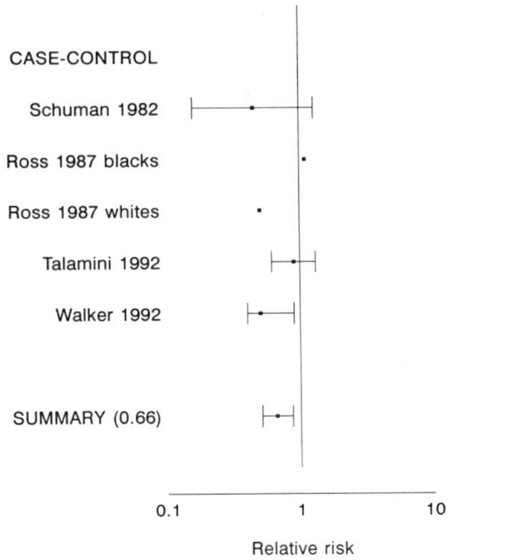

Fig. 6. Carrot consumption and prostate cancer. Risk for highest v. lowest intake group

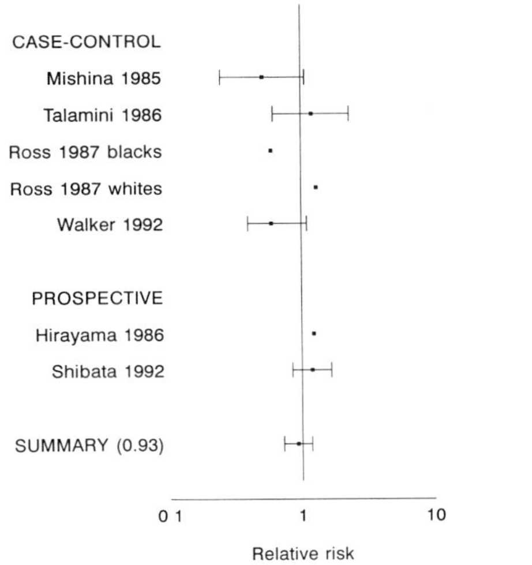

Fig. 7. Green vegetables and prostate cancer. Risk for highest v. lowest intake group

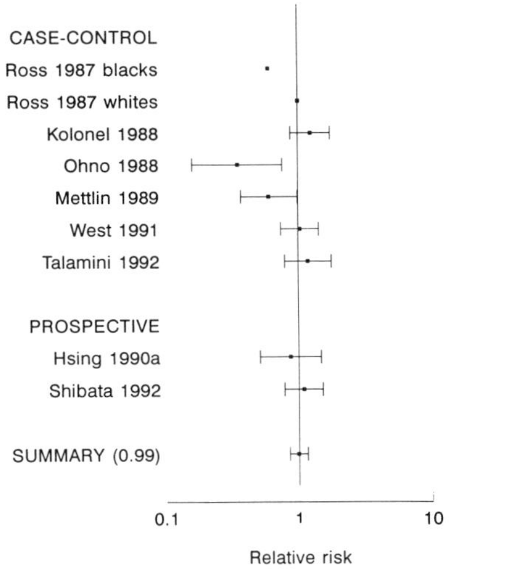

Fig. 8. Carotene intake and prostate cancer. Risk for highest v. lowest intake group

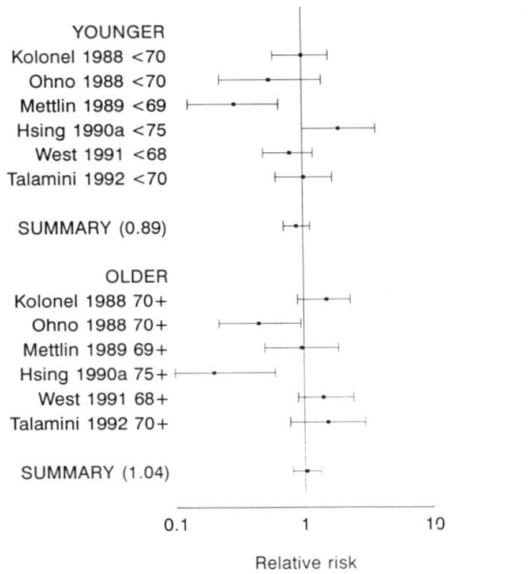

Fig. 9. Carotene intake and prostate cancer by age. Risk for highest v. lowest intake group

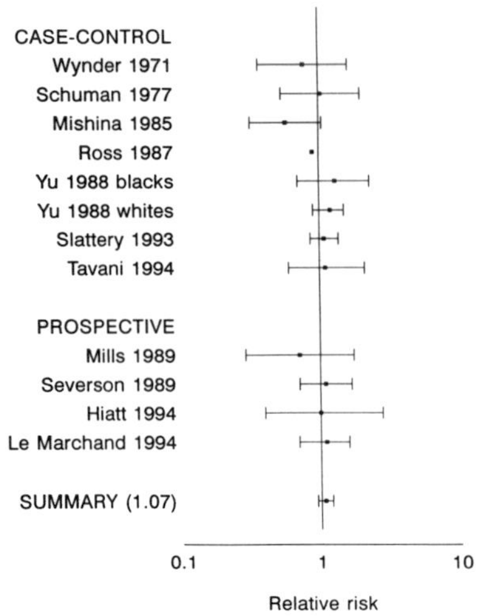

Fig. 10. Alcohol consumption and prostate cancer. Risk for highest v. lowest intake group

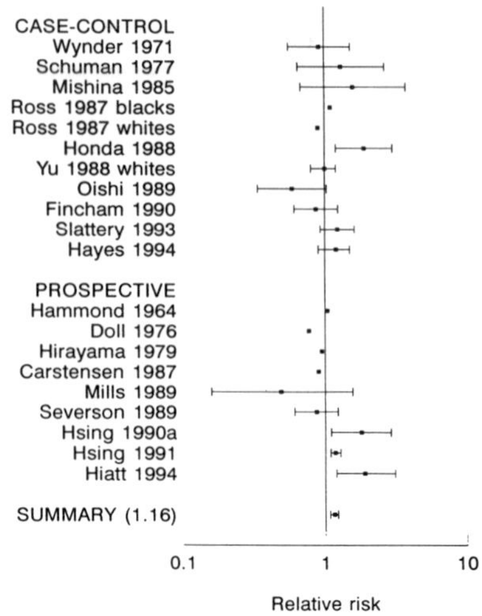

Fig. 11. Smoking and prostate cancer. Risk for current or ex-smokers v. non-smokers

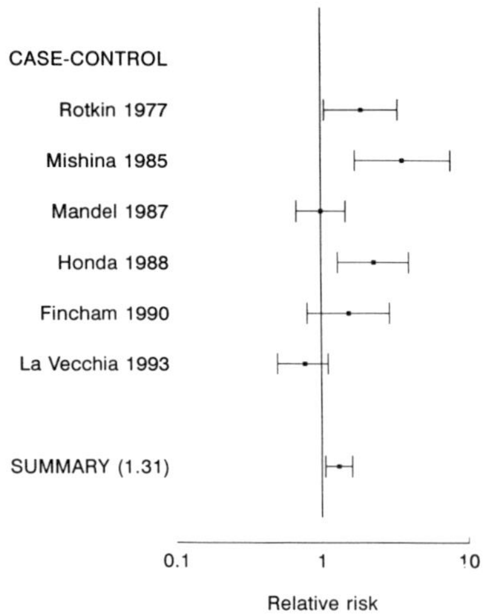

Fig. 12. Age at first intercourse and prostate cancer. Risk for early v. late first intercourse

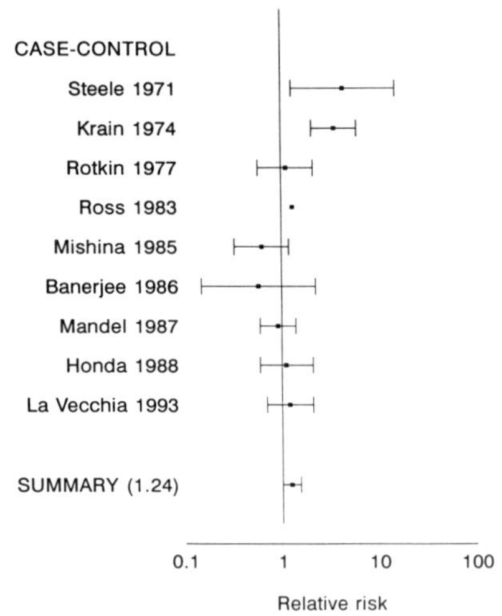

Fig. 13. Number of sexual partners and prostate cancer. Risk for most v. least number of partners

TABLE 2. Summary of overview of sexual behaviour risk factors for prostate cancer (see Figs. 12–17)

	Relative Risk[a]
Early age of first intercourse	1.31 (1.06–1.61)
Large number of sexual partners	1.24 (1.00–1.54)
History of any sexually acquired infection	1.86 (1.43–2.42)
History of syphilis	0.77 (0.53–1.11)
History of gonorrhoea	1.22 (0.92–1.62)
Vasectomy	1.54 (1.34–1.77)

[a]Estimate of summary relative risk, with 95% confidence interval in brackets

with number of sexual partners is due to the early studies of Steele *et al* (1971) and Krain (1974).

Sexually transmitted disease

The summary relative risk for men reporting any previous sexually transmitted disease is 1.86 (Fig. 14). As for the previous variable, much of this elevation in risk is due to the early studies. However, the summary relative risks for syphilis (0.77; Fig. 15) and gonorrhoea (1.22; Fig. 16) are close to 1 and are not statistically significant.

Vasectomy

The summary relative risk for vasectomy is 1.54, but the results of the individual studies vary somewhat (Fig. 17).

Discussion of Systematic Review

Although this is a systematic review of published data on the variables selected, considerable caution is needed in interpreting the results presented, particularly the summary relative risks. It is likely that the results for all the variables suffer from publication bias, in that studies with positive results are more likely to be published (Easterbrook *et al,* 1991). Furthermore, even within the published studies, there is biased reporting of results, in that variables that were not significantly associated with risk are sometimes dismissed with a comment in the text and therefore cannot be used in the review. Another problem is that when investigators select cut off points for continuous variables, there is a temptation to choose categories that maximize the estimated relative risks. Therefore, summarizing published data may give a distorted view.

Obesity appears to be associated with a small increase in the risk for prostate cancer. This might be due to the physiological effects of obesity (eg

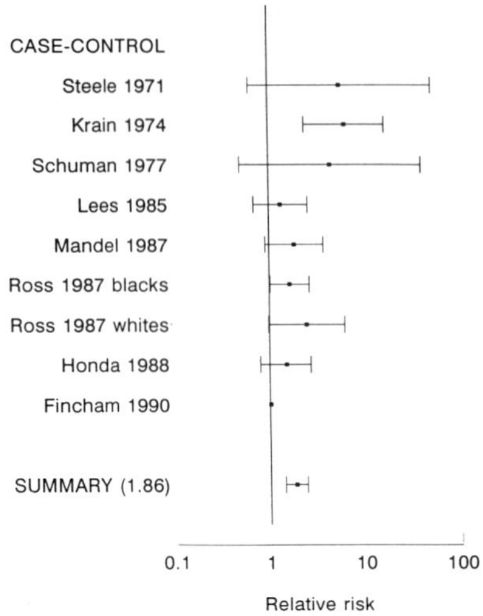

Fig. 14. History of sexually transmitted disease and prostate cancer. Risk for ever having had a sexually transmitted disease

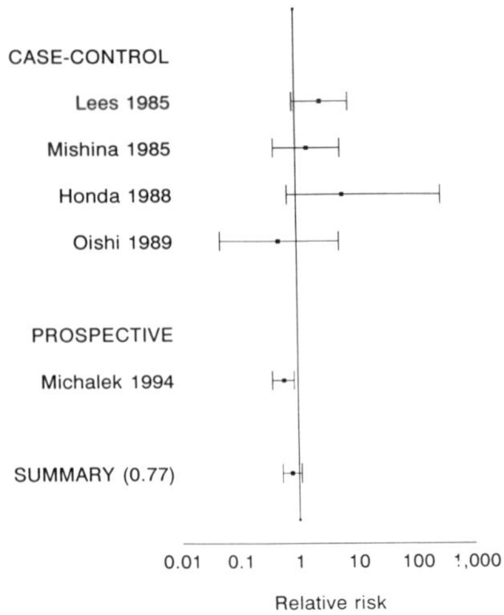

Fig. 15. History of syphilis and prostate cancer. Risk for ever having had syphilis

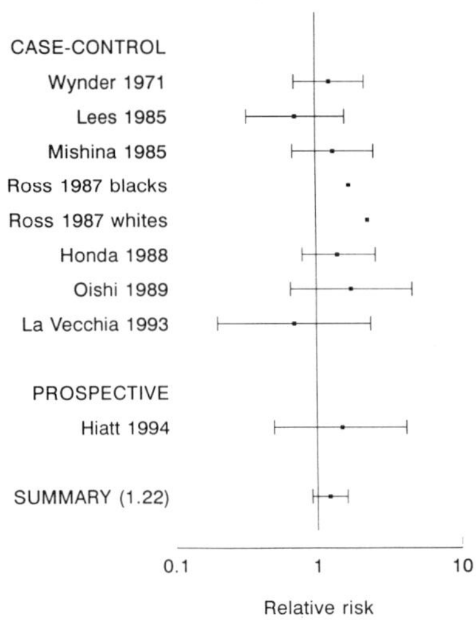

Fig. 16. History of gonorrhoea and prostate cancer. Risk for ever having had gonorrhoea

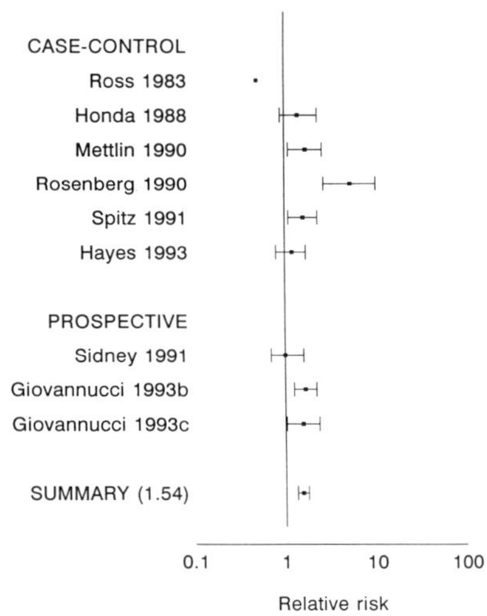

Fig. 17. Vasectomy and prostate cancer. Risk for vasectomy v. no vasectomy

on sex hormone metabolism) or to an association of obesity with a particular dietary pattern. It might also be due in part to publication bias because several studies reported that obesity was not associated with prostate cancer but did not report relative risks (Graham *et al,* 1983; Whittemore *et al,* 1985; Ross *et al,* 1987; Kolonel *et al,* 1988). There is also some evidence that the risk of prostate cancer is associated with increased height, although this variable has not been systematically reviewed here (Albanes *et al,* 1988; Albanes and Taylor, 1990; Le Marchand *et al,* 1994).

The evidence that meat, dairy products, total fat and animal fat are associated with an increase in the risk for prostate cancer is quite consistent. The size of the estimated increase in risk is only about 30–50%, but this does not mean that it can be disregarded because inaccuracies in measuring dietary intake can cause substantial underestimation of relative risks. The true relative risk might be much larger and further studies with more accurate measurement of dietary intake are needed.

The summary relative risk for carrots suggests a significant protective effect, but the studies of green vegetables and of dietary, serum and supplementary carotene are uniformly negative. It appears to be unlikely that carotene intake has an important effect on the risk of prostate cancer; the observation for carrots might be due to a constituent of carrots other than carotene or may be due simply to chance or publication bias. The report from the recently published intervention trial of a lower incidence of prostate cancer in men receiving supplementary α-tocopherol is interesting and should be investigated further. Alcohol intake is not associated with risk of prostate cancer. More data are needed on other constituents of fruits and vegetables such as fibre and phyto-oestrogens, and also on other factors related to diet such as vitamin D, since a recent prospective study reported a lower risk for subsequent prostate cancer in men with high serum concentrations of 1,25-dihydroxyvitamin D (Corder *et al,* 1993).

The summary relative risk for cigarette smoking is elevated, but the risk is so small (for an exposure measured quite accurately), and the studies are so inconsistent, that it is unlikely that the association is causal.

The relative risks for early first intercourse, large number of sexual partners and a history of any sexually transmitted disease are all elevated. These observations might be due to an infectious agent increasing risk or might be due to an underlying hormonal factor causing both increased sexual activity and increased prostate cancer risk. The highest summary relative risk (for all factors examined) was for a history of any sexually transmitted disease, but this variable is susceptible to both recall bias and selection bias and must be unreliable; this observation needs to be examined further in prospective studies utilizing biological markers of previous infections.

The elevation in relative risk associated with vasectomy is of great interest but some of the studies may suffer from bias in ascertainment, and further careful examination of this topic is needed.

SUMMARY

The risk for prostate cancer increases with age, with a family history of the disease and with living in a Westernized society, especially for blacks. Although there is no doubt that genetic factors are important, and might explain some of the geographical variation in rates, the differences between populations are so large that environmental factors must also be important.

The evidence suggesting that dietary fat and/or meat may increase risk is quite consistent. The observed relative risks are small (about a 30% increase for high v. low consumption) but may have been underestimated because of inaccurate measurement of diet and further study of this topic is needed. The evidence does not support the hypothesis that carotene intake is associated with risk.

There is reasonably consistent evidence suggesting that an increased risk for prostate cancer is associated with a high level of sexual activity and/or a history of sexually transmitted disease, and with vasectomy. These observations need further investigation to eliminate the possibility that they are due to biases.

Much more information is needed. Prospective studies, with dietary and lifestyle questionnaires and stored blood samples, are needed to answer the outstanding questions.

Acknowledgements

I thank Gillian Reeves for statistical advice, Gwyneth Davey for assistance with calculations and Valerie Beral for commenting on the manuscript.

References

Albanes D and Taylor PR (1990) International differences in body height and weight and their relationship to cancer incidence. *Nutrition and Cancer* **14** 69–77

Albanes D, Jones DY, Schatzkin A, Micozzi MS and Taylor PR (1988) Adult stature and risk of cancer. *Cancer Research* **48** 1658–1662

Alpha-Tocopherol, Beta Carotene Cancer Prevention Study Group (1994) The effect of vitamin E and beta carotene on the incidence of lung cancer and other cancers in male smokers. *New England Journal of Medicine* **330** 1029–1035

Banerjee AK (1986) Carcinoma of prostate and sexual activity. *Urology* **28** 159

Bravo MP, Castellanos E and del Rey Calero J (1991) Dietary factors and prostatic cancer. *Urology International* **46** 163–166

Carstensen J, Pershagen G and Eklund G (1987) Mortality in relation to cigarette and pipe smoking: 16 years' observation of 25 000 Swedish men. *Journal of Epidemiology and Community Health* **41** 166–172

Carter BS, Beaty TH, Steinberg GD, Childs B and Walsh PC (1992) Mendelian inheritance of familial prostate cancer. *Proceedings of the National Academy of Sciences of the USA* **89** 3367–3371

Carter BS, Bova GS, Beaty TH, Steinberg GD, Childs B, Isaacs WB and Walsh PC (1993) Hereditary prostate cancer: epidemiologic and clinical features. *Journal of Urology* **150** 797–802

Corder EH, Guess HA, Hulka BS *et al* (1993) Vitamin D and prostate cancer: a prediagnostic study with stored sera. *Cancer Epidemiology, Biomarkers & Prevention* **2** 467–472

Doll R and Peto R (1976) Mortality in relation to smoking: 20 years' observations on male British doctors. *British Medical Journal* **2** 1525–1536

Easterbrook PJ, Berlin JA, Gopalan R and Matthews DR (1991) Publication bias in clinical research. *Lancet* **337** 867–872

Fincham SM, Hill GB, Hanson J and Wijayasinghe C (1990) Epidemiology of prostatic cancer: a case-control study. *Prostate* **17** 189–206

Garfinkel L (1986) Overweight and mortality. *Cancer* **58** 1826–1829

Giovannucci E, Rimm EB, Colditz GA *et al* (1993a) A prospective study of dietary fat and risk of prostate cancer. *Journal of the National Cancer Institute* **85** 1571–1579

Giovannucci E, Ascherio A, Rimm EB, Colditz GA, Stampfer MJ and Willett WC (1993b) A prospective cohort study of vasectomy and prostate cancer in US men. *Journal of the American Medical Association* **269** 873–877

Giovannucci E, Tosteson TD, Speizer FE, Ascherio A, Vessey MP and Colditz GA (1993c) A retrospective cohort study of vasectomy and prostate cancer in US men. *Journal of the American Medical Association* **269** 878–882

Graham S, Haughey B, Marshall J *et al* (1983) Diet in the epidemiology of carcinoma of the prostate gland. *Journal of the National Cancer Institute* **70** 687–692

Hammond EC (1964) Smoking in relation to mortality and morbidity: findings in first thirty-four months of follow-up in a prospective study started in 1959. *Journal of the National Cancer Institute* **32** 1161–1188

Hayes RB, de Jong FH, Raatgever J *et al* (1992) Physical characteristics and factors related to sexual development and behaviour and the risk for prostatic cancer. *European Journal of Cancer Prevention* **1** 239–245

Hayes RB, Pottern LM, Greenberg R *et al* (1993) Vasectomy and prostate cancer in US blacks and whites. *American Journal of Epidemiology* **137** 263–269

Hayes RB, Pottern LM, Swanson GM *et al* (1994) Tobacco use and prostate cancer in blacks and whites in the United States. *Cancer Causes and Control* **5** 221–226

Heshmat MY, Kaul L, Kovi J *et al* (1985) Nutrition and prostate cancer: a case-control study. *Prostate* **6** 7–17

Hiatt RA, Armstrong MA, Klatsky AL and Sidney S (1994) Alcohol consumption, smoking, and other risk factors and prostate cancer in a large health plan cohort in California (United States). *Cancer Causes and Control* **5** 66–72

Hirayama T (1979) Epidemiology of prostate cancer with special reference to the role of diet. *National Cancer Institute Monograph* **53** 149–155

Hirayama T (1986) A large scale cohort study on cancer risks by diet–with special reference to the risk reducing effects of green-yellow vegetable consumption, In: Hayashi Y *et al* (eds). *Diet, Nutrition and Cancer,* pp 41–53, Japanese Scientific Society Press, Tokyo/VNU Science Press, Utrecht

Honda GD, Bernstein L, Ross RK, Greenland S, Gerkins V and Henderson BE (1988) Vasectomy, cigarette smoking, and age at first sexual intercourse as risk factors for prostate cancer in middle-aged men. *British Journal of Cancer* **57** 326–331

Hsing AW, McLaughlin JK, Schuman LM *et al* (1990a) Diet, tobacco use, and fatal prostate cancer: results from the Lutheran Brotherhood cohort study. *Cancer Research* **50** 6836–6840

Hsing AW, Comstock GW, Abbey H and Polk BF (1990b) Serologic precursors of cancer: retinol, carotenoids, and tocopherol and risk of prostate cancer. *Journal of the National Cancer Institute* **82** 941–945

Hsing AW, McLaughlin JK, Hrubec Z, Blot WJ and Fraumeni JF (1991) Tobacco use and prostate cancer: 26-year follow-up of US veterans. *American Journal of Epidemiology* **133** 437–441

Kaul L, Heshmat MY, Kovi J *et al* (1987) The role of diet in prostate cancer. *Nutrition and Can-*

cer **9** 123–128

Knekt P, Aromaa A, Maatela J *et al* (1990) Serum vitamin A and subsequent risk of cancer: cancer incidence follow-up of the Finnish mobile clinic health examination survey. *American Journal of Epidemiology* **132** 857–870

Kolonel LN, Yoshizawa CN and Hankin JH (1988) Diet and prostatic cancer: a case-control study in Hawaii. *American Journal of Epidemiology* **127** 999–1012

Krain LS (1974) Some epidemiologic variables in prostatic carcinoma in California. *Preventive Medicine* **3** 154–159

La Vecchia C, Franceschi S, Talamini R, Negri E, Boyle P and D'Avanzo B (1993) Marital status, indicators of sexual activity and prostatic cancer. *Journal of Epidemiology and Community Health* **47** 450–453

Lees REM, Steele R and Wardle D (1985) Arsenic, syphilis and cancer of the prostate. *Journal of Epidemiology and Community Health* **39** 227–230

Le Marchand L, Kolonel LN, Wilkens LR, Myers BC and Hirohata T (1994) Animal fat consumption and prostate cancer: a prospective study in Hawaii. *Epidemiology* **5** 276–282

Mandel JS and Schuman LM (1987) Sexual factors and prostatic cancer: results from a case-control study. *Journal of Gerontology* **42** 259–264

Mettlin C, Selenskas S, Natarajan N and Huben R (1989) Beta-carotene and animal fats and their relationship to prostate cancer risk. *Cancer* **64** 605–612

Mettlin C, Natarajan N and Huben R (1990) Vasectomy and prostate cancer risk. *American Journal of Epidemiology* **132** 1056–1061

Michalek AM, Mahoney MC, McLaughlin C, Murphy D and Metzger BB (1994) Historical and contemporary correlates of syphilis and cancer. *International Journal of Epidemiology* **23** 381–385

Mills PK, Beeson WL, Phillips RL and Fraser GE (1989) Cohort study of diet, lifestyle, and prostate cancer in Adventist men. *Cancer* **64** 598–604

Mishina T, Watanabe H, Araki H and Nakao M (1985) Epidemiological study of prostatic cancer by matched-pair analysis. *Prostate* **6** 423–436

Nomura AMY and Kolonel LN (1991) Prostate cancer: a current perspective. *American Journal of Epidemiology* **13** 200–227

Ohno Y, Yoshida O, Oishi K, Okada K, Yamabe H and Schroeder FH (1988) Dietary β-carotene and cancer of the prostate: a case-control study in Kyoto, Japan. *Cancer Research* **48** 1331–1336

Oishi K, Okada K, Yoshida O *et al* (1989) Case-control study of prostatic cancer in Kyoto, Japan: demographic and some lifestyle risk factors. *Prostate* **14** 117–122

Rooney C, Beral V, Maconochie N, Fraser P and Davies G (1993) Case-control study of prostatic cancer in employees of the United Kingdom Atomic Energy Authority. *British Medical Journal* **307** 1391–1397

Rosenberg L, Palmer JR, Zauber AG, Warshauer ME, Stolley PD and Shapiro S (1990) Vasectomy and the risk of prostate cancer. *American Journal of Epidemiology* **132** 1051–1055

Ross RK, Paganini-Hill A and Henderson BE (1983) The etiology of prostate cancer: what does the epidemiology suggest? *Prostate* **4** 333–344

Ross RK, Shimizu H, Paganini-Hill A, Honda G and Henderson BE (1987) Case-control studies of prostate cancer in blacks and whites in Southern California. *Journal of the National Cancer Institute* **78** 869–874

Rotkin ID (1977) Studies in the epidemiology of prostatic cancer: expanded sampling. *Cancer Treatment Reports* **61** 173–180

Schuman LM, Mandel J, Blackard C, Bauer H, Scarlett J and McHugh R (1977) Epidemiologic study of prostatic cancer: preliminary report. *Cancer Treatment Reports* **61** 181–186

Schuman LM, Mandel JS, Radke A, Seal U and Halber F (1982) Some selected features of the epidemiology of prostatic cancer: Minneapolis-St Paul, Minnesota case-control study 1976-1979, In: Magnus K (ed). *Trends in Cancer Incidence*, pp 345–354, Hemisphere, Washington

Severson RK, Grove JS, Nomura AMY and Stemmermann GN (1988) Body mass and prostatic cancer: a prospective study. *British Medical Journal* **297** 713–715

Severson RK, Nomura AMY, Grove JS and Stemmermann GN (1989) A prospective study of demographics, diet, and prostate cancer among men of Japanese ancestry in Hawaii. *Cancer Research* **49** 1857–1860

Shibata A, Paganini-Hill A, Ross RK and Henderson BE (1992) Intake of vegetables, fruits, beta-carotene, vitamin C and vitamin supplements and cancer incidence among the elderly: a prospective study. *British Journal of Cancer* **66** 673–679

Shimizu H, Ross RK and Bernstein L (1991) Possible underestimation of the incidence rate of prostate cancer in Japan. *Japanese Journal of Cancer Research* **82** 483–485

Sidney S, Quesenberry CP Jr, Sadler MC, Guess HA, Lydick EG and Cattolica EV (1991) Vasectomy and the risk of prostate cancer in a cohort of multiphasic health-checkup examinees: second report. *Cancer Causes and Control* **2** 113–116

Slattery ML and West DE (1993) Smoking, alcohol, coffee, tea, caffeine, and theobromine: risk of prostate cancer in Utah (United States). *Cancer Causes and Control* **4** 559–563

Snowdon DA, Phillips RL and Choi W (1984) Diet, obesity, and risk of fatal prostate cancer. *American Journal of Epidemiology* **120** 244–250

Spitz MR, Fueger JJ, Babaian RJ and Newell GR (1991) Vasectomy and the risk of prostate cancer. *American Journal of Epidemiology* **134** 108–109

Steele R, Lees REM, Kraus AS and Rao C (1971) Sexual factors in the epidemiology of cancer of the prostate. *Journal of Chronic Diseases* **24** 29–37

Talamini R, La Vecchia C, Decarli A, Negri E and Franceschi S (1986) Nutrition, social factors and prostatic cancer in a Northern Italian population. *British Journal of Cancer* **53** 817–821

Talamini R, Franceschi S, La Vecchia C, Serraino D, Barra S and Negri E (1992) Diet and prostatic cancer: a case-control study in Northern Italy. *Nutrition and Cancer* **18** 277–286

Tavani A, Negri E, Franceschi S, Talamini R and La Vecchia C (1994) Alcohol consumption and risk of prostate cancer. *Nutrition and Cancer* **21** 25–31

Walker ARP, Walker BF, Tsotetsi NG, Sebitso C, Siwedi D and Walker AJ (1992) Case-control study of prostate cancer in black patients in Soweto, South Africa. *British Journal of Cancer* **65** 438–441

West DW, Slattery ML, Robinson LM, French TK and Mahoney AW (1991) Adult dietary intake and prostate cancer risk in Utah: a case-control study with special emphasis on aggressive tumours. *Cancer Causes and Control* **2** 85–94

Whittemore AS, Paffenbarger RS, Anderson K and Lee JE (1985) Early precursors of site-specific cancers in college men and women. *Journal of the National Cancer Institute* **74** 43–51

Wynder EL, Mabuchi K and Whitmore WF (1971) Epidemiology of cancer of the prostate. *Cancer* **28** 344–360

Yu H, Harris RE and Wynder EL (1988) Case-control study of prostate cancer and socioeconomic factors. *Prostate* **13** 317–325

The author is responsible for the accuracy of the references.

Geographical Epidemiology of Prostate Cancer: Is There an Association with Infection?

FREDDY SITAS

National Cancer Registry, South African Institute for Medical Research, PO Box 1038, Johannesburg 2000

INTRODUCTION

There have been numerous epidemiological studies on cancer of the prostate, emphasizing the role of dietary fat, hormonal levels, vasectomy, smoking and occupational exposure, but very few have focused on whether cancer of the prostate is caused at least in part by an infectious agent (see eg reviews in Nomura and Kolonel, 1991; Pienta and Esper, 1993; Walker, 1986). Herpesvirus (Centifanto *et al,* 1973) and cytomegalovirus have shown some association with prostate cancer (Sanford *et al,* 1977), but the evidence to date appears to be tenuous. However, a positive association seems to be evident between cancer of the prostate and sexual history, even though some of these studies are based on retrospective recall of sexual history and may be prone to recall bias (see Key, this volume). There have been a few studies on the relationship between human papillomavirus (HPV) and cancer of the prostate, but the evidence is again weak (see Cuzick, this volume).

If prostate cancer is in part caused by a sexually transmitted agent, then populations that have high rates of sexually transmitted diseases would be expected to have high rates of prostate cancer as well. If a geographical association between prostate cancer and sexually transmitted diseases is not found, then the hypothesis is either incomplete or wrong. Cancer of the cervix is a sexually transmitted disease, so in an attempt to unravel the epidemiology of prostate cancer and the role of infection, worldwide incidence rates or proportions for prostate cancer were compared with rates of cervical cancer using

 0-87969-466-1/95. $5.00 + .00

TABLE 1. International variation in prostate cancer incidence

Region	Rate/100 000	Regional variation
Africa	1.2–6.3	5.25
S America and Carribbean	20–64	3
Canada	28–64	2.25
US White	47–83	1.8
US Black	65–**102**	1.6
US Oriental	20–33	1.7
Hawaii, Hawaiian	43	–
Hawaii, Oriental	28–34	1.2
China and Hong Kong	**0.83**–810	
India	2–73.5	
Japan	4–82	
Middle East	4–19	4.8
Eastern Europe	9–30	3.3
Northern Europe	36–52	1.4
Western Europe	11–51	4.6
UK	23–32	1.4
Australia and New Zealand	28–40	1.4
All	0.8–101	126

Source: Parkin *et al* (1992)

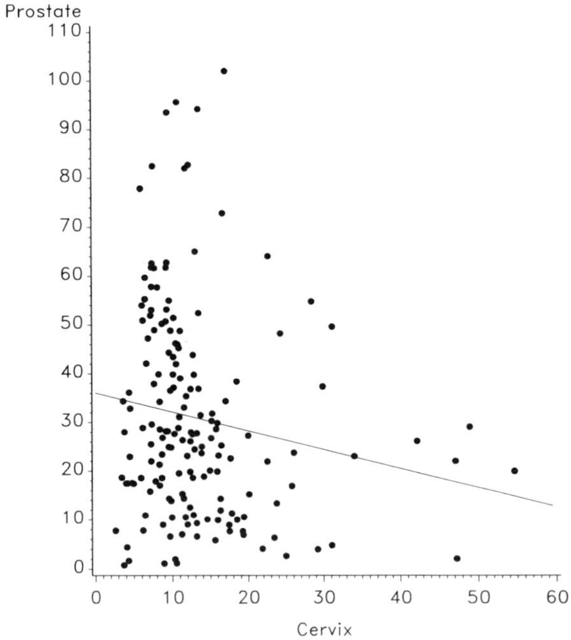

Fig. 1. Recent data (ie after the introduction of widespread screening of women for cancer of the cervix) show a significant negative association between incidence (per 100 000) of cancers of the prostate and cervix ($r = -0.15$, $p = 0.04$) (source: Parkin *et al*, 1992). Each point represents age adjusted incidence rates from one cancer registry

data from published sources such as the International Agency for Research on Cancer's *Cancer Incidence in Five Continents* reports, cancer mortality reports and cancer occurrence data from Africa.

Problems abound, however, in the comparison between rates of prostate cancer and rates of cervical cancer. The first problem is the level of underdiagnosis of prostate cancer. Autopsy series invariably show a large discrepancy between histological and clinical evidence of prostate cancer—that is, any change in intensity with which men are examined will result in significant increases in the apparent incidence of this condition (Walker, 1986; Pienta and Esper, 1993). As for cancer of the cervix, countries that have organized screening programmes may show artificially reduced incidence rates if screening succeeds in curing those with pre-malignant lesions.

INTERNATIONAL VARIATION

Table 1 illustrates the enormous international variation—about 120-fold—in the latest incidence figures for cancer of the prostate (Parkin *et al*, 1992). Blacks in Atlanta, USA, have the highest age standardized incidence rate ([ASIR], 102.0 per 100 000) and Chinese in Quidong have the lowest ASIR (0.8 per 100 000). Obviously, such striking variations suggest that manipulable determinants of this cancer do exist (Doll and Peto, 1983).

Figure 1 shows the geographical association between recent figures for incidence of cancer of the prostate and incidence of cancer of the cervix (Parkin *et al*, 1992). There is a significant negative association ($r = -0.15$, $p = 0.04$) between cancers of the prostate and cervix, but this could be accounted for by lowered incidence rates for cervical cancer, resulting from the introduction of screening.

To circumvent the effect of overinvestigation, earlier series (eg from before the start of mass screening) need to be examined. In Segi and colleagues' (1966) series of cancer mortality in 24 countries, there is a positive but statistically non-significant geographical association between cancers of the prostate and uterus ($r = 0.16$, $p = 0.4$) (Fig. 2). Similarly, in *Cancer Incidence in Five Continents* volume 1, there is again a weakly positive but statistically non-significant geographical association between incidence of cancer of the prostate and incidence of cancer of the cervix ($r = 0.1$, $p = 0.6$) (Fig. 3) (Doll *et al*, 1966).

AFRICA

An additional problem in unravelling the international epidemiology of prostate cancer is the strong positive geographical association between prostate cancer and per caput fat consumption (Nomura and Kolonel, 1991). Ideally, countries ought to be stratified according to fat consumption. Fat consumption is lower in sub-Saharan Africa than in western industrialized coun-

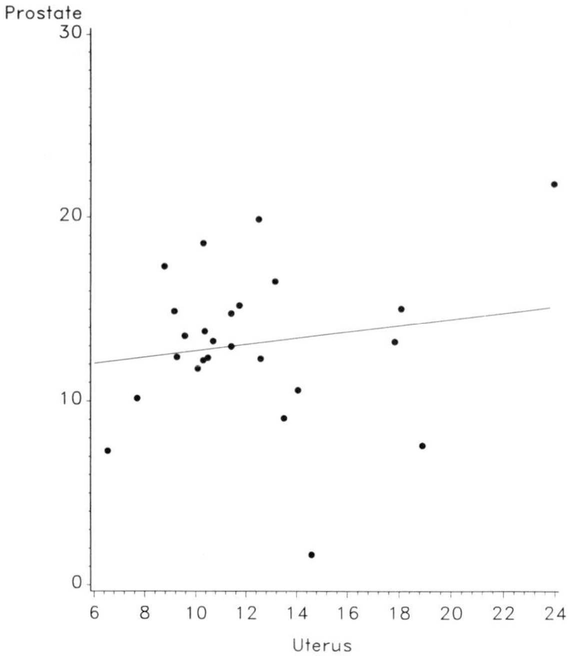

Fig. 2. Mortality data (deaths per 100 000) from 1966 show a positive but non-significant association between cancer of the prostate and cancers of the uterus in 24 countries ($r = 0.16$, $p = 0.44$) (source: Segi *et al*, 1966)

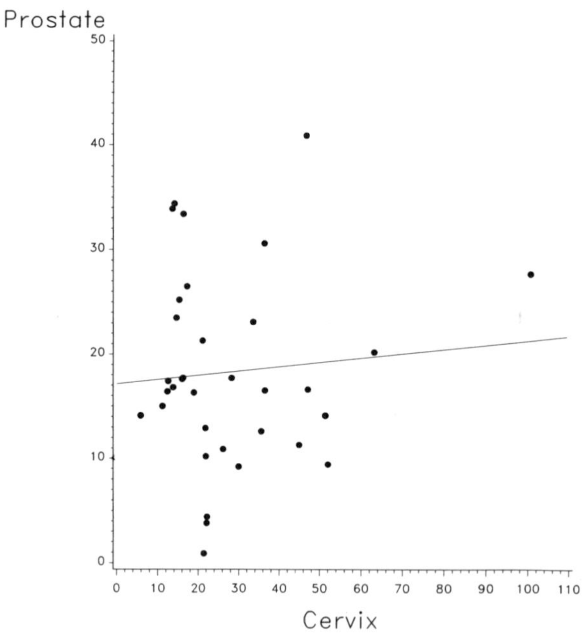

Fig. 3. Incidence data (per 100 000) from 1966 show a weakly positive but non-significant association between cancer of the prostate and cancer of the cervix ($r = 0.1$, $p = 0.6$) (source: Doll *et al*, 1966). Each point represents age standardized incidence rates from one cancer registry

tries, and the intensity of investigation of cancers of both prostate and cervix is minimal. For these reasons, data from Africa might point to some clues about a possible infectious aetiology for cancer of the prostate.

There have been sporadic attempts to register cancers in sub-Saharan Africa, but only a few regions have been able to estimate cancer incidence rates from population based registries, albeit over restricted time periods. Table 2 shows all the published information on cancer incidence emanating from population based cancer registries in sub-Saharan Africa between 1955 and 1994. There is a fair degree of variation in rates for cancer of the prostate, from 2.1 per 100 000 in the Gambia to 32.3 per 100 000 in Bulawayo, Zimbabwe. Cancer of the cervix varies less, about fourfold, from 10 per 100 000 in the Gambia to 43.6 per 100 000 in Uganda. Again, there is a positive (but weak) association between incidence of cancers of the prostate and cervix (r = 0.48, p = 0.09) (Fig. 4). There is a two- to threefold increase in both cancer of the prostate (from 4.4 to 12.3 per 100 000) and cervix (from 22.2 to 43.6 per 100 000) in Uganda between 1954–1960 and 1989–1991 (Table 2). It is possible that the two cancers have a common aetiology, but prostate cancer has been known in addition to increase in urbanized societies, possibly owing to changes in diet. Cancer of the cervix may increase in urban areas for different reasons, such as changes of sexual lifestyles. In Uganda, the presence of human immunodeficiency virus (HIV) might also have influenced the increase of both cancers, as illustrated by the tenfold increase in the incidence of Kaposi's sarcoma between the 1950s and 1989–1991, coinciding with the onset of AIDS (Wabinga *et al,* 1993). If an infectious agent is involved in the aetiology of both cervix and prostate cancers, then immune suppression caused by HIV may cause an increase in the incidence of infection associated cancers. Data from a case-control study of the relationship between HIV and cancer in South Africa might shed some light on this issue once the study is complete.

Some regions in Africa have published data on cancer from histopathology series (Parkin, 1986). Figure 5 shows the relative frequency of prostate and other cancers (skin cancers excluded) standardized for age. No association is evident between the relative frequencies of cancers of the prostate and cervix (r = 0.02, p = 0.9).

SOUTH AFRICA

In South Africa, a national histopathology based cancer registry was established in 1986, consisting of a network of all public and private pathology laboratories. In 1988, 45 570 cancers were recorded. Cancer of the prostate is the commonest cancer in the white population (ASIR = 27 per 100 000) and the second commonest cancer in the black population (ASIR = 14 per 100 000) (basal and squamous cancers excluded) (Sitas, 1994). To look at the geographical association between cancers of the prostate and cervix, cancer registrations were grouped into 11 regions according to the address of the

TABLE 2. Incidence (per 100 000) of cancer of the prostate and cervix in sub-Saharan African registeries

Region	Rate/100 000	Reference	Prostate	Cervix
South Africa, Johannesburg	1953–1955	Higginson and Oettlé (1966)	4.3	35.6
Uganda, Kampala	1954–1960	Parkin *et al* (1986)	4.4	22.2
Mozambique	1956–1960	Doll *et al* (1966)	9.2	30.0
South Africa, Durban	1964–1966	Schonland and Bradshaw (1968)	15.7	38.9
Uganda, Kampala	1968–1970	Parkin *et al.* (1986)	6.0	24.6
Zimbabwe, Bulawayo	1968–1972	Skinner *et al* (1993)	32.3	28.4
Senegal, Dakar	1969–1974	Tuyns and Quenum (1982)	4.3	17.2
Nigeria, Ibadan	1970–1976	Parkin *et al* (1986)	10.0	21.6
Swaziland	1979–1983	Parkin (1986)	3.1	28.2
Zaire, Kivu	1983–1986	Bourdeaux *et al* (1988)	3.3	3.3
Mali, Bamako	1987–1988	Bayo *et al* (1990)	4.7	20.8
Gambia	1986–1988	Bah *et al* (1990)	2.1	10.5
Uganda, Kampala	1989–1991	Wabinga *et al* (1993)	12.3	43.6

pathology laboratory and the population group. These are southern, northern, eastern and western Transvaal, northern, western and eastern Cape, Transkei, Orange Free State, Natal coast (Durban) and the Natal interior.

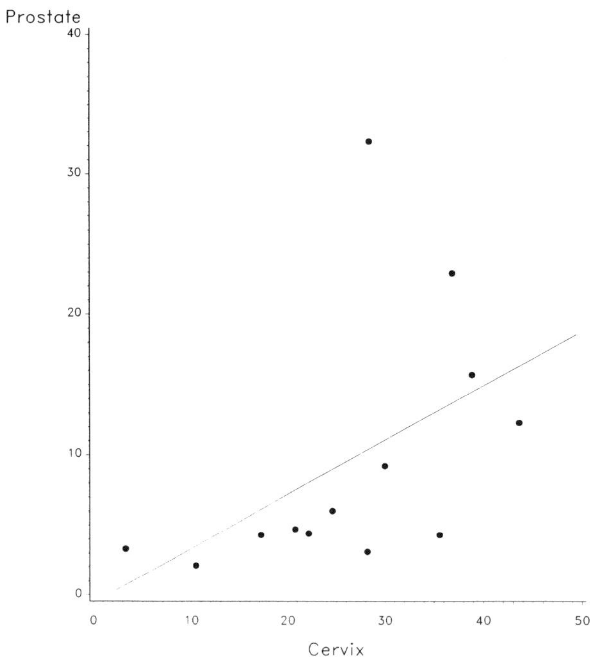

Fig. 4. Data reported to cancer registries in African countries show a positive but non-significant association between incidence (per 100 000) of cancers of the prostate and cervix ($r = 0.48$, $p = 0.09$)

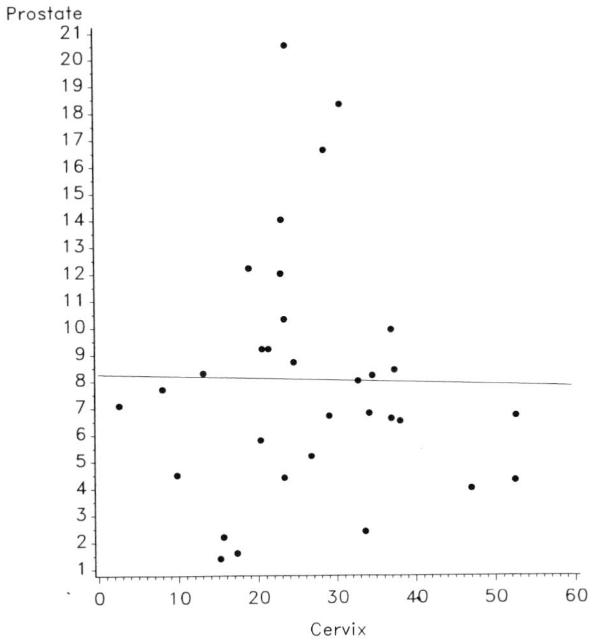

Fig. 5. Age standardized frequency data from available African histopathology series show no association between cancers of the prostate and cervix ($r = 0.02$, $p = 0.9$) (source: Parkin, 1986)

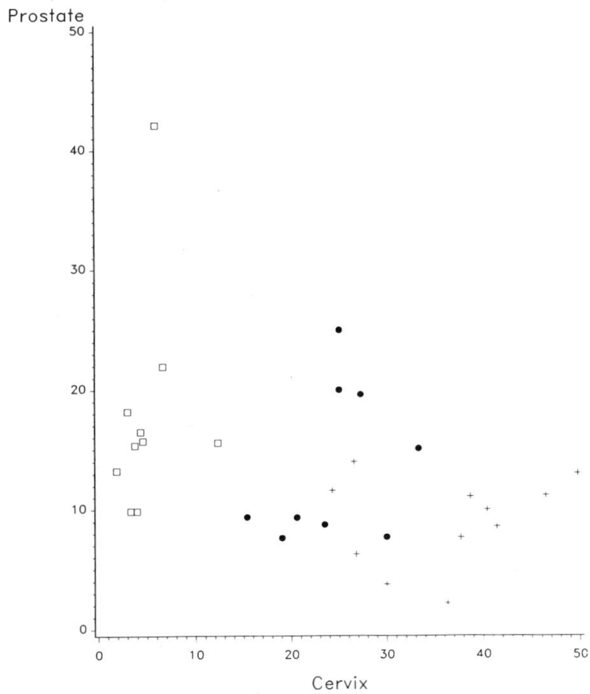

Fig. 6. Relative frequency of cancers of the prostate and cervix in white (*open box*), black (+) and coloured (*closed circle*) populations of South Africa

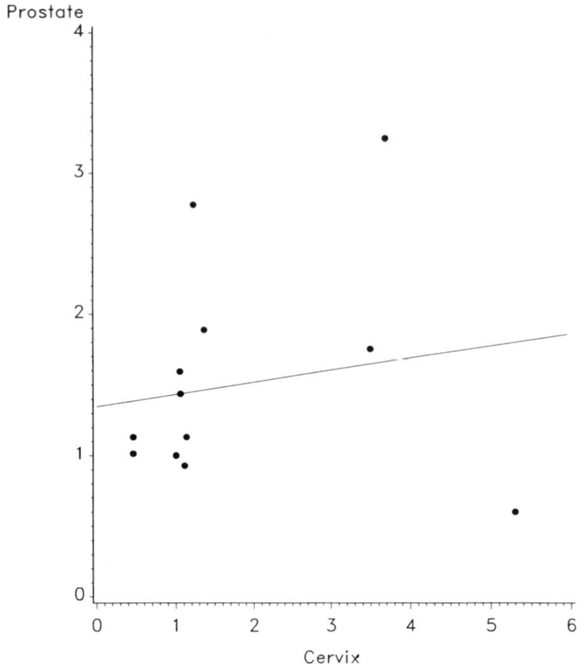

Fig. 7. Age adjusted odds ratios for cancers of the prostate and cervix in the white populations of 11 South African regions

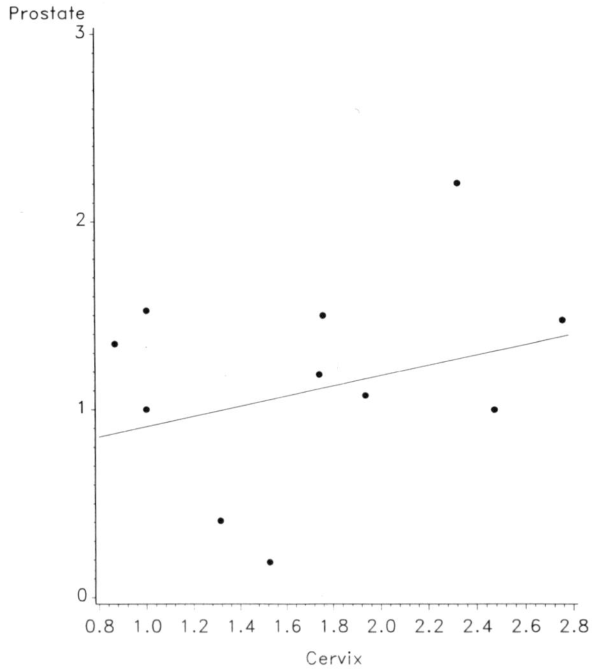

Fig. 8. Age adjusted odds ratios for cancers of the prostate and cervix in the black populations of 11 South African regions

Crude relative frequencies of cancers of the prostate and cervix by population group are shown in Fig. 6 (regions with no cases of cancers of the cervix or prostate excluded), illustrating the wide variation in occurrence of these two cancers. Age adjusted odds ratios were calculated for each region, using the southern Transvaal as baseline. Figures 7 and 8 show the distribution of the odds of developing cancers of the prostate and cervix in 11 regions in white and black groups, respectively. In the black population, the odds of developing prostate cancer varies about tenfold across regions, and among whites, about fivefold. Correlating the odds of cancers of the prostate and cervix yielded, again, positive but statistically weak associations ($r = 0.16$, $p = 0.6$ for whites; $r = 0.3$, $p = 0.2$ for blacks). Data for the mixed race (coloured) and Asian (Indian) populations are concordant with those found in whites and blacks.

DISCUSSION

Even in sub-Saharan Africa, where screening for cancer of the cervix and prostate is minimal, the geographical association between cancers of the cervix and prostate is weak. As with all geographical studies, even a strong association may be fortuitous, so case-control studies looking at the risk of a range of possible infectious agents in relation to prostate cancer are clearly required. An excellent study opportunity exists for using stored serum of men screened for prostate specific antigen (PSA). Serum could be tested for a range of antibodies against sexually transmitted agents such as *Chlamydia,* herpes simplex viruses, human papillomaviruses (HPV) and others. The prevalence of such infections in men with high and low levels of PSA could be then compared for potential associations. Such a study would avoid differential recall—that is, those with a prostate cancer remembering their past sexual history more clearly than a control group without reproductive organ problems.

In the geographical analyses discussed above, cancer of the cervix was used as a proxy for sexual activity and HPV infection. However, HPV has been mostly associated with squamous carcinoma (cervix, skin, oesophagus), whereas prostate cancer is predominantly an adenocarcinoma, so the search for infectious agents may have to be widened to include other viruses and bacteria.

In conclusion, the evidence for an infectious cause of prostate cancer based on geographical associations with cancer of the cervix is weak and as yet unconvincing. Nevertheless, these clues ought to be investigated further. Even 5 years ago, an infectious aetiology for stomach cancer would have been unthinkable, but the finding of moderate geographical association between *Helicobacter pylori* antibody prevalence and gastric cancer mortality in 1990 (Forman *et al,* 1990) was soon followed by a series of definitive cohort studies (Forman *et al,* 1991). The quest for an infectious aetiological agent in prostate cancer must continue, because even weak geographical associations are the building blocks of new hypotheses, notwithstanding the influence of other lifestyle factors, which must also be taken into account.

SUMMARY

Incidence and mortality data from the 1960s, when screening for cancers of the cervix and prostate was minimal, reveal a positive but statistically non-significant geographical association between the two diseases. Data on cancer incidence from African cancer registries and from the South African National Cancer Registry also show weak but positive associations. To determine whether infection is a cause of prostate cancer, case-control studies need to be conducted on individuals with and without prostate cancer or prostate cancer precursors. The screening of serum for prostate specific antigen provides an excellent opportunity to test for sexually transmitted agents.

References

Bah E, Hall AJ and Inskip HM (1990) The first 2 years of the Gambian cancer registry. *British Journal of Cancer* **62** 647–650

Bayo S, Parkin DM, Koumaré AK, Diallo AN, Ba T, Soumare S and Sangaré S (1990) Cancer in Mali 1987–88. *International Journal of Cancer* **45** 679–684

Bourdeaux L, Renard F, Gigase PL, Mukolo-Ndjolo, Maldague P and De Muynck A (1988) L'incidence des cancers à l'hôpital de Katana, Kivu est Zaire de 1983 à 1986. *Annales de la Société belge de médicine tropicale* **68** 141–156

Centifanto YM, Kaufmann HE, Zam ZS, Drylie DM and Dendourff SL (1973 Herpesvirus particles in prostatic carcinoma cells. *Journal of Virology* **12** 1608–1611

Doll R and Peto R (1983) *The Causes of Cancer,* Oxford Medical Publications, Oxford

Doll R, Payne P and Waterhouse J (eds) (1966) *Cancer Incidence in Five Continents: A Technical Report,* Springer, New York

Forman D, Sitas F, Newell DG *et al* (1990) Geographic association of *Helicobacter pylori* antibody prevalence and cancer mortality in rural China. *International Journal of Cancer* **46** 608–611

Forman D, Newell DG, Fullerton *et al* (1991) Association between infection with *Helicobacter pylori* and the risk of gastric cancer: evidence from a prospective investigation. *British Medical Journal* **302** 1302–1305

Higginson J and Oettlé AG (1966) Johannesburg, South Africa, In: Doll R (ed). *Cancer Incidence in Five Continents,* UICC, Geneva

Nomura AM and Kolonel LN (1991) Prostate cancer: a current perspective. *Epidemiological Reviews* **13** 200–227

Parkin DM (ed) (1986) *Cancer Occurrence in Developing Countries,* International Agency for Research on Cancer, Lyon

Parkin DM, Muir CS, Whelan SL, Gao YT, Ferlay J and Powell J (eds) (1992) *Cancer Incidence in Five Contients,* Vol VI (IARC Scientific Publications No 120), International Agency for Research on Cancer, Lyon

Pienta KJ and Esper P (1993) Risk factors for prostate cancer. *Annals of Internal Medicine* **118** 793–803

Sanford EJ, Geder L, Laychock A, Rohner TJ and Rapp F (1977) Evidence for the association of the cytomegalovirus with carcinoma of the prostate. *Journal of Virology* **12** 1608–1611

Schonland M and Bradshaw E (1968) Cancer in the Natal African and Indian. *International Journal of Cancer* **3** 304–316

Segi M, Kurihara M, Matsuyama T *et al* (1966) *Cancer Mortality for Selected Sites in 24 Countries: No 5 (1962-1963),* Department of Public Health, Tohoku

Sitas F (1994) Histologically diagnosed cancer in South Africa, 1988. *South African Medical Journal* **84** 344–348

Skinner MEG, Parkin DM, Vizcaino AP and Ndhlovu A (1993) *Cancer in the African Population of Bulawayo, Zimbabwe, 1963-1977: Incidence, Time Trends and Risk Factors* (IARC Technical Reports No 15), International Agency for Research on Cancer, Lyon

Tuyns AJ and Wuenum C (1982) Senegal, Dakar, In: Waterhouse J, Muir C, Shanmugaratnam K and Powell J (eds). *Cancer Incidence in Five Continents* Vol IV (IARC Scientific Publications No 42), International Agency for Research on Cancer, Lyon

Wabinga HR, Parkin DM, Wabwire-Mangen F and Mugerwa JW (1993) Cancer in Kampala, Uganda in 1989–1991: changes in incidence in the era of AIDS. *International Journal of Cancer* **54** 26–36

Walker ARP (1986) Prostate cancer—some aspects of epidemiology, risk factors, treatment and survival. *South African Medical Journal* **69** 44–47

The author is responsible for the accuracy of the references.

Human Papillomavirus Infection of the Prostate

JACK CUZICK
Imperial Cancer Research Fund, PO Box 123, Lincoln's Inn Fields, London WC2A 3PX

INTRODUCTION

The role of the human papillomavirus (HPV) in the genesis of anogenital cancers is well established, especially for cervix cancer (Durst *et al,* 1983; Munoz and Bosch, 1992), but also for cancers of the vulva (Daling *et al,* 1992), vagina (Daling *et al,* 1992), penis (McCance *et al,* 1986; Villa and Lopes, 1986) and anus (Beckmann *et al,* 1989; Scholefield *et al,* 1992). Specific types are important for these sites and most cancers are associated with one or more of types 16, 18, 33, 35, 39, 45, 51, 52 and 56. Type 16 is by far the most common in most populations. Given this range of well established sites, it is natural to ask if there is any involvement with cancers of nearby sites. The bladder is the next most likely site, but the uterus, kidney and prostate clearly are also possible areas of involvement. The currently available results for prostate are summarized in this chapter. Altogether eight series have been published and they are briefly summarized in Table 1. A more detailed summary follows.

In 1990, McNicol and Dodd reported on 16 fresh frozen biopsy samples, 14 of these were from transurethral resection and two from suprapubic prostatectomies for benign prostatic hypertrophy (BPH). Human papillomavirus types 16 and 18 were assayed by Southern blot hybridization after standard DNA extraction procedures. Altogether, 4 of 12 BPH samples were positive for HPV 16 or 18 and three of four prostate cancer (CaP) samples were positive. It is stated that positivity for both 16 and 18 was found in the study, but no details of the number of samples positive for each type were given.

In the following year, McNicol and Dodd published a new larger series of 88 samples. This time, both Southern blot and polymerase chain reaction (PCR) were used to assay the material. The PCR used probes and primers in the E6 region. No cases were positive for type 18 alone, but four (three BPH,

TABLE 1. Details of studies summarized

Study	HPV types	Material and HPV method	Population and number	HPV positivity (%)	Comments
Canada McNicol and Dodd (1990)	16, 18	Fresh frozen Southern blot mostly TURP	CaP (n=4) BPH (n=12)	16 and /or 18 CaP 3(75) BPH 4(25)	
Canada McNicol and Dodd (1991)	16, 18	Fresh frozen PCR mostly TURP	CaP (n=27) BPH (n=56) Normal autopsy (n=5)	16 only / 16 & 18 CaP 13(48) / 1(4) BPH 31(55) / 3(5) Normal 1(20) / 0(0)	
Japan Anwar *et al* (1992)	16, 18, 33	Paraffin blocks PCR	CaP (n=68) BPH (n=10) Normal (n=10)	Neg / 16 / 18 / 33 / Any CaP 40 / 11(16) / 17(25) / 5(7) / 28(41) BPH 10 / 0 / 0 / 0 / 0 Normal 10 / 0 / 0 / 0 / 0	*ras* mutations also studied HPV and *ras* correlated with late stage
Italy Rotola *et al* (1992)	6/11, 16	Fresh frozen biopsies PCR	CaP (n=8) BPH (n=17)	16 / 6/11 CaP 6(75) / 4(50) BPH 14(82) / 11(65)	High % also found in bladder, ureter, and kidney
North Carolina Ibrahim *et al* (1992)	16	Paraffin blocks (n=46) Frozen (n=23) PCR (also ISH on paraffin samples)	CaP (n=40) BPH (n=12) Normal (n=17)	CaP 6(15) BPH 0(0) Normal 2(12)	Only 1 sample positive by in situ hybridization
Florida Serfling *et al* (1992)	6, 11, 16, 18,33	Fresh frozen PCR	BPH and CaP (n=30)	0/30	
North Carolina Effert *et al* (1992)	16, 18	Paraffin PCR and Southern blot	CaP (n=30)	0/30 by both methods	
Canada Dodd *et al* (1993)	16	Fresh frozen PCR for RNA transcripts in HPV positives	CaP (n=7) BPH (n=10)	3/7 CaP and 5/10 BPH found to have transcripts	HPV positive samples from McNichol and Dodd (1991) used. No evidence for high transcription

TURP = Transurethral resection of the prostate; PCR = polymerase chain reaction; ISH = in situ hybridization; CaP = prostate cancer; BPH = benign prostatic hypertrophy

one CaP) were positive for both types and 45 (one normal autopsy, 31 BPH, 13 CaP) were positive for type 16 alone. Most of the specimens were obtained by transurethral resections, but similar positivity rates (7 of 12) were found after suprapubic prostatectomy, suggesting that the results were not a result of contamination with penile tissue.

Anwar *et al* (1992) reported on 75 paraffin embedded specimens from 68 Japanese patients with cancer and assayed for HPV types 16, 18 and 33 using type specific primers and probes. Twenty tissues from non-malignant cases obtained by transurethral resections or suprapubic prostatectomy were also examined. None of the ten normal or ten BPH specimens were found to contain HPV DNA, but 28 (41%) of the cancer cases showed one of the three types, with type 18 being most prevalent (17 of 68 = 25%). These authors suggest that HPV infection (as well as Ha-*ras* mutation at codon 61.2) might be related to progression of disease.

Rotola *et al* (1992) looked at HPV 6/11 and 16 by PCR in fresh frozen biopsy material. They found HPV 16 in six of eight CaP cases and 14 of 17 BPH cases; HPV 6/11 was found in four of eight CaP cases and 11 of 17 BPH cases. They also looked at samples from the bladder, ureter and kidney and found similar positivity rates at these sites. They examined integration of HPV by Southern blot hybridization and found that in most cancers, it appeared episomal, although evidence of integration was found in one cancerous tissue and one normal tissue. Rotola *et al* concluded that HPV 16 does not seem to be associated with urinary tract and prostate oncogenesis, but these tissues may be an important reservoir for the transmission of HPV types that normally infect the genital tract.

Much lower positivity rates were reported by Ibrahim *et al* (1992) on 69 samples assayed by PCR for HPV 16 using Manos L1 consensus primers. The material was a mixture of frozen and paraffin embedded tissues, but only 12% were positive. More specifically, 15% of cancers, none of the BPH tissues and 12% of the normal samples were positive. All of the positive normal samples were obtained by transrectal resection, and the authors suggested that positivity could have been due to anorectal contamination. Positivity rates were similar in paraffin embedded and frozen tissues.

Two more recent studies by Serfling *et al* (1992) and Effert *et al* (1992) each looked at 30 samples by PCR. In the former case, fresh frozen material was assayed for types 6, 11, 16, 18 and 33 as by the Manos consensus system, and in the latter case, types 16 and 18 were studied by type specific primers (and also by Southern blot). No positive cases were found in either study.

The last study by Dodd *et al* (1993) looked at transcription of HPV 16 E6/E7 in samples from their previous study (McNicol and Dodd, 1991) which were known to be positive. Evidence of transcription was found in about half of the samples studied: five of ten with BPH and three of seven with CaP. The lack of specificity of transcription left the authors to conclude "that the prostate may act as a site of HPV replication, but that HPV is unlikely to be involved in the transformation of prostatic cells".

TABLE 2. Positivity for high risk types: Summary

Reference	Normal	BPH		CaP
McNicol and Dodd (1990)	–	4/12		3/4
McNicol and Dodd (1991)	1/5	34/56		14/27
Anwar *et al* (1992)	0/10	0/10		28/68
Rotola *et al* (1992)	–	14/17		6/8
Ibrahim *et al* (1992)	2/17	0/12		6/40
Serfling *et al* (1992)			0/30	
Effert *et al* (1992)				0/30
Total	3/32	52/107	0/30	57/177
	(9)	(49)		(32)
			109/314	
			(35%)	

DISCUSSION

The positivity rates in the studies surveyed are shown in Table 2. Only the first four studies show an appreciable HPV positivity rate in prostatic cancers, and two of these were from the same authors. In most studies, the positivity rates are at least as high in BPH as in invasive cancer, and, overall, the evidence does not suggest a direct role for HPV in prostatic cancer.

There is considerable heterogeneity in the results across studies that cannot easily be accounted for by different methods of biopsy, different storage conditions or different assay systems. However, because of the enormous variability in the sensitivity that is used in PCR assays, it would have been helpful to have some rough quantification of the amount of HPV present.

The possibility that the prostate may serve as a reservoir for HPV in some cases is more tenable, but samples from multiple sites in the same individuals are needed to see if the prostate can act as the sole reservoir of infection. Rates of positivity in BPH and CaP are higher than in controls, and if this is not an artefact of collection methods, it could be due to a stimulatory effect on viral growth rates related to the higher rate of cell proliferation in both of these conditions. Thus, if very low level HPV infection was endemic, BPH or CaP may be the stimulus needed to raise the levels sufficiently for detection.

Conclusive proof of the relevance of the prostate as an important reservoir for HPV would require partner studies in women with cervical neoplasia to show that the prostate was the main or only reservoir of infection in her partner. Such studies will be difficult to carry out.

SUMMARY

Seven studies that have reported on the prevalence of anogenital types of the human papillomavirus in prostate cancer, benign prostatic hypertrophy and normal prostatic tissue are reviewed. When the data were combined, 32% of the cancers were positive, compared to 49% of the benign lesions and 9% of the normal tissue. The highest positivity rates were found in the earlier studies, and the more recent results have been more negative. The finding of higher rates in benign compared to malignant tissue and the failure of confirmatory studies to support earlier reports make it unlikely that the common anogenital papillomaviruses have an important role in prostate carcinogenesis. More work is needed to decide if the prostate is a significant reservoir for the papillomavirus in the male.

References

Anwar K, Nakakuki K, Shiraishi T, Naiki H, Yatani R and Inuzuka M (1992) Presence of *ras* oncogene mutations and human papillomavirus DNA in human prostate carcinomas. *Cancer Research* **52** 5991–5996

Beckmann AM, Daling JR, Sherman KJ *et al* (1989) Human papillomavirus infection and anal cancer. *International Journal of Cancer* **43** 1042–1049

Daling JR, Sherman KJ, Hislop TG *et al* (1992) Cigarette smoking and the risk of anogenital cancer. *American Journal of Epidemiology* **135** 180–189

Dodd JG, Paraskevas M and McNicol PJ (1993) Detection of human papillomavirus 16 transcription in human prostate tissue. *Journal of Urology* **149** 400–402

Durst J, Gissman L, Ikenberg H and zur Hausen H (1983) A papillomavirus DNA from a cervical carcinoma and its prevalence in cancer biopsy samples from different geographic regions. *Proceedings of the National Academy of Sciences of the USA* **80** 3812–3815

Effert PJ, Frye RA, Neubauer A, Liu ET and Walther PJ (1992) Human papillomavirus types 16 and 18 are not involved in human prostate carcinogenesis: analysis of archival human prostate cancer specimens by differential polymerase chain reaction. *Journal of Urology* **147** 192–196

Ibrahim GK, Gravitt PE, Dittrich KL *et al* (1992) Detection of human papillomavirus in the prostate by polymerase chain reaction and in situ hybridization. *Journal of Urology* **148** 1822–1826

McCance DJ, Kalache A and Ashdown K (1986) Human papillomavirus types 16 and 18 in carcinomas of the penis from Brazil. *International Journal of Cancer* **37** 55–59

McNicol PJ and Dodd JG (1990) Detection of papillomavirus DNA in human prostatic tissue by Southern blot analysis. *Canadian Journal of Microbiology* **36** 359–362

McNicol PJ and Dodd JG (1991) High prevalence of human papillomavirus in prostate tissues. *Journal of Urology* **145** 850–853

Munoz N and Bosch FX (1992) HPV and cervical neoplasia: review of case-control and cohort studies, In: Munoz N, Bosch FX, Shah KV and Meheus A (eds). *The Epidemiology of Cervical Cancer and Human Papillomavirus*, pp 251–261, International Agency for Research on Cancer, Lyon

Rotola A, Monini P, Di Luca D *et al* (1992) Presence and physical state of HPV DNA in prostate and urinary-tract tissues. *International Journal of Cancer* **52** 359–365

Scholefield JH, Hickson WGE, Smith JHF, Rogers K and Sharp F (1992) Anal intraepithelial neoplasia: part of a multifocal disease process. *Lancet* **340** 1271–1273

Serfling U, Ciancio G, Shu W-Y, Leonardi C and Penneys NS (1992) Human papillomavirus and herpes virus DNA are not detected in benign and malignant prostatic tissue using the polymerase chain reaction. *Journal of Urology* **148** 192–194

Villa LL and Lopes A (1986) Human papillomavirus DNA sequences in penile carcinomas in Brazil. *International Journal of Cancer* **37** 853–855

The author is responsible for the accuracy of the references.

Early Diagnosis and Treatment of Early Prostate Cancer

Screening Strategies: A Clinical Perspective

EDWARD P DeANTONI

Division of Urology, University of Colorado Health Sciences Center, Denver, Colorado 80262

INTRODUCTION: DEBATE PARAMETERS

Prostate cancer is a disease of old men: more than 80% of cases appear in men aged over 65. Two opposing views have emerged regarding the issues of screening and early detection of prostate cancer. One point of view argues that significant disease happens in this aged population and that physicians should address only the clinical manifestations of the disease, which is likely to be advanced at diagnosis. From this perspective, the primary objective is to identify state of the art treatments that prolong survival and allow an acceptable quality of life for the patient. A contrasting point of view argues that clinicians should pursue early detection and effective intervention to avoid progression to advanced disease. Necessarily, younger men would be recruited for prostate cancer screening and early detection initiatives. The primary objective here is the elimination of prostate cancer as a cause of morbidity and mortality for an ever larger percentage of men diagnosed earlier with the disease.

Advocates of the first position anticipate a relatively stable incidence of clinically diagnosed prostate cancer. Any increase in incidence is likely to be simply a reflection of an increased detection rate. These clinicians believe that cancer control efforts need to focus on clinical disease rather than on occult

Cancer Surveys Volume 23: *Preventing Prostate Cancer: Screening versus Chemoprevention*

disease. One fundamental assumption is that much more prostate cancer exists than will become clinically evident. Supporters of screening and early detection expect that certain epidemiological factors have contributed to a naturally occurring increase in prostate cancer. These clinicians believe that strategies that result in an increased incidence of earlier stage disease are in fact appropriate and advantageous, because thereby more curable cancers will be diagnosed and receive definitive therapy. In fact, the dynamics of early detection strategies have considerably reduced the prevalence of advanced prostate cancer. An underlying assumption here is that attempting to halt disease progression is for the individual good as well as for society.

DIMENSIONS OF THE PROBLEM

Prostate cancer is now the most common non-skin cancer among American men and the second leading cause of cancer death; yet, until recently, it was largely an ignored disease. The American Cancer Society (ACS) predicts 200 000 new cases of prostate cancer in the USA in 1994 and 38 000 deaths from the disease (Boring *et al,* 1994). This estimate represents a greater than 20% increase from 1993. The ACS states that the 50% increase in prostate cancer incidence between 1980 and 1990 was "largely due to improved detection" (American Cancer Society, 1994). From 1973 to 1990, age adjusted incidence rates increased 3.3% per year, rising more rapidly among Caucasian men than African-American men and more rapidly in Caucasians under 65 years of age, although the incidence is higher among African-American men (163.6 per 100 000) than Caucasians (128.5). Nevertheless, the aging of the US population and advances in cardiovascular disease control suggest a real increase in the incidence of prostate cancer and an increasingly serious public health problem (Davis *et al,* 1994).

The US National Cancer Institute (NCI) attributes the rise in incidence between 1973 and 1986 to a more complete reporting of prostate cancer found incidentally to transurethral resection of the prostate (TURP) (Miller *et al,* 1993b). Since 1986, the incidence of prostate cancer has increased 24% despite a declining rate of TURP, the increase being again attributed to better diagnostic tools, particularly the prostate specific antigen (PSA) blood test, transrectal ultrasound (TRUS) and TRUS guided biopsy.

The ACS has plotted a continuing rise in prostate cancer mortality, but 5 year survival rates have also improved. In fact, comparisons of breast and prostate cancer incidence and mortality demonstrate the important advances made in the early detection and treatment of prostate cancer. In the latest period for which comparable national data have been collected from the surveillance program of the NCI, 58% of prostate cancers were diagnosed as localized (T_1, T_2), compared with 53% of breast cancers. More breast cancers than prostate cancers were diagnosed as regional (T_3), 36% and 14%, respectively; but more prostate cancers than breast cancers were diagnosed as distant (T_4),

18% and 7%, respectively. Five year relative survival rates for 1983–1987 were equivalent for localized prostate and breast cancers, 91.9% and 93.2%. Prostate cancer had higher 5 year relative survival rates than breast cancer for both regional (81.7% v. 72.2%) and distant (28.1% v. 18.2%) disease (Miller *et al,* 1993b). Overall, 5 year relative survival for prostate cancer (all stages) has increased from 67% to 77%, whereas rates for breast cancer have increased from 74% to 79%, increases of 16.3% and 6.7%, respectively.

The NCI also notes the levelling of breast cancer incidence in the late 1980s, attributed to the widespread adoption of mammography screening. It will indeed be interesting to see whether or when this same phenomenon will occur with prostate cancer incidence.

PROSTATE CANCER AWARENESS WEEK

Prostate Cancer Awareness Week (PCAW) began in 1989 as an experiment to recruit symptom free men to prostate screening exams using digital rectal examination (DRE) and PSA testing. A national random survey sponsored in 1988 by the Prostate Cancer Education Council (PCEC) found that nearly two thirds of men aged over 40 who were surveyed had not had a physical examination within the past year and that fewer than half (48.8%) of those who ever had a physical exam had had DRE as part of it. Prostate cancer was rarely discussed with a physician and ranked eighth on the list of important health concerns. The PCEC concluded from these results that prostate cancer was indeed the "ignored male disease". Factors that might help explain this phenomenon are only beginning to be identified with the advent of psychosocial research among prostate cancer patients.

After 5 years and 1500 000 men screened during PCAW, together with the successful research efforts of many clinicians and increasing publicity given to prostate cancer and a few well known victims of the disease, some say prostate cancer is now getting unnecessary and unjustifiable public awareness.

Screening Finds Early Disease Sooner

One measure, albeit controversial, of the efficacy of a cancer screening and early detection programme is the stage distribution of diagnosed cancers. The rationale is that screening will detect earlier, organ confined lesions. Since earlier stage disease is usually more effectively treated than advanced disease, is often more cost effective in its treatment (Littrup *et al,* 1993) and is believed to result in better survival, early detection is therefore efficacious. Ten years ago, the distribution by stage for clinically diagnosed prostate cancer was approximately 10% stage A (T_0, T_1), 15–20% stage B (T_2), 40% stage C (T_3) and the remainder stage D (T_4) (DeVita *et al,* 1989). Since the 1970s, stage D_2 ($T_4N_{2-3}M_1$) lesions have decreased from approximately 40% to 25% (of T_4 cases) nationwide. In 1993, localized disease (T_0-T_2) represented 58% of all newly diagnosed cases (Miller *et al,* 1993b).

TABLE 1. Stage of prostate cancer at diagnosis, Prostate Cancer Awareness Week, 1989–1992

Year	Stage (no/%)								Total
	A		B			C	D		
1989	(4/11.4)		(20/57.0)			8/22.9)	(3/8.9)		35
	A_1	A_2	B_1	B_2	B_3	C	D_1	D_2	
1990	(25/6.7)	(15/4.0)	(115/30.8)	(104/27.9)	(19/5.1)	(51/13.7)	(24/6.4)	(20/5.4)	373
1991	(45/20.2)	(19/8.5)	(64/28.7)	(37/16.6)	(10/4.5)	(31/13.9)	(9/4.0)	(8/3.6)	223
1992	(25/11.7)	(43/20.2)	(55/25.8)	(45/21.1)	(7/3.3)	(29/13.6)	(6/2.8)	(3/1.4)	213

Source - Prostate Cancer Education Council (unpublished)

From 1989 to 1992, where stage was reported, PCAW consistently demonstrated superior results in the detection of early stage disease (Table 1). An important finding from PCAW is the distribution of prostate cancer by stage and age. Our data confirm that a majority of prostate cancer cases occur in men age 60–65, but the distribution by stage demonstrates that local disease occurs with proportional frequency among these men (Table 2). With curative therapy possible for local disease, early detection strategies among older men should be pursued aggressively. Moreover, the likelihood of advanced disease among younger men demands identification of those factors that lead to faster disease progression in this age group. A family history of prostate cancer suggests an important variable in the occurrence of the disease among younger men (Steinberg *et al,* 1990; Carter *et al,* 1993).

Acceptable Biopsy Performance

Many critics of prostate cancer screening claim that unnecessary morbidity results from high false positive biopsy rates (Gerber and Chodak, 1993a). However, the data shown in Table 3 suggest that with the exception of men aged of 45–55, positive biopsy rates are consistently 24–25% or higher. Given the purported prevalence of prostate cancer among older men, biopsy rates overall are reasonable. The distribution of detected cancers by race reflected racial percentages of the screened cohort: Caucasian, 90%; African-American, 6.4%; Latin, 2.4%; Asian, 0.2%. Some screening centres successfully recruited large numbers of minority participants.

In a cohort of more than 50 000 participants screened during PCAW 1992, 590 malignancies were confirmed. If extrapolated to the entire 1992 PCAW screened population of approximately 500 000 participants, this 1.2% detection rate would yield 5900 cancers. This would represent 4.5% of projected new 1992 cases, only a small fraction of the estimated increase due to screening and improved detection. A biopsy rate of 4.3% (n=2119) is reasonable for the estimated prevalence of prostate cancer in the population, as is a positive biopsy rate of 26.3%.

Prostate Cancer Awareness Week has consistently demonstrated the greater positive predictive value of the combination of DRE and PSA testing (Table 4)

IMPROVING THE EFFICACY OF PSA AS A SCREENING TEST

Prostate specific antigen is the most clinically useful tumour marker for prostate cancer (Oesterling, 1991), but it has not been perfected as a screening test for prostate cancer. Although specific for prostatic tissue, it is not prostate cancer specific, so an elevated serum concentration does not always denote prostate cancer. In fact, approximately 25% of men with benign prostatic hyperplasia (BPH) and no evidence of a prostate malignancy have an elevated serum PSA concentration. Conversely, not all prostate cancers give rise to an

TABLE 2. Stage of prostate cancer at diagnosis by age, Prostate Cancer Awareness Week, 1992

Stage at diagnosis: Whitemore-Jewett (TNM)	% of total	Age <60 years (%)	Age ≥60 years (%)
A_1 (T_1)	11.7	16	84
A_2 (T_1b)	20.2	21	79
B_1 (T_2)	25.8	16	84
B_2 (T_2a, T_2b)	21.1	20	80
B_3 (T_2c)	3.2	–	100
C (T_3N_0)	13.6	21	79
D_1 ($T_4N_{1\text{-}3}M_0$)	2.8	33	67
D_2 ($T_4N_{2\text{-}3}M_1$)	1.4	–	100

Source: Prostate Cancer Education Council

TABLE 3. Positive biopsies by age, Prostate Cancer Awareness Week, 1992

Age cohort	Positive biopsy number	Positive biopsy rate (%)	% of all biopsies
≥44	33	(28)	5.6
45–49	11	(16)	1.9
50–54	22	(15)	8.1
55–59	55	(24)	12.0
60–64	87	(25)	14.7
65–69	126	(27)	21.0
70–74	135	(33)	22.8
≥75	121	(29)	20.4

99% (590/593) of biopsies reported. Source: Prostate Cancer Education Council

TABLE 4. Positive biopsy rates (%) by DRE and PSA results, Prostate Cancer Awareness Week, 1989–1993

Year	+DRE –PSA	+DRE no PSA	–DRE +PSA	+DRE +PSA
1989	5	9	36	62
1990	7	18	28	44
1991	11	23	33	53
1992	18	n/a	26	54
1993	22	n/a	16	41

–DRE = normal; +DRE = abnormal; –PSA = ≥4 ng/ml; +PSA = >4 ng/ml; n/a = not available. Source: Prostate Cancer Education Council

elevated serum PSA concentration. Approximately 40% of men with organ confined prostate cancer who undergo radical prostatectomy for potential cure have a normal serum PSA concentration by the currently recommended reference range of 0–4.0 ng/ml. Thus, as currently used, PSA is neither specific enough nor sensitive enough to be a perfect screening test.

To study the efficacy of PSA testing, the Prostate Cancer Education Council instituted in 1992 a longitudinal study of PSA as a test for the early detection of prostate cancer. This study recruited 300 screening centres, and these screened over 75 000 men in 1992 and 1993, an estimated 45% of whom have been screened in both years. The computerized database for each year has more than 55 000 records containing demographic, medical history and clinical information.

PSA Density

Several methods have been offered to improve the specificity of serum PSA for prostate cancer. Benson *et al* (1992a,b) suggested adjusting the serum PSA concentration for the size of the prostate gland and developed the concept of PSA density (PSAD). Earlier studies suggested that PSAD, which is the serum PSA concentration divided by the volume of the prostate gland, can help distinguish men with early prostate cancer from those with BPH only. More recent studies based on whole mount sectioning attribute considerable predictive value to PSAD in identifying significant cancers (Blackwell *et al,* 1994; Epstein *et al,* 1994b). But this method is not yet well suited for clinical practice because of the difficulty in the precise determination of prostatic volume, whether by DRE, TRUS or magnetic resonance imaging. The coefficient of variation can be as great as 25% by either imaging modality.

Relationship between PSA and Age

Another technique for enhancing the clinical usefulness of serum PSA is to monitor change in serum PSA over a defined unit of time. Termed "PSA velocity" or "longitudinal change in serum PSA", this concept may provide useful information since more and more patients are returning every year for a serum PSA determination and DRE. In the initial study on this topic, analysis was presented to suggest that the rate of change in serum PSA could be more useful than the actual serum PSA level for detecting prostate cancer (Carter *et al,* 1992). A recent prospective study examined the characteristics of PSA in 471 healthy men aged between 40 and 79 years without clinical evidence of prostate cancer (Oesterling *et al,* 1993). From this investigation, the serum PSA concentration was found to correlate directly with age (r=0.43). These authors postulate that serum PSA concentration increases approximately 3.2% per year, or 0.04 ng/ml for a 60 year old man.

A relationship between age and PSA has been noted in data from the PCEC longitudinal study. The analysis of 1992 data was conducted on 47 286

TABLE 5. Age specific PSA reference ranges,[a] Prostate Cancer Awareness Week, 1992–1993

Age group	1992	1993	1992/1993[b]
40–49	0–2.0	0–2.3	0–2.3
50–59	0–3.3	0–3.3	0–3.5
60–69	0–4.8	0–4.9	0–4.9
70–79	0–5.6	0–5.9	0–5.8
No of records available for analysis	49 073	14 649	35 657

[a]Mean +2(1.96) standard deviations for upper limits (95% confidence interval).
[b]Mean screened in both 1992 and 1993. Source: Prostate Cancer Education Council

PSA values, after removal of all results from men reported with a positive diagnosis of cancer. The PSA results were reported by a reference laboratory using the Abbott IMx assay. A natural log transformation of PSA results established a normal distribution data model. Pearson correlation coefficient between age and PSA was 0.33 ($p=0.0001$; $R^2=0.11$). In 44 073 men (93.2%), the PSA concentration was <4 ng/ml; in 2729 (5.8%) 4–10 ng/ml; in 340 (0.7%) 10.1–20 ng/mg; in 58 (0.1%) 20.1–30.1 ng/ml; and in 86 (0.2%) >30.1 ng/ml. Of men with PSA concentrations above 10 ng/ml, 47 (0.09%) were aged 60 or less. Mean PSA concentrations were established for 10 year age cohorts. Upper normal values were established at +2 (1.96) standard deviations.

A similar relationship between age and PSA concentration was found from analysis of 1993 data from the same study. Table 5 presents age specific PSA ranges. The first column represents men screened in 1992, the second column men screened in 1993 but not in 1992, and the third column men screened in both 1992 and 1993. The age specific PSA reference ranges from 1992 data were used in a clinical study conducted during PCAW 1993 to determine prospective clinical validity.

In a retrospective analysis of 1066 biopsies performed in the group of 1992 participants, the sensitivity of the PSA test was increased for the 40–49 and 50–59 age cohorts, but specificity was decreased. The specificity was increased in the 60–69 and 70–75 age cohorts, but sensitivity was decreased. The establishment of age specific PSA reference ranges may improve the sensitivity and specificity of PSA as a test for the early detection of prostate cancer, but additional risk variables will need to be included in the algorithm for optimum sensitivity and specificity for PSA to be achieved.

PSA Velocity: Serial Screening and Rising PSA as a Risk Factor

Where no palpable abnormality is noted on DRE, serial PSA determinations can identify cancers with greater malignant potential from rising PSA concentrations. In a recent retrospective longitudinal study, a significant dif-

TABLE 6. Annual change in PSA by age, Prostate Cancer Awareness Week, 1992–1993

Age cohort	% Δ PSA	(95% CI)	Δ PSA (ng/μl)	(95% CI)
40–49 (n=867)	29	(2, 54)	0.13	(0.02, 0.25)
50–59 (n=2795)	32	(18, 47)	0.22	(0.15, 0.28)
60–69 (n=3656)	28	(16, 41)	0.26	(0.20, 0.31)
70–79 (n=1955)	42	(24, 59)	0.32	(0.25, 0.40)
Total (n=9273)				

Source: Prostate Cancer Education Council

ference was demonstrated in the age adjusted rate of change in PSA concentrations among men with prostate cancer, men with BPH and a control group (Carter *et al,* 1992). Subjects with BPH had a gradual rise in PSA, but those with prostate cancer had an exponential increase approximately 10 years before diagnosis. The rate of PSA change among the controls approximated 0.0 ng/ml per year, consistent with the concept that normal prostate glands exhibit no growth. An average annual rate of change of 0.75 ng/ml was able to increase to 90% the specificity of PSA in differentiating prostate cancer from BPH. This was a statistically significant greater specificity than that for a single PSA test.

In a prospective study of change in PSA concentrations in 1 year, Brawer used as a follow up criterion an arbitrary 20% rise in PSA among men whose PSA had originally been >4.0 ng/μl (Brawer *et al,* 1993). This study detected a high percentage of surgically determined organ confined disease among those whose PSA increased >20% but remained in the reference range for normal.

In a cohort of over 9000 men tested in 1992 and 1993, the average PSA change was 30% among men under age 70 and over 40% in men aged 70 and older. The absolute change ranged from a mean of 0.13 ng/μl in the youngest age group to 0.32 ng/μl in the oldest (Table 6).

Although the meaning and interpretation of PSA velocity (or ΔPSA) remain equivocal, continued elevations or significant interval increases in PSA over time may thus be more important than absolute PSA values. Velocity of PSA change permits continued investigation of interval screening of symptom free men. When used in conjunction with DRE, PSA as a screening test for prostate cancer should be considered an appropriate community based health care practice.

Serial PSA testing assumes a direct correspondence of PSA level to tumour volume and growth rate; yet pathological correlation with clinically benign specimens suggests that PSA concentrations do not increase significantly until tumours reach a size of cm^3 (Brawn *et al,* 1991). Consequently, the same conundrums regarding a "reference range" of PSA concentrations continue to plague use of PSA velocity as an aid to prostate cancer screening. Nevertheless, serial testing would, at this point, allow an initial indexing of disease risk, and perhaps the rate of PSA increase together with age, prostatism symptom score and other factors may recommend variable screening intervals and appropriate follow up diagnostic procedures.

THE CRITIQUE OF SCREENING

The combination of improved detection methods for prostate cancer and increased public awareness of the disease (in a culture where the belief exists that any disease can and should be cured) has impinged on health services and costs and has raised scientific and health care policy questions about the merit of screening and early detection initiatives (Kramer *et al,* 1993). The two primary areas of scientific criticism directed at screening for prostate cancer focus on theoretical issues of screening and the natural history of prostate cancer.

The theory of screening demands that efficacy be proven by a reduction in disease specific mortality. Such a hypothesis can be examined properly only in a randomized controlled trial (Prorok *et al,* 1990; Gerber and Chodak, 1993b). The NCI has embarked on such a study, the Prostate, Lung, Colorectal and Ovarian (PLCO) Cancer Screening Trial. This trial began in 1993 and will recruit and randomize 148 000 men and women who will be screened for 4 years. A 10 year follow up period has been established. The issue of PSA testing contamination among men in the control group is a major concern for the trial.

A NEW PARADIGM AS RETORT

The explosion of new knowledge about prostate cancer and its markers, and the rush of clinical advances in the diagnosis and treatment of prostate cancer, will probably make the findings of the long drawn out PLCO clinical trial marginally important when they appear. Moreover, the findings of any such clinical trial are likely to be analysed and debated for some additional length of time.

Older Models of the Natural History of Prostate Cancer

New research findings and clinical advances raise the question "Which model is correct for a clinical understanding and response to prostate cancer?". The classic initiation→promotion→progression paradigm supports the orthodox view that a natural process of tumour growth and spread occurs, that pathogenic characteristics—if left to their own devices—follow a predetermined course of development. In this light, classic studies in prostate cancer have suggested that poorly differentiated tumours evolve from well differentiated tumours, that mutations accumulate (McNeal, 1992). Furthermore, such studies recommend the analysis of prognostic factors that are self defined by this paradigm. For example, the doubling time of PSA has been suggested as one such critical prognostic factor (Schmid *et al,* 1993). Thus, definitive treatment can be postponed until or unless a rise in PSA levels begins to approach some specific threshold.

This particular model supports the criticism of lead time bias in prostate cancer screening. In fact, classical theories of screening for chronic disease are premised on this very model of disease progression (Zelen and Feinleib, 1969). Lead time bias argues that any increase in survival that results from detecting an early lesion is specious because that benefit simply represents a preclinical phase before the lesion becomes clinically evident. With prostate cancer, that progression has been viewed as essentially problematic. The interval during which "latent" disease is transformed to clinical disease is thought to be considerable. Unless progression is inevitable and cure definitively proven, treatment of preclinical disease is unnecessary and irrelevant to treatment for clinical disease.

Autopsy studies have provided the basis for a two disease paradigm of prostate cancer (Franks, 1954; Wynder *et al,* 1971; Breslow *et al,* 1977; Yatani *et al,* 1982). A significant difference is observed between the high prevalence of undetected (occult) disease, estimated at 40% in men over age 50 and nearly 80% in men over age 80, and the low clinical manifestation of prostate cancer, representing only 2.5% of all deaths in males. This discrepancy provides the underpinning for a paradigm of "occult" or "latent" disease versus "clinical" disease. A very slow and generally harmless growth rate has therefore been postulated for most prostate cancers. More men are predicted to die with prostate cancer than from it, supporting the belief that many would benefit from deferred treatment (expectant management) for localized disease rather than attempted definitive therapy if normal life expectancy from the time of diagnosis would be 10 years or less (Handley *et al,* 1988; Smith, 1990; Whitmore *et al,* 1991).

Until PSA and TRUS became widely used as early detection modalities, DRE was the "gold standard" of prostate cancer detection. The physical limitations of DRE resulted in most tumours being clinically diagnosed as locally advanced and incurable. Few if any localized tumours were clinically diagnosed and treated. This paradigm has been codified in the famous dictum that "those for whom treatment is necessary cannot be helped, and those who can be helped do not need treatment" (Whitmore, 1990). This seemingly unresolvable dilemma has promoted an essentially nihilistic attitude that nothing can or should be done: advanced (clinical) disease cannot be cured whereas localized (latent) disease should not be aggressively detected and should be managed expectantly since nothing more serious is likely to result before death from other causes. Some studies have suggested no significantly greater benefit from definitive therapy than from deferred treatment for localized disease (Fleming *et al,* 1993; Wasson *et al,* 1993).

A recent attempt to synthesize these models has led to the conception of prostate cancers as either "turtles" or "birds". That is, there may be some fundamental biological distinction between slow growing (or non-growing "latent") tumours and fast growing tumours. From one perspective, this model has lent credence to the length bias criticism of prostate cancer screening. This criticism claims that in screening and early detection initiatives among symptom free men, a majority of those tumours detected are harmless occult tumours, whereas fast growing tumours always present clinically at advanced stages when current treatment methods, while lengthening survival, are ineffective in significantly decreasing mortality (Stamey, 1983; Whitmore, 1990; Hinman, 1991; Johansson, 1992).

Critics of screening suggest that morbidity and mortality are significantly increased when the "turtle" tumours are detected and treated, particularly in men whose life expectancy is equal to or shorter than current prostate cancer survival rates. One need not search the literature very far before encountering the hypothetical "case" of the 70 year old man for whom treatment of a low grade indolent prostate cancer would cause more damage than the disease itself (Gerber and Chodak, 1990).

A New Paradigm Suggests an Efficacious Use for Screening

This last model has encouraged the investigation of different phenomena, which may explain the heterogeneity of prostate cancer (Aihara *et al,* 1994b). The natural history of the disease is becoming clearer and an effective clinical strategy more evident. Recent studies, along with analysis of previous studies of observation versus treatment, suggest that the two (latent and clinical) diseases are distinct.

Comparing non-palpable PSA detected (T_{1c}) prostate cancers with T_{1a} lesions found incidentally to TURP and clinically palpable (T_2) tumours, researchers at Johns Hopkins University have developed a model to predict whether a tumour warrants expectant management or definitive therapy (Epstein *et al,* 1994b). These T_{1c} tumours are of intermediate extent compared with the others, most are moderate or advanced in terms of PSAD and Gleason grade and many may become incurable before they are palpable. Thus, preoperative clinical and pathological findings can determine which patients would benefit from treatment or from observation.

Gleason grade has become an increasingly important prognostic factor in separating latent indolent tumours from aggressive deadly tumours. Grades 1 and 2 are associated with indolent tumours, whereas grade 3 is the predominant pattern in clinically localized cancer (Aihara *et al,* 1994a). However, small high grade tumours do appear independently of low grade lesions, thus suggesting that a one disease model does not explain the heterogeneity found in prostate cancer. The growth advantage of poorly differentiated tumours, which produce less PSA, may help explain why many clinically detected tumours have already advanced yet are associated with low PSA (Partin *et al,* 1990; Epstein *et al* 1994a). Tumours causing elevated PSA are more likely to have greater volume, higher grade (poorly differentiated) and a more advanced pathological stage than tumours with normal PSA (Blackwell *et al,* 1994). Older studies, based on clinically detected disease, may not be appropriate any longer to explain the parameters of a new disease paradigm being formulated.

Screening and early detection of prostate cancer, therefore, can be most efficacious when a diagnostic workup is performed on the basis of DRE, PSA test results (performed serially) and histological data (Catalona *et al,* 1993; Partin *et al,* 1993). Favourable predictive factors (low PSA, low PSAD, low Gleason grade) are more likely to identify latent or non-aggressive disease. Unfavourable predictive factors, identified through PSA testing and histological examination, clearly identify a subset of candidates for definitive therapy. The clinician can determine the degree to which these prognostic variables warrant immediate treatment and whether age, co-morbidity and life expectancy should moderate the recommendation of definitive therapy.

A reduction in prostate cancer specific mortality is the only definitive evidence of the efficacy of prostate cancer screening. However, a simultaneous reduction of mortality with increased screening cannot be reasonably expected, except over an extended time period. Survival time is correlated with a number of critical prognostic factors, and prostate cancer mortality in 1994 is related to the particular mix of these factors. Studies of breast cancer incidence and mortality suggest that cohort analysis is an appropriate method to demonstrate screening efficacy (Feuer *et al,* 1993; Miller *et al,* 1993a). Comparisons of screened and unscreened men who have been diagnosed with prostate cancer may suggest particular advantages of screening and early detection in the face of constant or even increasing mortality (Weiss *et al,* 1992). If a significant outcome of screening and early detection of prostate cancer is the cure of clinically localized disease, such analyses should demonstrate reduced mortality from screening. Otherwise, earlier detection would only substantiate a lead time bias of longer survival and unchanged mortality over time (Morrison, 1982; Weiss, 1983).

SUMMARY

Prostate cancer is increasing in incidence, particularly because of the control of competing causes of death and the lengthening life span of western men. Screening and early detection initiatives among symptom free men show that the disease can be detected at earlier stages when hope for cure is reasonable. Prostate specific antigen is the most useful marker for prostate cancer. Analytical methods to improve its sensitivity and specificity include PSA density, age specific PSA reference ranges and PSA velocity or the rate of change in PSA. Older paradigms of the natural history of prostate cancer have been heavily influenced by characteristics of clinical disease. However, improved detection of the disease through better diagnostic tools and heightened public awareness may be changing the dynamics of the disease. The prevalence of advanced disease is falling, and more knowledge is accumulating on the identification of clinically significant disease. The most appropriate definition of clinically significant disease today must be based on a new paradigm, one that can build on but not be bound by older models.

References

Aihara M, Lebovitz RM, Wheeler TM *et al* (1994a) Prostate specific antigen and gleason grade: an immunohistochemical study of prostate cancer. *Journal of Urology* **151** 1558–1564

Aihara M, Wheeler TM, Ohori M *et al* (1994b) Heterogeneity of prostate cancer in radical prostatectomy specimens. *Urology* **43** 60–66

American Cancer Society (1994) *Cancer Facts and Figures 1994,* p 10, American Cancer Society, Atlanta, Georgia

Benson MC, Whang IS, Pantuck A *et al* (1992a) Prostate specific antigen density: a means of distinguishing benign prostatic hypertrophy and prostate cancer. *Journal of Urology* **147** 815–816

Benson MC, Whang IS, Olsson CA *et al* (1992b) The use of prostate specific antigen density to enhance the predictive value of intermediate levels of serum prostate specific antigen. *Journal of Urology* **147** 817–821

Blackwell KL, Bostwick DG, Myers RP *et al* (1994) Combining prostate specific antigen with cancer and gland volume to predict more reliably pathological stage: the influence of prostate specific antigen cancer density. *Journal of Urology* **151** 1565–1570

Boring CC, Squires TS, Tong T and Montgomery S (1994) Cancer Statistics, 1994. *CA-A Cancer Journal for Clinicians* **44** 7–26

Brawer MK, Beatie J, Wender MH *et al* (1993) Screening for prostatic carcinoma with prostate specific antigen: results of the second year. *Journal of Urology* **150** 106–109

Brawn PN, Speights VO, Kuhl D *et al* (1991) Prostate-specific antigen levels from completely sectioned, clinically benign, whole prostates. *Cancer* **68** 1592–1599

Breslow N, Chan CW, Dhom G *et al* (1977) Latent carcinoma of the prostate at autopsy in seven areas. *International Journal of Cancer* **20** 680–688

Carter HB, Pearson JD, Metter EJ *et al* (1992) Longitudinal evaluation of prostate-specific antigen levels in men with and without prostate disease. *Journal of the American Medical Association* **267** 2215–2220

Carter BS, Bova GS, Beaty TH *et al* (1993) Hereditary prostate cancer: epidemiologic and clinical features. *Journal of Urology* **150** 797–802

Catalona WJ, Smith DS, Ratliff TL *et al* (1993) Detection of organ-confined prostate cancer is increased through prostate-specific antigen-based screening. *Journal of the American Medical Association* **270** 948–954

Davis DL, Dinse GE and Hoel DG (1994) Decreasing cardiovascular disease and increasing cancer among whites in the United States from 1973 through 1987. *Journal of the American Medical Association* **271** 431–437

DeVita Jr VT, Hellman S and Rosenberg SA (1989) *Cancer: Principles and Practice of Oncology,* p 1035, JB Lippincott, Philadelphia

Epstein JI, Carmichael MJ, Partin AW *et al* (1994a) Small high grade adenocarcinoma of the prostate in radical prostatectomy specimens performed for nonpalpable disease: pathogenetic and clinical implications. *Journal of Urology* **151** 1587–1592

Epstein JI, Walsh PC, Carmichael M *et al* (1994b) Pathologic and clinical findings to predict tumor extent of nonpalpable (stage T1c) prostate cancer. *Journal of the American Medical Association* **271** 368–374

Feuer EJ, Lap-Ming W, Boring CC *et al* (1993) The lifetime risk of developing breast cancer. *Journal of the National Cancer Institute* **85** 892–897

Fleming C, Wasson JH and Albertsen PC (1993) A decision analysis of alternative treatment strategies for clinically localized prostate cancer. *Journal of the American Medical Association* **269** 2650–2658

Franks LM (1954) Latent carcinoma of the prostate. *Journal of Pathology and Bacteriology* **68** 603–616

Gerber GS and Chodak GW (1990) Digital rectal examination in the early detection of prostate cancer. *Urologic Clinics of North America* **17** 739–744

Gerber GS and Chodak GW (1993a) Early diagnosis of prostate cancer, In: DeVita VT, Hellman S and Rosenberg SA (eds). *Important Advances in Oncology 1993*, pp 93–101, JB Lippincott, Philadelphia

Gerber GS and Chodak GW (1993b) Value of prostate cancer screening. *European Urology* **24** 161–165

Handley R, Carr TW, Travis D *et al* (1988) Deferred treatment for prostate cancer. *British Journal of Urology* **62** 249–253

Hinman F (1991) Screening for prostatic carcinoma. *Journal of Urology* **145** 126–129

Johansson J-E, Adami H-O, Andersson S-O *et al* (1992) High 10-year survival rate in patients with early, untreated prostatic cancer. *Journal of the American Medical Association* **267** 2191–2196

Kramer BS, Brown ML and Prorok PC (1993) Prostate cancer screening: what we know and what we need to know. *Annals of Internal Medicine* **119** 914–923

Littrup PJ, Goodman AC and Mettlin CJ (1993) The benefit and cost of prostate cancer early detection. *CA—A Cancer Journal for Clinicians* **43** 135–149

McNeal JE (1992) Cancer volume and site of origin of adenocarcinoma in the prostate: relationship to local and distant spread. *Human Pathology* **23** 258–266

Miller BA, Feuer EJ and Hankey BF (1993a) Recent incidence trends for breast cancer in women and the relevance of early detection: an update. *CA-A Cancer Journal for Clinicians* **43** 27–41

Miller BA, Ries LAG, Hankey BF *et al* (eds) (1993b) *SEER Cancer Statistics Review: 1973-1990*, Publication No 93-2789, National Cancer Institute NIH

Morrison AS (1982) Case definition in case-control studies of the efficacy of screening. *American Journal of Epidemiology* **115** 6–8

Oesterling JE (1991) Prostate-specific antigen: a critical assessment of the most useful tumor marker for adenocarcinoma of the prostate. *Journal of Urology* **145** 907–923

Oesterling JE, Jacobsen SJ, Chute CG *et al* (1993) Serum prostate-specific antigen in a community-based population of healthy men: establishment of age-specific reference ranges. *Journal of the American Medical Association* **270** 860–864

Partin AW, Carter HB, Chan DW *et al* (1990) Prostate-specific antigen in the staging of localized prostate cancer: influence of tumor differentiation, tumor volume, and benign hyperplasia. *Journal of Urology* **143** 747–752

Partin AW, Yoo J, Carter HB *et al* (1993) The use of prostate antigen, clinical stage, and gleason score to predict pathological stage in men with localized prostate cancer. *Journal of Urology* **150** 110–114

Prorok PC, Connor RJ and Baker SG (1990) Statistical considerations in cancer screening programs. *Urologic Clinics of North America* **17** 699–708

Schmid HP, McNeal JE and Stamey TA (1993) Observations on the doubling time of prostate cancer. *Cancer* **71** 2031–2040

Smith PH (1990) The case for no initial treatment of localized prostate cancer. *Urologic Clinics of North America* **17** 827–834

Stamey TA (1983) Cancer of the prostate: an analysis of some important contributions and dilemmas. *Monographs in Urology* **4** 65–92

Steinberg GD, Carter BS, Beaty TH *et al* (1990) Family history and the risk of prostate cancer. *Prostate* **17** 337–347

Wasson JH, Cushman CC and Bruskewitz RC (1993) A structured literature review of treatment for localized prostate cancer. *Archives of Family Medicine* **2** 487–493

Weiss NS (1983) Control definition in case-control studies of the efficacy of screening and diagnostic testing. *American Journal of Epidemiology* **118** 457–460

Weiss NS, McKnight B and Stevens NG (1992) Approaches to the analysis of case-control studies of the efficacy of screening for cancer. *American Journal of Epidemiology* **135** 817–823

Whitmore Jr WF (1990) Natural history of low-stage prostatic cancer and the impact of early detection. *Urologic Clinics of North America* **17** 689–697

Whitmore WF, Warner JA and Thompson IM (1991) Expectant management of localized prostatic cancer. *Cancer* **67** 1091–1096

Wynder EL, Mabuchi K and Whitmore W (1971) Epidemiology of cancer of the prostate. *Cancer* **28** 344–360

Yatani R, Chigusa I, Akazaki K *et al* (1982) Geographic pathology of latent prostatic carcinoma. *International Journal of Cancer* **29** 611–616

Zelen M and Feinleib M (1969) On the theory of screening for chronic diseases. *Biometrika* **56** 601–614

The author is responsible for the accuracy of the references.

Screening in General Practice

MARK R FENELEY[1] • MICHAEL G KIRBY[3] • TOM McNICHOLAS[4]
ALISON McLEAN[2] • JUDITH A W WEBB[2] • ROGER S KIRBY[1]

[1]Departments of Urology and [2]Diagnostic Radiology, St Bartholomew's Hospital, West Smithfield, London EC1A 7BE; [3]The Surgery, Nevells Road, Letchworth, Hertfordshire SG6 4TS; [4]Department of Urology, Lister Hospital, Stevenage SG1 4AB

INTRODUCTION

Carcinoma of the prostate is now the second commonest cause of death from cancer in males in many developed countries. The incidence in England and Wales is 0.72 new cases per 1000 men between 55 and 70 years of age, and in 1991, 8500 men died from the disease (Office of Population Censuses and Surveys, 1991). In the European Community as a whole, it was estimated that 85 000 new cases were diagnosed in 1980, and 35 084 men die annually from prostate cancer (Moller-Jensen *et al,* 1990).

The progression of prostate cancer is insidious, and many patients already have locally advanced or metastatic disease at the time of presentation (Murphy *et al,* 1982). For these individuals, treatment remains palliative and has advanced little since hormone sensitivity was recognized by Huggins and Hodges more than 50 years ago (Huggins *et al,* 1941). Approximately 70% of cases will respond to anti-androgen treatment; however, more than half of these will suffer relapse within 2 years, and the mean survival even with maximal androgen blockade is only 36 months (Crawford *et al,* 1989).

The limited efficacy of current therapy for advanced malignancy and the rising disease mortality have led to calls for the introduction of prostate cancer screening to facilitate the diagnosis of localized disease (Yamanaka, 1993). Others have suggested the need for large scale controlled studies of screening (Schroder, 1993). Such efforts have been made fuelled by the characterization of a new tumour marker, prostate specific antigen (PSA). This is a glycoprotein secreted exclusively by prostatic epithelial cells and is present in large amounts in seminal and prostatic fluid; it is the most useful serum marker for prostatic malignancy, and its value for the monitoring of established disease has been

Cancer Surveys Volume 23: *Preventing Prostate Cancer: Screening versus Chemoprevention*

proved (Stamey *et al*, 1987). It also provides the means by which screening might be achieved (Oesterling, 1992).

The criteria that need to be fulfilled in order for screening for a given disease to be acceptable were set out by Wilson and Jungner in 1969. There is no doubt that prostate cancer is a significant public health problem, since it is already common and the incidence appears to be rising steadily. With the projected demographic shifts towards greater longevity, the death rate from prostate cancer is likely to increase markedly over the next two decades. Screening for prostate cancer may be achieved by digital rectal examination (DRE), serum PSA determination and transrectal ultrasound (TRUS).

METHODS

We undertook a pilot study to evaluate critically the performance and acceptability of the three detection methods in a general practice setting (Kirby *et al*, 1994). Altogether, 856 men between the ages of 55 and 70 who were registered with a single general practice and had no previous history of prostatic cancer were invited by letter to attend the surgery for a health check including prostatic evaluation; 568 (66%) men accepted this invitation. At the first visit, blood was drawn for PSA determination and assayed using the Hybritech Tandem R (Hybritech Corp, San Diego, CA) immunoassay. A careful DRE was then performed by the general practitioner. The findings from the DRE were recorded as normal, benign enlargement or suspicious of malignancy (ie nodularity or asymmetry). Patients with a normal or a benign enlarged prostate on palpation and a PSA level of 4.0 ng/ml or less were reassured and will be re-evaluated; those with suspicious findings of nodularity or asymmetry on DRE or a PSA level greater than 4.0 ng/ml were referred for TRUS.

In 69 patients, TRUS was performed by one of two radiologists at St Bartholomew's Hospital, London, who were experienced in the technique (JAWW and AM). Forty nine patients (71%) were examined with an ATL Ultramark 5 machine and a 5 MHz biplanar transducer. The remainder were examined with an Acuson 128 XP machine with Doppler and 7.5 MHz transverse and linear transducers. Nine patients who were unwilling to travel to St Bartholomew's Hospital were scanned at the Lister Hospital by a urologist (TM) experienced in the technique using a Siemens Sonoline 2051 with a biplanar variable frequency (5.0–7.5 MHz) transducer. A further two patients had TRUS elsewhere, one with a Siemens Sonoline AC machine with a biplanar variable frequency (5.0–7.5 MHz) transducer, and one with a Bruel and Kjaer 1846 machine with a multifrequency (up to 7.0 MHz) probe. The prostate was scanned in the transverse and longitudinal planes with the patient in the left lateral decubitus position. With the Acuson machine, a colour Doppler examination was also performed. Transrectal ultrasound guided biopsies were obtained from any focal peripheral zone abnormality: masses 6 mm or more in diameter, areas of inhomogeneity or areas of increased Doppler colour flow. If the PSA was greater than 10.0 ng/ml, random biopsies of the right and left peripheral zones and of the mid-gland (peripheral plus transition zones) were performed even if no focal abnormality was seen. Biopsy guided by TRUS was also performed in areas of palpable abnormality even when a focal abnormality was not seen on the TRUS.

All biopsies were performed with an 18G Bard Biopsy-cut needle in a Biopty gun (Bard, Covington GA). With the ATL Ultramark 5, transperineal biopsy specimens were obtained after infiltration with 10–15 ml of 1% lignocaine, and no antibiotic prophylaxis was used. At St Bartholomew's Hospital and the Lister Hospital, transrectal biopsies were performed after intravenous gentamicin 120 mg. At St Bartholomew's Hospital, co-amoxiclav 625 mg was given three times daily for the first 24 hours after the procedure unless there was a history of penicillin sensitivity, when co-trimoxazole two tablets twice daily were given in the 24 hours following biopsy. At the Lister Hospital, a 1 g metronidazole suppository was given after biopsy, followed by a 3 day course of co-trimoxazole two tablets twice daily.

The acceptability of these procedures was evaluated by means of a postal questionnaire sent to the 568 men screened for prostate cancer. They were asked to indicate none, a little or considerable discomfort associated with DRE, venesection, TRUS and biopsy, and concern about the screening exercise. The results were analysed using a relational database (Paradox 4.0, Borland Int., Scott's Valley, CA). Histopathological examination of prostatic biopsy specimens was the reference test for demonstrating the presence of malignancy. Subjects with a negative DRE and a PSA level equal to or less than 4.0 ng/ml, those with a PSA of less than 10.0 ng/ml and negative findings on TRUS and those with negative prostatic biopsies were considered for the purpose of the evaluation not to have prostatic cancer.

RESULTS

Of the 856 men invited for screening, 568 (66%) complied. Table 1 shows the results of DRE examination and PSA ranges in the 568 men screened: 476 (85%) had a normal PSA and no evidence of malignancy on DRE and were consequently reassured. A total of 81 (14%) had a PSA level greater than 4.0 ng/ml. In 62 of these, the PSA level was greater than 4.0 ng/ml and less than 10.0 ng/ml, whereas in 19, the level was 10.0 ng/ml or greater. In a further patient whose PSA level was less than 4.0 ng/ml, there were suspicious findings on the DRE and he was referred for TRUS. Of the 80 men who consented to undergo TRUS, 29 (5% of the screened population) underwent prostatic biopsy, and in 11 of these (2% of the screened population), carcinoma was detected. The ages of these men and their PSA levels, DRE findings and clinical stage of cancer detected are listed in Table 2. Six of these

TABLE 1. Results of digital rectal examination (DRE) and serum prostate specific antigen (PSA) determination in 568 screened men

PSA level	DRE results: Normal	BPH	CAP	Not done	All
≤4	312 (0)	164 (0)	1 (0)	6 (0)	483 (0)
4–10	13 (1[a])	48 (3[b])	1 (0)	0 (0)	62 (4)
≥10.0	0 (0)	7 (2)	12 (8)	0 (0)	19 (10)
Not done	1 (0)	2 (0)	0 (0)	1 (0)	4 (0)
All	326 (1)	221 (5)	14 (8)	7 (0)	568 (14)

Figures in parentheses show the number of prostate cancers known in each group
BPH = benign prostatic hyperplasia on palpation; CAP = carcinoma of the prostate on palpation
[a]Includes one incidental cancer found at subsequent biopsy
[b]Includes two incidental cancers found at subsequent transurethral resection of the prostate

tumours were clinically confined to the prostate with no evidence of bone metastases; the remaining five were clinically T_3, and three of these were associated with metastatic disease. Following either radiotherapy or hormone manipulation, PSA levels in all patients except one with bone metastases have normalized within 6 months; follow up is continuing.

Notably, 10 of the 11 cases detected were in men with a PSA level greater than 10.0 ng/ml. Eight of these showed focal abnormality at TRUS. However, in three, TRUS was considered entirely normal both at the time of the original scan and on review of the scan images. Only one cancer was detected in a man with a PSA level of between 4.0 ng/ml and 10.0 ng/ml. He had no focal abnormality at TRUS, but there was a diffuse increase in Doppler colour flow, which led to the biopsy being performed. Of the remaining eight men with a PSA level of between 4.0 ng/ml and 10.0 ng/ml who were biopsied, all had focal abnormalities at TRUS and all had negative biopsies.

Three men who had been considered cancer free on screening were subsequently found to have carcinoma of the prostate. Two were diagnosed following transurethral resection of the prostate (TURP): both had palpably benign prostatic enlargement with a PSA of less than 10.0 ng/ml. The third had a palpably benign prostate, a PSA level of 6.0 ng/ml, suspicious ultrasound findings and negative biopsies; previous TURP had revealed atypical adenomatous hyperplasia and subsequent repeat biopsy showed the presence of malignant disease.

Table 3 shows the screening performance of the tests in different combinations. It can be seen that raising the PSA cut off level from 4.0 ng/ml to 10.0 ng/ml lowers the false positive rate from 12% (67/550) to 2% (9/550), although the corresponding reduction in the detection rate, especially of localized tumours, cannot be calculated. Since not all men were scanned, the use of TRUS as a primary screening test has not been assessed. Nor can this study shed light on the detection rate (sensitivity) as the true disease status in all the men is unknown: not all were biopsied and the results of long term follow-up are still unknown.

TABLE 2. Test results for individuals with prostate cancer identified on initial screening

Age (years)	DRE result	PSA result (ng/ml)	TRUS result	Cancer stage	
62	BPH	5	Positive	T_1	M0
59	BPH	10.1	Negative	T_1	M0
64	CAP	16.7	Positive	T_2	M0
65	CAP	23.1	Negative	T_3	M+
62	CAP	24.8	Positive	T_2	M0
70	CAP	66.2	Positive	T_2	M0
60	CAP	66.1	Positive	T_3	M0
65	BPH	72.5	Negative	T_2	M0
70	CAP	84	Positive	T_3	M+
59	CAP	252	Positive	T_3	M+
62	CAP	356	Positive	T_3	M+

BPH = benign prostatic hyperplasia; CAP = carcinoma of the prostate

The postal questionnaire was sent to all those who accepted the original invitation for screening. There were 472 (83%) replies: 327 (69%) men reported no concern, 141 (30%) reported a little concern and only 3 (1%) indicated considerable concern about the screening exercise. The main source of anxiety was not the actual performance of the tests but the wait for the results. Of the 80 patients who had undergone TRUS, 67 (84%) replied to the questionnaire: 21 (31%) reported no discomfort associated with TRUS, 43 (64%) indicated a little discomfort, but only 3 (5%) reported considerable discomfort. Of the 24 patients who replied to the questionnaire and had undergone TRUS guided biopsy, 5 (21%) reported no discomfort, 16 (67%) reported a little discomfort and 3 (12%) reported considerable discomfort. However, 448 of the 472 respondents (94%) said that they would be prepared to undergo the examination again. These results are summarized in Table 4.

DISCUSSION

This study demonstrated that screening for prostate cancer in a general practice setting is feasible. Digital rectal examination is cheap and has almost no morbidity, and patients do not find it unpleasant. However, the number of cancers detected is very low when performed by non-urologists (Faul, 1993). Even when specialists perform the examination, more than half of the tumours detected are found on pathological staging to be locally advanced (Thompson *et al,* 1984; Chodak *et al,* 1989). Nevertheless, most screening or case finding studies report that a proportion of clinically significant cancers are detected by DRE despite a normal PSA level (Mettlin *et al,* 1991).

Serum PSA may be determined by a simple blood test. Using a cut off

TABLE 3. Performance of different combinations of primary (PSA and DRE) and secondary (TRUS) screening tests

Definition of positive result for primary test	Total no of men tested with primary screening test (PSA, DRE or both)	Approximate proportion of men without prostate cancer who had positive test results (approximate false positive rate) (%)	No of prostate cancers detected by test	Total number of known prostate cancers to date	Odds of being affected given by positive test result
PSA only	564				
PSA > 4 ng/ml		12 (67/550)	14	14	1:5
PSA ≥ 10 ng/ml		2 (9/550)	10	14	1:1
PSA > 4 ng/ml *followed* by TRUS positive		2 (10/550)	8	14	1:1
PSA ≥ 10 ng/ml *followed* by TRUS positive		0.4 (2/550)	7	14	7:2
DRE only	561				
DRE positive		1 (6/547)	8	14	1:1
PSA and DRE	558				
PSA > 4 ng/ml *and* DRE positive		1 (5/544)	8	14	2:1
PSA ≥ 10 ng/ml *and* DRE positive		1 (4/544)	8	14	2:1
PSA > 4 ng/ml *and* DRE positive *followed* by TRUS positive		0.2 (1/544)	7	14	7:1
PSA ≥ 10 ng/ml *and* DRE positive *followed* by TRUS positive		0 (0/544)	7	14	7:0

TABLE 4. Acceptability of the screening process, DRE, serum PSA determination, TRUS and biopsy

	Test				
	DRE	venesection for PSA	TRUS	biopsy	Screening process
Total no of patients	561 (99)	564 (99)	80 (15)	29 (5)	568 (100)
Respondents	472 (83)	472 (83)	67 (84)	24 (83)	472 (83)
Patient response	**Discomfort**	**Discomfort**	**Discomfort**	**Discomfort**	**Concern**
None	262 (56)	403 (86)	21 (31)	5 (21)	327 (69)
A little	194 (41)	63 (13)	43 (64)	16 (67)	141 (30)
Considerable	11 (2)	1 (0)	3 (5)	3 (12)	3 (1)
Not answered	5 (1)	5 (1)	0 (0)	0 (0)	1 (0)

Patients were asked by questionnaire to indicate discomfort associated with these investigations and overall concern as none, a little or considerable. Percentages in parentheses

point at 4.0 ng/ml (Hybritech), the currently recommended upper limit of normal, Catalona *et al* (1991) reported a detection rate in a study population of 79% with a false positive rate of 41%. When the cut off point was 10.0 ng/ml, the detection rate fell to 48%, with a reduction in the false positive rate to 9%; however, on clinical staging, many of these patients appeared to have locally extensive disease for which curative therapy may not always be possible. Patients with a PSA level of between 4.0 ng/ml and 10.0 ng/ml seem more likely to have localized disease, but unfortunately, this degree of PSA elevation may also be present in as many as 25% of men with benign prostate hyperplasia (Oesterling, 1991), a disease that may be present in symptomatic form in up to 43% of the screened population (Garraway *et al,* 1991). It must also be presumed that some patients have prostate cancer despite a PSA level of 4.0 ng/ml or less. The exact proportion of patients with prostatic cancer whose PSA level is within the normal range is currently unknown; however, in most series of radical prostatectomy, approximately 30% of patients are reported to have a PSA of less than 4.0 ng/ml. In the study by Catalona *et al* (1991), 21% of patients were discovered on biopsy to have prostate cancer despite having a normal PSA.

Because of these difficulties, efforts have been made to reduce the biopsy rate in patients with minor rises in PSA level by adjusting the PSA for prostate volume to calculate a PSA density (Benson *et al,* 1992) or by sequential estimations to detect rises in PSA over time (Carter *et al,* 1992). A further promising development is the observation that the PSA level appears to rise predictably with age, allowing an age specific adjustment to be made (Oesterling *et al,* 1993).

Although TRUS is capable of detecting small cancers of less than 1.5 cm in the peripheral portion of the prostate gland (Lee *et al,* 1988), Catalona *et al*

(1993b) reported that it may miss up to 40% of cancers subsequently detected by random quadrant biopsy. The disappointing sensitivity of TRUS in part relates to its difficulty in detecting the approximately 30% of cancers that originate in the transition and central zones. Thus, Seth *et al* (1991) found that TRUS had only 55% sensitivity in detecting stage A cancers. In addition, up to 24% of prostate cancers may be isoechoic, with no difference in echogenicity between them and adjacent normal tissue (Dahnert *et al,* 1986). However, the detection rate may be improved by the use of colour Doppler, which shows increased colour flow in some cancers not detected by greyscale ultrasound (Rifkin *et al,* 1993). In addition to having insufficient sensitivity for use as a first line screening test, TRUS also has a high false positive rate. Thus, of the nine patients in this study with a PSA level between 4.0 ng/ml and 10.0 ng/ml and focal TRUS abnormalities, eight had no malignancy detected at biopsy. Chronic inflammation in the peripheral zone of the prostate may produce masses identical to those found in carcinoma, and Rifkin and Choi (1988) found that only 20% of hypoechoic masses of less than 1.5 cm in the peripheral gland were malignant. Unfortunately, this poor specificity increases the biopsy rate for no extra yield of cancers.

We identified on screening only one patient with cancer with a PSA level of between 4.0 ng/ml and 10.0 ng/ml. This may reflect our rather conservative biopsy policy, since cancer was subsequently diagnosed in three men with a PSA level in this range, two at TURP and one at repeat biopsy. Other investigators who have biopsied a much greater proportion of screened subjects have reported a greater incidence of cancers in this PSA range, and moreover, these tumours have usually been confined to the gland (Brawer *et al,* 1992; Labrie *et al,* 1992).

Had a biopsy been performed in all our patients with a PSA level of over 4.0 ng/ml, a greater number of localized cancers would almost certainly have been detected, potentially including those in the two patients, originally negative on screening in whom stage A tumour was diagnosed at TURP. Such a policy would, however, have meant that 14% of the patients we screened would have undergone biopsy of the prostate. About three quarters of our patients noted discomfort with the biopsy and the technique carries a small but significant morbidity. A short period of bleeding into the urine, semen and faeces (for transrectal biopsies) is common (Clements *et al,* 1993; Webb *et al,* 1993). However, sepsis is uncommon after transrectal biopsy provided adequate antibiotic prophylaxis is used (Cooner *et al,* 1990; Clements *et al,* 1993).

The high prevalence rates detected in many screening studies are somewhat disconcerting, bearing in mind that prostate cancer is a disease of older men, many of whom die with, rather that from, the disease (Johansson *et al,* 1992). The detection prevalence of 2.0% in our study is about 28 times greater than the present reported incidence of 0.72/1000 men aged 55 to 70 in England and Wales (Office of Population Censuses and Surveys, 1991). A more aggressive biopsy policy advocated by some has yielded an even higher detection rate of 3% in the 50–59 year age group, rising to as much as 15% in those over

80 (Catalona *et al,* 1993a), further increasing the disparity between the numbers of cases detected at screening and those presenting with symptoms or dying of the disease in the community.

The central question in screening for prostate cancer is whether early diagnosis and treatment will reduce disease specific mortality, as many older men die with prostate cancer rather than because of it. The natural history of prostate cancer is unpredictable, and it is difficult to be certain whether or not a lesion once identified will become the cause of clinical disease in an individual patient (Johansson *et al,* 1992). This problem is confounded by the fact that screening for prostate cancer occurs most frequently in elderly men in whom there are many competing causes of death. Autopsy studies have shown that microfoci of prostate cancer that show little tendency to progress may be present in 20–30% of men over 50 years of age, and many patients with prostatic malignancy will not die from their disease (Franks, 1954; Breslow *et al,* 1997). By detecting such tumours, screening may lead to overdiagnosis and overtreatment of cancers that would not cause clinical disease within the natural lifespan of the host.

McNeal *et al* (1986) have suggested that the clinical course of prostate cancer may be predicted by the volume of the primary tumour. Tumours of less than 0.5 cc constitute little threat to the individual, but cancers greater than 4.5 cc are associated with extraprostatic disease in more than half of the cases. Since the tumour doubling time for adenocarcinoma of the prostate may be as long as 2 years, a window of opportunity may exist when a growing tumour remains confined within the prostate and therefore potentially curable. Nevertheless, there is still considerable controversy over the management of localized disease. There have been no properly conducted, randomized long term studies that compare the results of radical prostatectomy and external beam radiotherapy with no treatment until disease progression. It is essential that prostate cancer be carefully evaluated before being introduced generally. A large scale controlled trial of screening is currently being organized in the USA (Prorok *et al,* 1991).

Our study of screening using DRE and serum PSA determination, followed by TRUS and biopsy in selected individuals, suggests that this is generally acceptable to patients and will detect a considerable number of cancers. Whether those detectable tumours would ever cause clinical disease cannot be determined in this small study, and a long term randomized controlled study will be required to demonstrate whether screening can achieve a reduction in the disease specific mortality of this common disease.

SUMMARY

Screening for prostate cancer in a general practice setting seems to be technically feasible and generally acceptable. In our study, 14 cancers were diagnosed among the 568 men screened, giving an overall detection rate of 2%;

five of these were either locally advanced or associated with metastatic disease. Although these results may reflect our somewhat conservative biopsy rate, there is a considerable false positive rate in the PSA range of 4–10 ng/ml, particularly among men with clinical evidence of benign prostatic hyperplasia. A large scale prospective controlled study will be necessary to establish the true benefit of screening.

References

Benson MC, Whang IS, Pantuck A *et al* (1992) Prostate specific antigen density: a means of distinguishing benign prostatic hypertrophy and prostate cancer. *Journal of Urology* **147** 815–816

Brawer MK, Chetner MP, Beattie J *et al* (1992) Screening for prostatic carcinoma with prostate specific antigen. *Journal of Urology* **147** 841–845

Breslow N, Chan CW, Dhom G *et al* (1977) Latent carcinoma of prostate of autopsy in seven areas. *International Journal of Cancer* **20** 680–688

Carter HB, Pearson JD, Metter EJ *et al* (1992) Longitudinal evaluation of prostate-specific antigen levels in men with and without prostate disease. *Journal of the American Medical Association* **267** 2215–2220

Catalona WJ, Smith DS, Ratliff TL *et al* (1991) Measurement of prostate-specific antigen in serum as a screening test for prostate cancer. *New England Journal of Medicine* **324** 1156–1161

Catalona WJ, Richie JP, Ahmann FR *et al* (1993a) A multicenter examination of PSA and digital rectal examination for early detection of prostate cancer in 6,374 volunteers. *Journal of Urology* **149** 412A

Catalona WJ, Richie JP, Ahmann FR *et al* (1993b) Patient age and the effectiveness of PSA and digital rectal examination for early detection of prostate cancer. *Journal of Urology* **149** 412A

Chodak GW, Keller P and Schoenberg HW (1989) Assessment of screening for prostate cancer using the digital rectal examination. *Journal of Urology* **141** 1136–1138

Clements R, Aideyan OU, Griffiths GH and Peeling WB (1993) Side effects and patient acceptability of transrectal biopsy of the prostate. *Clinical Radiology* **47** 125–126

Cooner WH, Mosley BR, Rutherford CL Jr *et al* (1990) Prostate cancer detection in a clinical urological practice by ultrasonography, digital rectal examination and prostate specific antigen. *Journal of Urology* **143** 1146–52

Crawford ED, Eisenberger MA, McLeod DG *et al* (1989) A controlled trial of leuprolide with and without flutamide in prostatic carcinoma. *New England Journal of Medicine* **321** 419–424

Dahnert WF, Hamper UM, Eggleston JC, Walsh PC and Saunders RC (1986) Prostatic evaluation by transrectal ultrasonography with histopathological correlation: the echopenic appearance of early carcinoma. *Radiology* **158** 97–102

Faul P (1993) Experience with the German annual check-up examination, In: Jacobi M and Hoffenfeller R (eds). *Prostate Cancer*, pp 57–70, Williams and Wilkins, Baltimore

Franks LM (1954) Latent carcinoma of the prostate. *Journal of Pathology and Bacteriology* **68** 603–616

Garraway WM, Collins GN and Lee RJ (1991) High prevalence of benign prostatic hypertrophy in the community. *Lancet* **338** 469–471

Huggins C and Hodges CV (1941) Studies of prostatic cancer: effect of castration, of estrogen and of androgen injection on serum phosphatases in metastatic carcinoma of the prostate. *Cancer Research* **1** 293–297

Johansson JE, Adami HO, Andersson SO, Bergstrom R, Holmberg L and Krusemo UB (1992)

High 10-year survival rate in patients with early, untreated prostatic cancer. *Journal of the American Medical Association* **267** 2191–2196

Kirby RS, Kirby MG, Feneley MR, McNicholas T, McLean A and Webb JAW (1994) Screening for carcinoma of the prostate: a GP based study. *British Journal of Urology* **74** 64–71

Labrie F, Dupont A, Suburu R *et al* (1992) Serum prostate specific antigen as pre-screening test for prostate cancer. *Journal of Urology* **147** 846–852

Lee F, Littrup PJ, Torp-Pedersen ST *et al* (1988) Prostate cancer: comparison of transrectal US and digital rectal examination for screening. *Radiology* **168** 389–394

McNeal JE, Bostwick DG, Kindrachuk RA, Redwine EA, Freiha FS and Stamey TA (1986) Patterns of progression in prostate cancer. *Lancet* **i** 60–63

Mettlin C, Lee F, Drago J and Murphy GP (1991) The American Cancer Society National Prostate Cancer Detection Project: findings on the detection of early prostate cancer in 2425 men. *Cancer* **67** 2949–2958

Moller-Jensen O, Esteve J, Moller H and Renard H (1990) Cancer in the European community and its member states. *European Journal of Cancer* **26** 1167–1256

Murphy GP, Natarajan N, Pontes JE *et al* (1982) The national survey of prostate cancer in the United States by the American College of Surgeons. *Journal of Urology* **127** 928–934

Oesterling JE (1991) Prostate specific antigen: a critical assessment of the most useful tumor marker for adenocarcinoma of the prostate. *Journal of Urology* **145** 907–923

Oesterling JE (1992) Prostate-specific antigen: improving its ability to diagnose early prostate cancer. *Journal of the American Medical Association* **267** 2236–2238

Oesterling JE, Jacobsen SJ, Chute CG *et al* (1993) The establishment of age-specific reference ranges for prostate-specific antigen. *Journal of Urology* **149** 510A

Office of Population Censuses and Surveys (1991) *1990 Mortality statistics,* Series DH2 No 17, Government Statistical Service, London

Prorok PC, Byar DP, Smart CR, Baker SG and Connor RJ (1991) Evaluation of screening for prostate, lung and colorectal cancers: the PLC trial, In: Miller AB, Chamberlain J, Day NE, Hakamaand M and Prorok PC (eds). *Cancer Screening,* pp 300–320, Cambridge University Press, Cambridge

Rifkin MD and Choi H (1988) Implications of small, peripheral hypoechoic lesions in endorectal ultrasound of the prostate. *Radiology* **166** 619–622

Rifkin MD, Sudakoff GD and Alexander AA (1993) Prostate: techniques, results and potential applications of colour Doppler US scanning. *Radiology* **186** 509–513

Schroder FH (1993) Prostate cancer: to screen or not to screen. *British Medical Journal* **306** 407–408

Seth S, Hamper UM, Walsh PC, Holtz PM and Epstein JI (1991) Stage A adenocarcinoma of the prostate: transrectal ultrasound and sonographic-pathologic correlation. *Radiology* **179** 35–49

Stamey TA, Yang N, Hay AR, McNeal JE, Freiha FS and Redwine E (1987) Prostate-specific antigen as a serum marker for adenocarcinoma of the prostate. *New England Journal of Medicine* **317** 909–916

Thompson IM, Ernst JJ, Gangai MP and Spence CR (1984) Adenocarcinoma of the prostate: results of routine urological screening. *Journal of Urology* **132** 690–692

Webb JAW, Shanmuganathan K and McLean A (1993) The complications of ultrasound guided transperineal prostate biopsy: a prospective study. *British Journal of Urology* **72** 775–777

Wilson JMG and Jungner G (1969) *Principles and Practice of Screening for Disease,* pp 1–34, World Health Organization, Geneva

Yamanaka H (1993) Incidence and prevention of prostate cancer. *Asian Medical Journal* **36** 91–95

The authors are responsible for the accuracy of the references.

An Epidemiologist's Viewpoint on Screening

CAROL A PARKES

Department of Environmental and Preventive Medicine, Wolfson Institute of Preventive Medicine, St Bartholomew's Hospital Medical College, Charterhouse Square, London EC1M 6BQ

INTRODUCTION

Prostate cancer is an important cause of morbidity and mortality among men in many westernized countries. Each year, there are about 12 500 new cases diagnosed in England and Wales and about 8700 deaths (OPCS, 1993, 1994). It is the third most common cause of cancer death among men (after lung and colorectal) and accounts for about 11% of cancer deaths in males (OPCS, 1994).

In the last decade, there has been increasing interest in screening for prostate cancer, and some countries have advocated screening programmes. Many published studies have investigated the three main screening methods: digital rectal examination, transrectal ultrasound examination and measurement of a tumour marker in venous blood—namely, prostate specific antigen. However, there is at present insufficient evidence to suggest that prostate cancer screening is worthwhile. This chapter discusses the main issues to consider when deciding whether screening for prostate cancer is worthwhile. It is a synopsis based on a more detailed analysis of published studies of prostate cancer screening tests to be submitted for publication elsewhere (Parkes C and Wald N, unpublished).

Cancer Surveys Volume 23: *Preventing Prostate Cancer: Screening versus Chemoprevention*

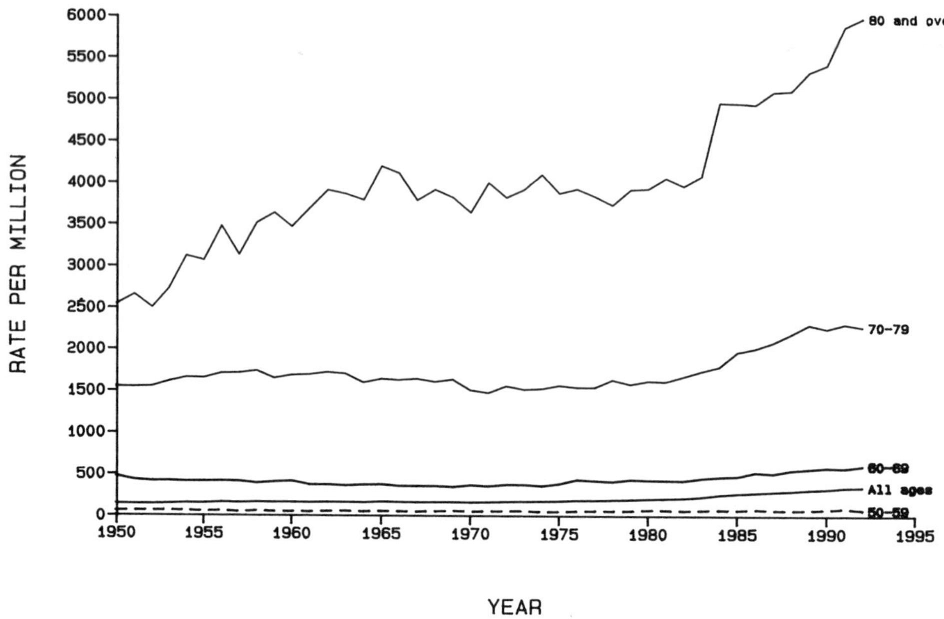

Fig. 1. Prostate cancer death rates (deaths per million population—England and Wales)

MAIN ISSUES TO CONSIDER WHEN ASSESSING WHETHER PROSTATE CANCER SCREENING IS WORTHWHILE

Importance of Prostate Cancer

In England and Wales, about a quarter of all male deaths is due to cancer and of these, about one in ten is due to prostate cancer (OPCS, 1994). There has been a rise in the age specific death rates for prostate cancer in the last 50 years among older men, particularly in the age group over 80 years old, where there was a fivefold increase between 1950 and 1992 (Fig. 1). Some of this rise may be due to increased diagnosis rather than an increased prevalence of the disease. Although prostate cancer is mainly a disease of older men with 88% of new cases occurring in men over the age of 65, it was responsible for 72 000 years of life lost among men in England and Wales in 1992 (OPCS, 1987, 1994). This compares with 226 000 and 35 000 years of life lost, respectively, from breast and cervical cancer deaths in 1992.

Stage Distribution and 5 Year Survival Rates

Prostate cancer has a poor overall 5 year survival rate of 54%, which increases to about 68% if it is diagnosed early when the cancer is still localized to the gland, suggesting that early detection may improve prognosis (Axtell *et al,* 1976; Norwegian Cancer Society, 1980). Table 1 shows the stage distribution and survival for prostate cancer in the absence of screening taken from data published by the Cancer Surveillance, Epidemiology and End Results (SEER)

TABLE 1. Stage distribution and survival data for prostate cancer

Stage	Stage distribution			Relative 5 year survival rate		
	SEER[a]	Norway[b]	average	SEER[a]	Norway[b]	average
Localized	61	70	67	70	65	68
Regional	14	5	10	61	39	50
Distant	22	25	23	20	18	19
All	100	100	100	57	51	54

[a]Cancer Surveillance, Epidemiology and End Results (SEER) Programme USA: white men diagnosed between 1965 and 1973 (Axtell *et al*, 1976)
[b]Cancer Registry of Norway: men diagnosed between 1968 and 1975 (Norwegian Cancer Society, 1980)

Program in the USA, and the Cancer Registry of Norway; 67% of cases are diagnosed in the localized stage even in the absence of screening.

Suitability of Screening Tests

Three main screening tests have been proposed.

(i) Digital Rectal Examination (DRE)

The examination of the prostate gland per rectum using the index finger has been part of the general patient examination for many years. A presumptive clinical diagnosis of prostate cancer is usually made if part or all of the prostate gland feels nodular, irregular or stony hard.

(ii) Transrectal Ultrasound (TRUS)

Transrectal ultrasound has been used in the investigation of prostatic disease for about 20 years (Watanabe, 1975). In more recent years, more refined scanning equipment has become available and the latest devices with 4–7 mHz ultrasound probes are now able to visualize smaller lesions in the prostate more consistently (Rifkin and Choi, 1988). Transrectal ultrasound is a relatively simple investigation that can be done in an outpatient office without the need for anaesthesia. It usually takes about 15–20 minutes to perform carefully (Waterhouse and Resnick, 1989). With the latest scanning equipment, transrectal prostatic biopsies or aspirations can be simply performed under ultrasound guidance.

The ultrasound appearances of prostate cancers vary, but they are generally seen in the peripheral zone (where 70% of prostatic cancers originate) and are hypoechoic in nature (Griffiths *et al*, 1987; Rifkin and Choi, 1988; Lee *et al*, 1989a,b,c). This appearance is the result of fewer sound waves being reflected to the transducer, because the sound waves are absorbed or deflected, thus appearing black on the screen. Currently, TRUS can usually only detect lesions of more than 5 mm in diameter (Cooner *et al*, 1987).

TABLE 2. Definition of parameters used in screening[a]

		True disease status: Cancer present	True disease status: Cancer not present	
Test result	Positive	a (true positive)	b (false positive)	a+b (all positive)
	Negative	c (false negative)	d (true negative)	c+d (all negative)
		a+c (all cancers)	b+d (all without cancer)	

Prevalence of cancer	=	$\frac{a+c}{a+b+c+d}$		
Detection rate (or sensitivity)	=	$\frac{\text{true positives}}{\text{all cancers}}$	=	$\frac{a}{a+c}$
False positive rate	=	$\frac{\text{false positives}}{\text{all without cancer}}$	=	$\frac{b}{b+d}$
Specificity	=	$\frac{\text{true negatives}}{\text{all without cancer}}$	=	$\frac{d}{b+d}$
Odds of being affected given positive result	=	true positives:false positives	=	a:b
Positive predictive value	=	$\frac{a}{a+b}$		

[a]The results of a cancer screening exercise can be considered in a 2 x 2 table, comparing the test results with the true disease status as defined from the "gold standard" method of diagnosis

(iii) Prostate Specific Antigen (PSA)

Prostate specific antigen is a glycoprotein produced exclusively by prostate epithelium, first described by Wang *et al* in 1979. It is not specific to prostate cancer, however, as it is also produced by the normal prostate, and levels are often considerably raised in benign prostatic hyperplasia. Clinically, PSA has been used as a marker for diagnosing, staging and monitoring response to treatment in advanced prostate cancer (Oesterling *et al*, 1988). Its use as a tumour marker in the diagnosis of early prostate cancer has been the subject of several studies; however, its value remains unclear.

When reviewing the efficacy of a potential screening test, three main parameters need to be assessed. These are (a) the detection rate (or sensitivity) of the test, (b) the false positive rate of the test and (c) the odds of being affected given a positive test (OAPR). The definitions and derivations of these screening parameters are shown in Table 2.

The detection rate is the proportion of men with prostate cancer at the time of the test who have been designated screen positive. In practice for cancer screening, however, it is often defined as the proportion of men who develop prostate cancer over a defined period of time who were designated screen positive.

The detection rate is important in that it is a measure of the test's ability to identify correctly men with prostate cancer; the lower the detection rate, the more cases of missed cancer. The false positive rate is the proportion of men without prostate cancer at the time of the test (or, in practice, the proportion of men who did not develop prostate cancer over the same interval of time used to define the detection rate) who have been incorrectly designated screen positive. Alternatively, the complement of the false positive rate, the specificity of a test, is often referred to. This measures the test's ability to identify correctly men without prostate cancer. The advantage in stating the false positive rate instead of the specificity arises because it is the screen positives, not the screen negatives, that are the focus of attention. The odds of being affected given a positive result is the ratio of the number of men with cancer to those without cancer among the screen positive men.

Many studies have been published in the last decade examining the efficacy of these three proposed screening tests. However, no studies have reported on asymptomatic men who had the tests and were all followed up to ascertain whether they had developed, or died of, prostate cancer, and so the performance of the tests in an asymptomatic population cannot be determined as shown in Table 2. Therefore, to make the best assessment of the performance of the proposed tests in an asymptomatic population, estimates of the detection rate, false positive rate and OAPR need to be taken from different sources:

(a) The detection rate: an estimate of this can be obtained from studies of symptomatic men who had the tests and who all had a subsequent histological examination, and this rate applied to a hypothetical asymptomatic population.

(b) The false positive rate: an approximate false positive rate can be obtained from studies of asymptomatic men who had the tests but only some men were followed up or biopsied. As prostate cancer is a rare disease in absolute terms, in a study of asymptomatic men, the number of men without the disease can be estimated as total tested – true positives. Therefore, approximate false positive rates in the studies of asymptomatic men can be estimated from false positives/total tested – true positives. (For example, if there were 1000 asymptomatic men screened, and the screening test detected two of the three prostate cancers present, and there were 50 false positive results among the 997 men without prostate cancer, then [i] the false positive rate would be 50/997 or 5% and [ii] if the disease status

TABLE 3. Summary of prostate cancer screening studies to show screening parameters and combined results

Screening test assessed	Studies of symptomatic men with a histological diagnosis		
	Study	**Age**	**Detection rate (%)**
DRE only	Guinan *et al*, 1980	50–90	69 (48/69)
	Allen and Embry, 1991	45–90	60 (45/75)
	Vallancien *et al*, 1989	46–89	82 (32/39)
	Hammerer *et al*, 1992++	54–76	88 (15/17)
	Hudson *et al*, 1954+	38–83	23 (9/39)
	Catalona *et al*, 1991	>50	86 (62/72)
	Lee *et al*, 1989a	36–89	68 (71/104)
	Combined total		**68 (282/415)**
TRUS only	Rifkin *et al*, 1990	40–76	66 (84/127)
	Carter *et al*, 1989 (i)	na	92 (54/59)
	(ii)	na	52 (13/25)
	Allen and Embry, 1991	45–90	87 (65/75)
	Vallancien *et al*, 1989	46–89	69 (27/39)
	Hammerer *et al*, 1992++	54–76	76 (13/17)
	Catalona *et al*, 1991	>50	92 (66/72)
	Combined total		**78 (322/414)**
PSA only cut off >4 μg/l	Catalona *et al*, 1991	>50	79 (48/61)
PSA only cut off >10 g/l	Catalona *et al*, 1991	>50	48 (29/61)
DRE and TRUS	Vallancien *et al*, 1989	46–89	64 (25/39)
	Hammerer *et al*, 1992++	54–76	71 (12/17)
	Catalona *et al*, 1991	>50	38 (14/37)
	Combined total		**55 (51/93)**

na = not available; + = some symptom free men were included; ++ = symptom free men urologically, but with diagnosed lung cancer

Table 3 (Continued)

Screening test assessed	Studies of asymptomatic men with a histological diagnosis in some			
	Study	**Age**	**Approximate false positive (%)**	**OAPR**
DRE only	Thompson *et al*, 1984	40–70	2 (48/1988)	1:3
	Chodak *et al*, 1989	45–80	5 (108/2094)	1:3
	Vihko *et al*, 1985	54–76	3 (21/762)	1:4
	Pederson *et al*, 1990	50–69	3 (32/1150)	1:3
	Waaler *et al*, 1988	45–67	5 (25/479)	1:25
	Lee *et al*, 1988	60–86	3 (19/762)	1:2
	Palken *et al*, 1991	50–86	10 (28/292)	1:2
	Nesbitt *et al*, 1989	55–70	na	na
	Chadwick *et al*, 1991	55–69	3 (12/400)	1:12
	Mettlin *et al*, 1991	55–70	5 (129/2368)	1:4
	Perrin *et al*, 1991	50–60	19 (163/860)	:54
	Muschenheim *et al*, 1991	na	12 (67/545)	1:4
	Combined total		**5 (643/11 700)**	**1:4**
TRUS only	Lee *et al*, 1988	60–86	6 (44/762)	1:2
	Palken *et al*, 1991	50–86	13 (38/292)	1:3
	Nesbitt *et al*, 1989	55–70	12 (26/221)	1:1
	Mettlin *et al*, 1991	55–70	12 (287/2368)	1:7
	Combined total		**11 (395/3643)**	**1:4**
PSA only cut off >4 μg/l	Catalona *et al*, 1991	>50	6 (100/1609)	1:3
	Chadwick *et al*, 1991	55–69	13 (56/430)	1:8
	Labrie *et al*, 1992	45–80	9 (83/945)	1:2
	Brawer *et al*, 1992	>50	12 (147/1209)	1:4
	Moon and Clejan, 1991	40–59	2 (9/409)	1:2
	Carter *et al*, 1992	56–87	25 (9/36)	2:1
	Perrin *et al*, 1991	50–60	4 (35/860)	1:2
	Muschenheim *et al*, 1991	na	8 (44/545)	1:3
	Combined total		**8 (483/6043)**	**1:3**
PSA only cut off >10 μg/l	Catalona *et al*, 1991	>50	1 (12/1609)	2:1
	Labrie *et al*, 1992	45–80	2 (17/945)	1:1
	Brawer *et al*, 1992	>50	2 (22/1210)	1:2
	Carter *et al*, 1992	56–87	0	
	Combined total		**1 (51/3764)**	**1:1**
DRE and TRUS	Lee *et al*, 1988	60–86	1 (8/762)	1:1
	Palken *et al*, 1991	50–86	2 (7/292)	1:1
	Mettlin *et al*, 1991	55–70	3 (63/2368)	1:3
	Combined total		**2 (78/3422)**	**1:2**

na = not available; + = some symptom free men were included; ++ = symptom free men urologically, but with diagnosed lung cancer were not known in the screen negatives, the apparent false positive rate would be 50/[1000-2], again 5%.) This will be a minimum estimate and a reasonable approximation to the true false positive rate among asymptomatic men.

(c) The OAPR can also be obtained directly from studies of asymptomatic men.

It would not be appropriate to obtain estimates of the false positive rate and OAPR from studies of symptomatic men and apply these to an asymptomatic population. This is because the false positive rate is likely to be higher in symptomatic men because they will have a higher prevalence of benign disorders, such as benign prostatic hyperplasia, which could cause a false positive result. In addition, the prevalence of cancer will be much higher in symptomatic men, and this will be reflected in a more favourable OAPR, despite a higher false positive rate.

Table 3 shows the detection rates, false positive rates and OAPR estimates for the proposed screening tests obtained in this way from the published literature up to September 1993. Summary data were obtained by adding together the data from each similar study within the same category. In this way, an overall average was produced that was weighted in favour of the larger studies. Some heterogeneity among the studies will remain within the groups even after categorization, but the effect of this on the combined estimates of the screening parameters is likely to be small. Table 4 shows the summary data only. These estimates suggest that DRE or measurement of PSA look the most promising since DRE has a 68% detection rate for a 5% false positive rate, and PSA (cut off >4 μg/l) has a 79% detection rate for an 8% false positive rate. Transrectal ultrasound appears to have too high a false positive rate (11%) to be acceptable in practice. Unfortunately, there are few data on combinations of screening tests—this may be the best approach to keep the false positive rate as low as possible.

There is an inevitable trade off between the detection rate and false positive rate of a screening test. The more extreme the definition of a positive test (eg in prostate cancer screening, raising the PSA cut off level to >10 μg/l instead of >4 μg/l), then the lower the false positive rate, but only at the expense of the detection rate and an increase in missed cancers. Similarly, by combining tests, such that both have to be positive for an overall positive test result, the false positive rate will be lower but again will be at the expense of the detection rate.

In the case of a quantitative biochemical marker such as PSA measurement, it is relatively easy to adjust the cut off level to alter the detection rate for a given false positive rate. For qualitative tests such as DRE and TRUS, altering the false positive rate would require a qualitative reassessment of what is considered to be a test indication of cancer.

The OAPR results shown from the studies of asymptomatic men are problematic because the prevalence of prostate cancer in the asymptomatic study

TABLE 4. Comparison of combined results of screening methods

	Symptomatic men with a histological diagnosis		Asymptomatic men with a histological diagnosis in some	
	PSA cut off level (μg/l)	detection rate	approximate false positive rate (%)	odds of being affected given positive result
DRE only		68 (282/415)	5 (643/11700)	1:4
TRUS only		78 (322/414)	11 (395/3643)	1:4
PSA only	>4	79 (48/61)*	8 (483/6043)	1:3
	>10	48 (29/61)*	1 (51/3764)	1:1
DRE *and* TRUS		55 (51/93)	2 (78/3422)	1:2

*Results of only one study

populations was considerably higher than that expected from known incidence and survival data (prevalence can be estimated from incidence multiplied by duration of survival). The mean prevalence in the studies of asymptomatic men (mainly aged 50–80) was 2.8%, which is about sixfold higher than that derived from observed incidence and duration of survival data (0.5%). (Incidence data were taken from OPCS cancer registrations [OPCS, 1994] and survival data from the USA SEER programme [Axtell *et al,* 1976].) Using a prevalence estimate of 0.5% makes the OAPR results less favourable for each of the screening methods.

The higher prevalence of prostate cancer in the reported studies may be a result of "overdiagnosis", a well recognized potential problem with prostate cancer screening. It has been shown from autopsy studies and coincidental findings at transurethral prostatectomy (Mebust *et al,* 1989) that the prevalence of clinically unapparent cancer is high. Estimates vary from 10% to 50% in autopsy studies (Franks, 1954; Breslow *et al,* 1977). If there are latent cancers that are insignificant and cannot be distinguished from small, potentially lethal cancers, then the detection of latent cancers becomes a cost of screening rather than a benefit. Not only will clinicians not know how to manage these patients, but the detection of these cancers will also cause inevitable anxiety in the person screened.

The combined results from the published studies shown are tentative, but they provide an indication of the potential for screening. Further substantive evidence is needed on the efficacy of the proposed screening tests, especially in combination. Studies would be needed in a group of asymptomatic men. Men with positive test results would be offered diagnostic biopsy and the remaining men would be followed up to determine disease status. However, the assessment of PSA performance can be done in an observational study using stored serum samples collected from disease free men and then measur-

TABLE 5. Relationship of stage distribution of cancers to expected reduction in mortality

(i) Effect of increasing the proportion of localized cancers

Proportion of localized prostate cancers diagnosed by screening (%)	Equivalent reduction in prostate cancer mortality at 5 years compared to unscreened population (%)
67[a]	0
75	7
90	20
100	29

(ii) Effect of increasing the proportion of localized clinically inapparent cancers

Proportion of localized *clinically inapparent* prostate cancers diagnosed by screening (%)	Equivalent reduction in prostate cancer mortality at 5 years compared to unscreened population (%)
23[b]	0
50	17
75	33
90	40
100	48

[a]Proportion of localized cancers observed in the absence of screening (average proportion from USA SEER Program [Axtell *et al*, 1976] and Norway Cancer Registry [Norwegian Cancer Society, 1980])
[b]Proportion of localized clinically inapparent cancers observed in the absence of screening (from National Survey of Prostate Cancer in USA by American College of Suregons [Murphy *et al*, 1982])

ing serum PSA in the group of men who eventually developed or died of prostate cancer (cases) and a matched group of men who did not develop prostate cancer (controls).

Effect of Screening on Mortality from Prostate Cancer

Before embarking on a screening programme for prostate cancer, evidence is needed that screening reduces mortality from this disease. A randomized controlled trial is needed to answer this. Not only would this avoid selection bias, but also by using mortality from prostate cancer as the measure of outcome rather than survival after diagnosis, two other biases can be avoided—bias as a result of increased survival in the screened men being due simply to detecting the tumour earlier without genuinely prolonging life (lead time bias) and bias due to detecting slower growing tumours in the screened men (length bias). A randomized trial would require the recruitment of at least 20 000 men and would take about 10 years before a result could be obtained. In the meantime, the effect that screening may have on mortality can be estimated by examining existing stage distribution and 5 year survival data. Table 5 shows the effect that screening may have on mortality, if screening increases the proportion of cancers diagnosed in (a) the localized stage and (b) the localized clinically inapparent stage. These calculations were done using the observed stage distribution and 5 year survival data published in Norway and the USA, as shown in Table 1.

Even if the effect of screening was such that all cases were diagnosed when the disease was in the localized stage (which would be almost impossible in practice), then the equivalent expected reduction in mortality would be only 29%. A greater effect on mortality (with a reduction of 48%) might be obtained if all cases were diagnosed in the localized clinically inapparent stage (by either TRUS or PSA measurement), but this would be even more difficult to achieve in practice.

It is unlikely that any future screening programme would be offered to men under 55 (since the number of prostate cancer deaths is too low in this younger group) or men over 74 (since they are unlikely to respond to screening invitations). There were approximately 3100 deaths from prostate cancer in 1992 in England and Wales in men aged 55–74, so a 29% reduction in deaths would represent only 900 lives saved per year, and a 48% reduction in deaths would represent 1500 lives saved per year (OPCS, 1993). To compare with breast cancer screening among 50–64 year old women, a 25% reduction in mortality is expected (based on the results of six randomized trials) representing about 1000 lives saved per year.

SUMMARY

Prostate cancer is an important disease causing a considerable number of new cases, deaths and premature loss of life each year. Three screening tests have been suggested: DRE, TRUS and PSA measurement in venous blood. From aggregated data from studies examining the performance of these tests, DRE or PSA measurement look the most promising with respect to their estimated detection rates and false positive rates (detection rate [DR] = 68%, false positive rate [FPR] = 5% for DRE and DR = 79%, FPR = 8% for PSA with a cut off of >4 μg/l). However, these results are tentative—more research is needed on the performance of these screening tests. In particular, the prevalence of prostate cancer in the studies was considerably higher than that expected in the general population and so the OAPR estimates derived are more favourable than predicted.

A randomized controlled trial of prostate cancer screening is needed to know whether screening reduces mortality from this disease, although this would take about 10 years to perform. Current stage distribution and 5 year survival data suggest that if screening could increase the proportion of cancers diagnosed at the localized clinically inapparent stage from 23% (currently diagnosed) to 100%, this would represent an equivalent reduction in mortality of 48%—about 1500 lives saved per year if screening were offered to 55–74 year old men.

When more substantive information is available on the potential screening tests, it may be appropriate to conduct a randomized controlled trial. In the meantime, any ad hoc screening should be strongly discouraged.

References

Allen MD and Embry B (1991) Biopsy of the prostate guided by transrectal ultrasonography: early experience in a teaching hospital. *Southern Medical Journal* **84** 579–586

Axtell LM, Asire AJ and Myers MH (eds) (1976) *Cancer Patient Survival* (report number 5), US Department of Health, Education and Welfare, Bethesda, Maryland

Babaian RJ, Miyashita H, Evans RB, von Eschenbach AC and Ramirez EI (1991) Early detection program for prostate cancer: results and identification of high-risk patient population. *Urology* **37** 193–197

Benson MC, Whang IS, Pantuck A *et al* (1992a) Prostate specific antigen density: a means of distinguishing benign prostatic hypertrophy and prostate cancer. *Journal of Urology* **147** 815–816

Benson MC, Whang IS, Olsson CA, McMahon DJ, Cooner WH (1992b) The use of prostate specific antigen density to enhance the predictive value of intermediate levels of serum prostate specific antigen. *Journal of Urology* **147** 817–821

Brawer MK, Chetner MP, Beatie J, Buchner DM, Vessella RL and Lange PH (1992) Screening for prostatic carcinoma with prostate specific antigen. *Journal of Urology* **147** 841–845

Breslow N, Chan CW and Dhom G (1977) Latent cancer of the prostate at autopsy in seven areas. *International Journal of Cancer* **20** 680–688

Brooman PJC, Peeling WB, Griffiths GJ, Roberts E and Evans K (1981) A comparison between digital examination and per-rectal ultrasound in the evaluation of the prostate. *British Journal of Urology* **53** 617–620

Cancer Research Campaign Press Release (1991) Top marks for first full year of breast screening programme. *Network* **1** (Oct) 1–4

Carter HB, Hamper UM, Sheth S, Sanders RC, Epstein JI and Walsh PC (1989) Evaluation of transrectal ultrasound in the early detection of prostate cancer. *Journal of Urology* **142** 1008–1010

Carter HB, Pearson JD, Metter J *et al* (1992) Longitudinal evaluation of prostate-specific antigen levels in men with and without prostate disease. *Journal of the American Medical Association* **267** 2215–2220

Catalona WJ, Smith DS, Ratliff TL *et al* (1991) Measurement of prostate-specific antigen in serum as a screening test for prostate cancer. *New England Journal of Medicine* **324** 1156–1161

Chadwick DJ, Kemple T, Astley JP *et al* (1991) Pilot study of screening for prostate cancer in general practice. *Lancet* **338** 613–616

Chodak GW, Wald V, Parmer E, Watanabe H, Hoe H and Saitoh M (1986) Comparison of digital examination and transrectal ultrasonography for the diagnosis of prostatic cancer. *Journal of Urology* **135** 951–954

Chodak GW, Keller P and Schoenberg HW (1989) Assessment of screening for prostate cancer using the digital rectal examination. *Journal of Urology* **141** 1136–1138

Cooner WH, Eggers GW and Lichtenstein P (1987) Prostate cancer: new hope for early diagnosis. *Journal of the Medical Association of the State of Alabama* **56** 13–16

Cooner WH, Mosley BR, Rutherford CL *et al* (1988) Clinical application of transrectal ultrasonography and prostate specific antigen in the search for prostate cancer. *Journal of Urology* **139** 758–761

Cooner WH, Mosley BR, Rutherford CL *et al* (1990) Prostate cancer detection in a clinical urological practice by ultrasonography, digital rectal examination and prostate specific antigen. *Journal of Urology* **143** 1146–1154

Faul P (1982) Experience with the German annual preventive checkup examination, In: Jacobi and Hoffenfeller (eds). *Prostate Cancer,* pp 57–70, Williams and Wilkins, Baltimore Maryland

Forrest P *et al* (1986) *Breast Cancer Screening: Report to the Health Ministers of England, Wales, Scotland and Northern Ireland,* HMSO, London

Franks LM (1954) Latent carcinoma of the prostate. *Journal of Pathology and Bacteriology* **68** 603

Griffiths GJ, Clements R, Jones DR, Roberts EE and Peeling WB (1987) The ultrasound appearances of prostatic cancer with histological correlation. *Clinical Radiology* **38** 219–227

Guinan P, Bush I, Ray V, Vieth R, Rao R and Bhatti R (1980) The accuracy of the rectal examination in the diagnosis of prostate cancer. *New England Journal of Medicine* **303** 499–503

Hammerer P, Loy V, Diereinger J and Huland H (1992) Prostate cancer in nonurological patients with normal prostates on digital rectal examination. *Journal of Urology* **147** 833–836

Hudson PB, Finkle AL, Hopkins JA, Sproul EE and Stout AP (1954) Prostatic cancer XI: early prostatic cancer diagnosed by arbitrary open perineal biopsy among 300 unselected patients. *Cancer* **7** 690–703

Labrie F, Dupont A, Suburu R *et al* (1992) Serum prostate specific antigen as pre-screening test for prostate cancer. *Journal of Urology* **147** 846–852

Lee F, Littrup PJ, Torp-Pedersen S *et al* (1988) Prostate cancer: comparison of transrectal US and digital rectal examination for screening. *Radiology* **168** 389–394

Lee F, Torp-Pedersen S, Littrup PJ *et al* (1989a) Hypoechoic lesions of the prostate: clinical relevance of tumor size, digital rectal examination, and prostate-specific antigen. *Radiology* **170** 29–32

Lee F, Torp-Pederson ST and Siders DB (1989b) Use of transrectal ultrasound in diagnosis, guided biopsy, staging and screening of prostate cancer. *Urology* **33** 7–12

Lee F, Torp-Pedersen S, Siders DB, Littrup PJ and McLeary RD (1989c) Transrectal ultrasound in the diagnosis and staging of prostatic carcinoma. *Radiology* **170** 609–615

Mebust WK, Holtgrewe HL and Cockett ATK (1989) TURP immediate and post operative complications: a cooperative study of 13 institutions evaluating 3,885 points. *Journal of Urology* **141** 243–247

Mettlin C, Lee F, Drago J and Murphy GP (1991) The American Cancer Society National Prostate Cancer Detection Project: findings on the detection of early prostate cancer in 2425 men. *Cancer* **67** 2949–2958

Moon TD and Clejan S (1991) Prostate cancer screening in younger men: prostate specific antigen and public awareness. *Urology* **38** 216–219

Murphy GP, Natarajan N, Pontes JE *et al* (1982) The national survey of prostate cancer in the United States by the American College of Surgeons. *Journal of Urology* **127** 928–934

Muschenheim F, Omarbasha B, Kardjian PM and Mondou EN (1991) Screening for carcinoma of the prostate with prostate specific antigen. *Annals of Clinical Laboratory Science* **21** 371–380

Nesbitt JA, Drago JR and Badalament RA (1989) Transrectal ultrasonography: early experience with use as prostate cancer detection tool. *Urology* **34** 120–123

Norwegian Cancer Society (1980) *Survival of Cancer Patients: Cases Diagnosed in Norway 1968-1975,* The Norwegian Cancer Society, Oslo

Oesterling JE, Chan DW, Epstein JI *et al* (1988) Prostate specific antigen and the preoperative and postoperative evaluation of localized prostatic cancer treated with radical prostatectomy. *Journal of Urology* **139** 766–772

OPCS (1987) *English Life Tables—1980-1982* (OPCS Series DS, No 7), Office of Population Censuses and Surveys, London

OPCS (1993) *Mortality Statistics—Cause, 1992* (OPCS Series DH2, No 19, Office of Population Censuses and Surveys, London

OPCS (1994) *Cancer Statistics—Registrations, 1988* (OPCS Series MB1, No 21), Office of Population Censuses and Surveys, London

Palken M, Cobb OE, Simons E, Warren BH and Aldape HC (1991) Prostate cancer: comparison of digital rectal examination and transrectal ultrasound for screening. *Journal of Urology* **145** 89–92

Pederson KV, Carlsson P, Varenhorst E, Lofman O and Berglund K (1990) Screening for carcinoma of the prostate by digital rectal examination in a randomly selected population. *British Medical Journal* **300** 1041–1044

Perrin P, Maquet JH, Bringeon G and Devonec M (1991) Screening for prostate cancer: comparison of transrectal ultrasound, prostate specific antigen and rectal examination. *British Journal of Urology* **68** 263–265

Rifkin MD and Choi H (1988) Implications of small, peripheral hypoechoic lesions in endorectal US of the prostate. *Radiology* **166** 619–622

Rifkin MD, Zerhouni EA, Gatsonis CA *et al* (1990) Comparison of magnetic resonance imaging and ultrasonography in staging early prostate cancer. *New England Journal of Medicine* **323** 621–626

Thompson IM, Ernst JJ, Gangai MP and Spence CR (1984) Adenocarcinoma of the prostate: results of routine urological screening. *Journal of Urology* **132** 690–692

Thompson IM, Rounder JB, Teague JL, Peek M and Spence CR (1987) Impact of routine screening for adenocarcinoma of the prostate on stage distribution. *Journal of Urology* **137** 424–426

Toms JR (1982) *Trends in Cancer Survival in Great Britain: Cases Registered Between 1960 and 1974,* Cancer Research Campaign, London

Vallancien G, Prapotnich D, Sibert L *et al* (1989) Comparison of the efficacy of digital rectal examination and transrectal ultrasonography in the diagnosis of prostatic cancer. *European Urology* **16** 321–324

Vihko P, Kontturi M, Lukkarinen O, Ervasti J and Vihko R (1985) Screening for carcinoma of the prostate: rectal examination, and enzymatic and radioimmunologic measurements of serum acid phosphatase compared. *Cancer* **56** 173–177

Waaler G, Ludvigsen TC, Runden TO, Stenehjem E, Ogreid P and Schei OM (1988) Digital rectal examination to screen for prostatic cancer. *European Urology* **15** 34–36

Wang MC, Valensuela LA, Murphy GP and Chu TM (1979) Purification of a human prostate specific antigen. *Investigations in Urology* **17** 159–163

Watanabe H, Igari D, Tanahashi Y, Harada K and Saitoh M (1975) Transrectal ultrasonotomography of the prostate. *Journal of Urology* **114** 734–739

Waterhouse RL and Resnick MI (1989) The use of transrectal prostatic ultrasonography in the evaluation of patients with prostatic carcinoma. *Journal of Urology* **141** 233–239

The author is responsible for the accuracy of the references.

Radical Prostatectomy, Radiotherapy or Deferred Treatment for Localized Prostate Cancer?

JAN ADOLFSSON
Department of Urology, Karolinska Hospital, S-171 76 Stockholm, Sweden

INTRODUCTION

Outcome results from the current literature indicate a slightly better outcome at 10 years' follow-up for patients subjected to radical prostatectomy compared with patients treated with external radiotherapy or managed conservatively by deferred treatment. A direct comparison between data compiled for radical prostatectomy, external radiation therapy and deferred treatment is, however, certainly biased. The magnitude of this bias cannot be resolved due to lack of data in the current literature.

Management of patients with prostate cancer localized to the prostate gland is still controversial. A patient may be advised anything from aggressive local treatment, such as radical prostatectomy or external radiotherapy, to more conservative treatment, such as initial surveillance followed by therapy if and when there is disease progression (deferred treatment), or even early endocrine therapy. Since there are no published data from reliable controlled studies, the prevailing opinions regarding the optimal treatment of patients with localized prostate cancer must be based on a combination of personal observations and data from reports of uncontrolled studies.

Cancer Surveys Volume 23: *Preventing Prostate Cancer: Screening versus Chemoprevention*

TABLE 1. Outcome data from a pooled analysis of original data from 820 patients with clinically localized prostate cancer with initial observation followed by treatment on progression (Chodak *et al*, 1994)

	10 year metastasis free survival (%) (95% CI)	10 year disease specific survival (%) (95% CI)
Well differentiated (n=492)	81 (75–86)	87 (81–91)
Moderately differentiated (n=265)	58 (49–66)	87 (80–92)
Poorly differentiated (n=63)	26 (13–41)	34 (19–50)

CI = confidence interval

OVERVIEW OF OUTCOME DATA

Randomized Studies

Despite the presumably very large number of patients treated for localized prostate cancer to date, only two randomized treatment studies have been reported (Paulson *et al,* 1982; Graverson *et al,* 1990). Together, these two series comprise less than 250 patients and both series have been criticized on methodological grounds.

Paulson *et al* (1982) in the Uro-Oncology Research Group compared radical prostatectomy with external radiation therapy and found a significantly lower disease progression rate after surgery. However, the randomization procedure was not entirely blinded, and there was an unexplained difference in the number of patients included in the treatment groups.

Graverson *et al* (1990) reported a Veterans Administration Cooperative Urological Research Group study randomizing deferred treatment versus radical prostatectomy. They found no difference in overall survival 15 years after inclusion. However, almost one third of the patients were lost to follow-up, and some patients were not analysed as "intention to treat".

Pooled Analysis

Recently, a pooled outcome analysis of deferred treatment was published (Chodak *et al,* 1994). Original patient data from six different series from Israel, Scotland, Sweden and the USA were reanalysed. The analysis comprised 828 patients with prostate cancer that was clinically confined to the prostate gland. Disease specific survival at 10 years was 87% for patients with well or moderately differentiated tumour, whereas patients with poorly differentiated tumours fared much worse (Table 1). Metastasis free survival at 10 years was lower for patients with moderately differentiated tumours compared with patients with well differentiated tumours (Table 1). This indicates that further follow-up beyond 10 years may show a higher mortality of prostate cancer in patients with moderately differentiated tumours than in patients with well differentiated tumours.

TABLE 2. Summary of the basic features of three recent literature reviews on outcome of treatment of localized prostate cancer

		No of articles				
Author	Period	reviewed	evaluable	Stage	Analysed endpoints	Analysed bias
Adolfsson *et al* (1993)	1980–	73	RP 14 RT 22 DT 7	T1-2	Compiled disease specific survival at 10 years, compiled incidences for developing metastasis, mortality of prostate cancer or intercurrent disease	Yes
Wasson *et al* (1991)	1966–1991	144	RP 23 RT 22 DT 23	A-B	Compiled median annual rate of developing metastasis, mortality of prostate cancer or of all causes	No
MS Austenfeld (personal communication)	?	?	?	B	Compiled disease specific survival at 10 years variance assessment	?

RP = radical prostatectomy, RT = external radiation therapy, DT = deferred treatment

Literature Reviews with Compilations of Data

During 1993, three separate reviews of current outcome data for radical prostatectomy, external radiation therapy and deferred treatment of patients with clinically confined prostate cancer have been presented (Adolfsson *et al,* 1993; Wasson *et al,* 1993; Austenfeld *et al,* 1994). Essentially, these reports were based on the same literature, but the authors used different techniques for compiling the data (Table 2). A common feature in both published reports was that only about half of the articles reviewed were regarded as evaluable, indicating a generally poor quality of the literature.

Adolfsson *et al* (1993) calculated a weighted mean of disease specific survival at 10 years as reported in the literature, with the number of patients in each study as weights. To expand the study base and thereby increase the precision of analysis, the number of patients, generated person-time and number of patients dying from prostate cancer in each evaluable study were used to calculate a disease specific survival at 10 years. The results of the two methods of estimating disease specific survival corresponded for radical prostatectomy and deferred treatment (Table 3). For external radiation therapy, the figures did not cohere. The compilation of the reported values of disease specific survival for radiotherapy included the largest number of patients and must therefore be regarded as most precise. The basic data in the literature were also used to calculate a weighted number of patients who, during 1000 person-years at risk, developed metastases and died from prostate cancer or from intercurrent disease, that is, an incidence for the various endpoints. The in-

TABLE 3. Disease specific survival at 10 years compiled from two reports

	Adolfsson *et al* (1993) weighted reported mean (%)	Adolfsson *et al* (1993) calculated (%)	MS Austenfeld (pers comm) (%)
Radical prostatectomy	93	93	89
External radiation therapy	74	62	67
Deferred treatment	84	83	86

cidence for developing metastases and mortality of prostate cancer was lowest for radical prostatectomy and highest for radiation therapy (Table 4).

Wasson *et al* (1993) in the Prostate Patient Outcomes Research Team (PORT) group calculated a median annual rate of distant metastasis, a median annual mortality rate from cancer specific causes and a median annual mortality rate from all causes. Their results were similar for radical prostatectomy and deferred treatment, but both rates were higher for external radiation therapy (Table 4). The rates were comparable to the incidence for developing metastases and mortality of prostate cancer reported by Adolfsson (Table 4) (Adolfsson *et al,* 1993).

Austenfeld *et al* (1994) have presented the work done by the American Urological Association guideline committee for prostate cancer. They recorded

TABLE 4. Compilation of incidence in the reports by Wasson *et al* (1993) and Adolfsson *et al* (1993)

Wasson *et al* (PORT)	Median annual rate of metastases (95% CI)	Median annual mortality rate of prostate cancer (95% CI)	Median annual mortality rate all causes (95% CI)
Radical prostatectomy	0.023(0.014–0.025)	0.009(0.007–0.013)	0.032(0.020–0.044)
External radiation therapy	0.050(0.030–0.095)	0.023(0.010–0.030)	0.045(0.040–0.053)
Deferred treatment	0.017(0.011–0.043)	0.009(0.006–0.012)	0.060(0.050–0.104)
Adolfsson *et al*	**Weighted number of patients per 1000 years at risk developing metastases (95% CI)**	**Weighted number of patients per 1000 years at risk of dying of prostate cancer (95% CI)**	**Weighted number of patients per 1000 years at risk of dying of intercurrent disease (95% CI)**
Radical prostatectomy	13(10–15)	7(5–9)	10(8–12)
External radiation therapy	29(25–33)	38(23–59)	36(22–57)
Deferred treatment	25(20–31)	17(13–21)	50(43–57)

CI = confidence interval

disease specific survival for each evaluable series and in addition estimated a variance based on the number of patients included. These data were subsequently "summarized" to a mean and a variance for the various treatments, thereby assessing not only the mean, but also the precision of the compiled data. The results regarding disease specific survival at 10 years were closely similar to the data presented by Adolfsson *et al* (Table 3), and the precision in their data was regarded as highest for radical prostatectomy and lowest for external radiotherapy.

The PORT group has also reported a decision analysis model for treatment of localized prostate cancer (Flemming *et al,* 1993). They used the outcome results available in the literature in the model and concluded that "Radical prostatectomy and radiation therapy may benefit selected groups of patients with localized prostate cancer, particularly younger patients with higher-grade tumours. However, our model shows that in most cases the potential benefits of therapy are small enough that the choice of therapy is sensitive to the patient's preferences for various outcomes and discounting". Results derived from decision analysis models must, however, be regarded with great caution since the outcome may vary with small changes in the modelling. The quality of the data coming out of such a model also totally depends on the quality of the data going in.

OVERVIEW OF VARIOUS BIASES AFFECTING OUTCOME DATA

It is important to understand that the data compiled on the various treatments from the studies mentioned above cannot be directly compared. This is due to various biases in the respective series. This aspect was addressed in one of the three literature reviews (Adolfsson *et al,* 1993) where data on possible sources of bias were extracted form the individual series considered evaluable for the review.

The total bias in a study can be understood as the sum of errors inferred during the inclusion, follow-up and analysis of the series. This therefore is the reason why the actual result of a series does not correspond with the "true" condition. According to Steineck and Ahlbom (1992), the total bias can be divided into confounding, misrepresentation, misclassification and calculating errors. Each of these biases can be related to the various stages of a study.

Confounding originates from the collection of individuals into a series. An important source for confounding is uneven distribution of prognostic factors, usually due to differences in selection criteria between the treatment groups to be compared. This can best be dealt with by a randomization procedure. Confounding was probably the most conspicuous bias in the literature reviewed on localized prostate cancer where several prognostic factors appeared to be unevenly distributed in the various series as well as for the different treatments (Adolfsson *et al,* 1993). Poorly differentiated tumours were more abundant in the series on radical prostatectomy and external radiation therapy than in those on deferred treatment. There seemed to be stage migration towards smaller tumours in the series on radical prostatectomy compared with external radiation therapy and deferred treatment. In some surgery series, only patients with pathologically confined tumours were included in the analysis, and it is also possible that patients with palpably large, but still clinically confined, tumours may have been considered unsuitable for surgery and given other therapy. Almost all patients included in the surgery series had been subjected to pelvic lymph node dissection and found to be without obvious lymph node metastases before the surgeon proceeded with the radical prostatectomy. Lymph node dissection was less commonly performed in the series on external radiation therapy and was not done at all in the series on deferred treatment. This undoubtedly resulted in the inclusion of an unknown but probably significant number of patients with lymph node metastases in the radiotherapy and deferred treatment series. Another apparent confounding factor in the literature was the inclusion of an unknown proportion of patients with prostate cancers that were not newly diagnosed in some radiotherapy series. This may indicate that in a certain number of patients in the radiation series, the disease may already have progressed and other treatments had even failed before radiotherapy.

Unbalanced observation periods with varying hazard rates over time may also be a source of confounding in the literature reviews. There was a marked difference in follow-up times for the various treatments, with the shortest for the radiation series and the longest for the surgery series. If, for instance, the hazard rate for dying of prostate cancer is not constant over time, the difference in follow-up times will mean that different intervals of the hazard rate curve are observed for the various treatments and the hazard rate may be different in these intervals. This will disturb all types of incidence compilations.

Age is a special problem. There was a marked difference in mean age for the various treatments. The mean age for the surgery series was approximately 10 years less than for the series on deferred treatment. If age is a prognostic factor—for instance, if the disease in younger men is more malignant than in older men—this difference in mean age represents a confounding factor related to an unbalanced distribution of prognostic factors.

Age may also be involved as a bias in another respect. Elderly men will each generate a shorter observation time due to a higher competing mortality than younger men. Thereby different age groups observe different intervals on the hazard rate curve. Older men with short observation times will only observe the first part of the hazard rate curve, whereas younger men with longer observation times will observe a larger part of the curve. If the hazard rate curve for prostate cancer mortality is not constant, this will mean that the hazard rates for various age groups are not equal and the difference of mean age for the various treatments will again be a confounder, but this time due to an imbalance in observation periods. The only way to correct for the possible effects of age is to compare patient groups with a similar mean or median age.

Misrepresentation occurs during the follow-up of the series and derives from loss of individuals from the population originally included. Loss to follow up is probably more common than can be understood from the literature and is especially serious if the loss is dependent on the outcome studied. For instance, patients developing metastases may be treated in other departments and fail to attend follow-up with the surgeon or radiotherapist. In the literature on treatment of localized prostate cancer, only a minority of the reports presented data on or even mentioned loss to follow-up. There was, however, no reason to believe that there was any difference in this respect between the various treatments for localized prostate cancer. In literature reviews, failure to include relevant reports represents a similar misrepresentation.

Misclassification occurs when data are not accurately measured or categorized in the analysis of a series. Various definitions of follow-up time was one such misclassification found. Some authors used time from inclusion of the patient to censoring for any reason or, if the patient was still at risk, the date of the last check up. This can be called the actual follow-up time of the patient. Other authors used time from inclusion of the patient to the follow-up date of the series irrespective of whether the patient was still at risk or not. The latter can be called the follow-up period and is by definition equal to or longer than the actual follow-up time. This difference in definitions of follow-up time does not influence a life-table analysis such as a Kaplan Meyer analysis but will disturb data compilations when total person-time in various series is used in the calculations. Other sources of misclassification in the literature on prostate cancer were various definitions of local and distant progression, which created problems with interpreting endpoints such as progression free or disease free survival (Steineck *et al*, 1991). For survival endpoints, the varying criteria for defining death from prostate cancer or intercurrent disease are a constant problem.

Lastly, the final calculation of the data in individual series may give rise to biases such as pure calculating errors, mistakes in modelling—for instance, when trying to adjust for covariates—and mistakes when attempting to control for confounding. In literature reviews and data compilations, these errors can be categorized as misclassifications.

Once again, there was no reason to believe that the two latter categories of bias were different for the various treatments of localized prostate cancer.

SUMMARY

Before considering the possible biases discussed above, the results as reported in the current literature may indicate an advantage for radical prostatectomy in disease specific survival at 10 years' follow-up when compared with external radiation therapy and deferred treatment. It appears that most of the obvious biases found in the literature work in favour of radical prostatectomy. The actual advantage of radical prostatectomy with respect to disease specific survival at 10 years may therefore be less than the data compilations suggest. The magnitude of these biases is, however, impossible to assess.

A probable but perhaps marginal benefit for the majority of the patients must, however, be put in relation to possible side effects and long term complications of the various treatments as well as the patient's preferences when choosing treatment. Reliable controlled data on outcome and quality of life for the various treatments of localized prostate cancer are needed, but we may have to wait for many years for such data.

It must also be remembered that the results presented in this overview derive from a series started in the late 1970s of patients treated with the surgical techniques and radiotherapy technology available at that time. Today, the frequent use of prostate specific antigen in early detection or screening programmes will definitely detect a larger number of low volume prostate cancers that may be more curable by surgery or radiotherapy. This, however, remains to be proved. Moreover, new technology in radiotherapy, such as conformal therapy, may enable radiotherapists to deliver higher local doses of radiation to the prostate, which in turn may improve the cure rate for radiotherapy.

Acknowledgements

The author is grateful to Gunnar Steineck, Department of Cancer Epidemiology and Oncology, Karolinska Hospital, Stockholm, Sweden, for valuable suggestions during the preparation of this manuscript.

References

Adolfsson J, Steineck G and Whitmore WF (1993) Recent results of management of palpable clinically localized prostate cancer. *Cancer* **72** 310–322

Austenfeld MS, Thompson Jr IM and Middleton RG for the American Urological Association Prostate Cancer Guideline Panel (1994) Meta-analysis of the literaure: Guideline development for prostate cancer treatment. *Journal of Urology* **152** 1866–1869

Chodak G, Thiested R, Gerber G *et al* (1994) Outcome following conservative management of patients with clinically localized prostate cancer. *New England Journal of Medicine* **330** 242–248

Flemming C, Wasson JH, Albertsen PC *et al* (1993) A decision analysis of alternative treatment strategies for clinically localized prostate cancer. *Journal of the American Medical Association* **269** 2650–2658

Graverson PH, Nielsson KT, Gasser TC *et al* (1990) Radical prostatectomy versus expectant treatment in stages I and II prostatic cancer: a fifteen-year follow up. *Urology* **36** 493–498

Paulson DF, Lin GH, Hinshaw W *et al* (1982) The Uro-Oncology Research Group. Radical surgery versus radiotherapy for adenocarcinoma of the prostate. *Journal of Urology* **128** 502–504

Steineck G, Adolfsson J and Whitmore WF Jr (1991) "Local recurrence" and "disease free survival"; doubtful parameters when comparing non-randomized studies of prostate cancer. *Scandinavian Journal of Urology and Nephrology* **138 (Supplement)** 121–126

Steineck G and Ahlbom A (1992) Definition of bias founded on the concept of the study base. *Epidemiology* **3** 477–482

Wasson JH, Cushman CC, Bruskewitz RC *et al* (1993) A structured literature review of treatment for localized prostate cancer. *Archives of Family Medicine* **2** 487–493

The author is responsible for the accuracy of the references.

Downstaging by Combination Therapy with Flutamide and an LHRH Agonist before Radical Prostatectomy

FERNAND LABRIE • LIONEL CUSAN • JOSÉ-LUIS GOMEZ
PIERRE DIAMOND • RAUL SUBURU • MARTIN LEMAY
BERNARD TÊTU • YVES FRADET • BERNARD CANDAS

Prostate Cancer Research Unit and Departments of Molecular Endocrinology, Medicine, Radiology, Pathology and Urology, CHUL Research Center and Laval University; Departments of Pathology and Urology, Hôtel-Dieu de Québec, Québec City, Canada

INTRODUCTION

Although little information is available on the best choice of therapy for early stage prostate cancer (Kolata, 1987), it is well recognized that the only opportunity for a cure of prostate cancer is at an early stage when the cancer is still localized to the prostate (Walsh and Jewett, 1980; Kolata, 1987; Labrie *et al*, 1992). The main objective in prostate cancer should thus be early diagnosis and treatment of organ confined disease since it is known that such patients treated by radical prostatectomy have a life expectancy comparable to that of men who do not have prostate cancer (Jewett *et al*, 1968; Walsh and Jewett, 1980).

Unfortunately, not all men who are thought to have organ confined prostate cancer at diagnosis are found to have organ confined disease at surgery. In fact, in 50–60% of cases, the pathological analysis of the specimen obtained at radical prostatectomy shows that the cancer is more advanced than originally predicted at diagnosis (Boxer *et al*, 1977; Veenema *et al*, 1977; Catalona and Stein, 1982; Elder *et al*, 1982; Lange and Narayan, 1983; Gibbons *et al*, 1989; Brawer and Lange, 1990).

A possible means of improving the proportion of patients with organ confined disease and cancer negative margins at surgery was clearly suggested by

 0-87969-466-1/95. $5.00 + .00

the observation that patients treated by combination therapy using a pure anti-androgen associated with medical or surgical castration for metastatic disease show a much more rapid and marked regression of their cancer in the prostatic area compared with distant metastatic disease (Labrie *et al,* 1982, 1985, 1993a).

Following an encouraging preliminary trial (Monfette *et al,* 1989), we have conducted a prospective, randomized clinical trial in order to assess precisely the potential advantages of neoadjuvant combination therapy with the pure anti-androgen flutamide and a luteinizing hormone releasing hormone (LHRH) agonist administered for 3 months before radical prostatectomy compared with surgery alone (Labrie *et al,* 1993b). This chapter is an update of this first randomized trial and an analysis of the data on organ confined disease and specimen confined disease and on the comparison of the final stage at histopathology of the surgical specimen with the clinical stage at diagnosis.

METHODS

Patients

A total of 161 men aged between 46 and 72 years with histopathology proven adenocarcinoma of the prostate took part in the study. Six patients were classified at diagnosis as having stage B_0 disease, defined as one localized nodule at digital rectal examination (DRE) and/or a lesion found on transrectal ultrasonography (TRUS) of <1.0 cm (mean TRUS diameter); 82 had stage B_1 disease, defined as one localized nodule at DRE and/or a lesion on TRUS of between 1.0 and 1.5 cm (mean TRUS diameter); 46 had stage B_2 disease, defined as more than one palpable nodule at DRE and/or a lesion >1.5 cm (mean TRUS diameter); 15 had stage C_1 disease, defined as minimal palpable extracapsular extension and/or invasion of the prostatic capsule seen at histopathology of biopsy specimen; and 12 had stage C_2 disease, defined as C_1 but with, in addition, invasion of seminal vesicles and/or neurovascular bundle seen at histopathology of biopsy specimen.

The median and average ages of the patients as well as the distribution of stages at diagnosis showed no significant difference between the two groups. Among patients assigned to have retropubic radical prostatectomy alone, 26 declined randomization; in the group assigned to neoadjuvant combination therapy for 3 months (leuprolide or [DTRP$_6$, des-GlyNH$_2^{10}$] LHRH ethylamide 7.5 mg intramuscularly every 28 days or 250 μg subcutaneously daily + flutamide 250 mg every 8 hours orally) before radical prostatectomy, only four refused. Therefore, a logistic regression analysis of randomized and non-randomized patients, including covariates for treatment and important prognostic factors (age and stage), was done for each group to assess and confirm the validity of the trial, in which all eligible patients were studied (Olschewski *et al,* 1992). All patients had liver function tests on a monthly basis for 3 months, as described previously (Gomez *et al,* 1992).

TABLE 1. Effect of 3 month neoadjuvant combination therapy with the anti-androgen flutamide and an LHRH agonist on positive margins at radical prostatectomy in stages B and C prostate cancer

Group	Negative margins	Positive margins	Total
Control	47 (66.2%)	24 (33.8%)	71
Combination therapy	83 (92.2%)	7 (7.8%)	90
Total			161

χ^2 test: $p<0.001$

RESULTS

As Table 1 shows, the incidence of cancer positive surgical margins was reduced in a highly significant way to only 7.8% (7 of 90) in the group of patients who received an LHRH superagonist and flutamide for 3 months before radical prostatectomy compared with 33.8% (24 of 71) in the group of men who had no endocrine therapy before radical prostatectomy (χ^2 test, $p<0.001$). The decrease in cancer positive surgical margins is of major amplitude at all stages of the disease except at stage B_0, where there were only three patients in each group. In fact, although cancer positive margins were found in the surgical specimen in 25.6% of stage B_1, 58.8% of stage B_2, and 80% of stage C_2 control patients, the incidence of positive margins decreased to 2.6% in stage B_1, 10.8% in stage B_2 and 14.3% in stage C_2 patients who received combination therapy for 3 months before surgery.

It is then of particular interest to examine the final staging at histopathological examination of the specimen obtained at surgery compared with clinical staging at diagnosis and to determine the effect of combination therapy at each stage of the disease. Upstaging is particularly striking at stages B_1 and B_2 in the control untreated group. In fact, of 39 cancers originally classified as B_1, 21 showed a more advanced stage at surgery, including 5 C_1 and 10 C_2 disease (Table 2). Similarly, of 17 cancers originally classified as B_2 disease in the control group, 3 became C_1, 8 became C_2 and 2 became D_1 disease. On the other hand, it can also be seen in Table 2 that downstaging following neoadjuvant combination therapy was frequent at all stages of the disease: in fact, in the patients originally classified as having B_1 disease, 14 of 43 (32.5%) tumours originally classified as having a mean diameter of 1.0–1.5 cm decreased to <1.0 cm, while no cancer was found in 6 patients after thorough examination of additional histological sections. Downstaging was seen in 13 of 29 (44.8%) of patients originally classified as having stage B_2 disease. Although the number of patients is small, the downstaging effect was particularly important in patients originally classified as having C_1 disease at diagnosis, where six of eight (75.0%) had downstaging, and in patients originally classified at diagnosis as stage C_2, where six of seven cancers (85.7%) were downstaged following neoadjuvant combination therapy.

TABLE 2. Effect of 3 month neoadjuvant combination therapy with flutamide and an LHRH agonist on the final histopathological stage at surgery compared with the initial clinical stage at diagnosis

Original stage		Final histopathological stage at surgery						
	No	NC	B_0	B_1	B_2	C_1	C_2	D_1
A. Control–untreated								
B_0	3	0	1	0	1	1	0	0
B_1	39	0	7	11	6	5	10	0
B_2	17	0	0	3	1	3	8	2
C_1	7	0	1	1	2	3	0	0
C_2	5	0	0	0	1	0	1	3
B. 3 month neoadjuvant combination therapy								
B_0	3	0	1	0	0	1	1	0
B_1	43	6	14	11	7	3	2	0
B_2	29	0	2	11	6	5	3	2
C_1	8	0	2	1	3	1	1	0
C_2	7	0	1	2	2	1	0	1

NC = No Cancer

Comparison of the initial clinical stage at diagnosis with the final stage at histopathological examination of the surgical specimen following radical prostatectomy can be more easily seen in Fig. 1. The downstaging effect of combination therapy is thus clearly seen at all stages of the disease except at stage B_0. The net advantages of combination therapy are best illustrated by the final stage at surgery, which was, on average, worsened by 35.9% (14 of 39) in stage B_1 disease, 58.8% (10 of 17) in stage B_2 disease and 40% in stage C_2 disease in patients who had radical prostatectomy alone, whereas the final stage of the disease, on the contrary, was improved following combination therapy by 18.5% (8 of 43) in stage B_1 disease, 10.3% (3 of 29) in stage B_2 disease, 62.5% (5 of 8) in stage C_1 disease and 71.4% (5 of 7) in stage C_2 patients.

After 3 months of combination therapy, average upstaging decreased to 28.9% (26 of 90) in patients who received neoadjuvant combination therapy compared to 54.9% (39 of 71) in the control group. Thus, net upstaging (difference between the number of patients who had upstaging and the number of those who had downstaging) occurred on average in 33.8% of control patients, whereas 21.1% of patients were downstaged at analysis of the surgical specimen in the group of patients who had combination therapy before surgery, for a net difference of 54.9% in favour of neoadjuvant combination therapy (Fig. 2).

The net effect of neoadjuvant therapy on specimen confined margins and organ confined disease can be clearly seen in Fig. 3. Since organ confined disease has such an important prognostic value, it is of major interest to see in Fig. 3A that organ confined disease increased from 49.3% (35 of 71) in the control group to 77.8% (70 of 90) for a 57.8% improvement in the group of

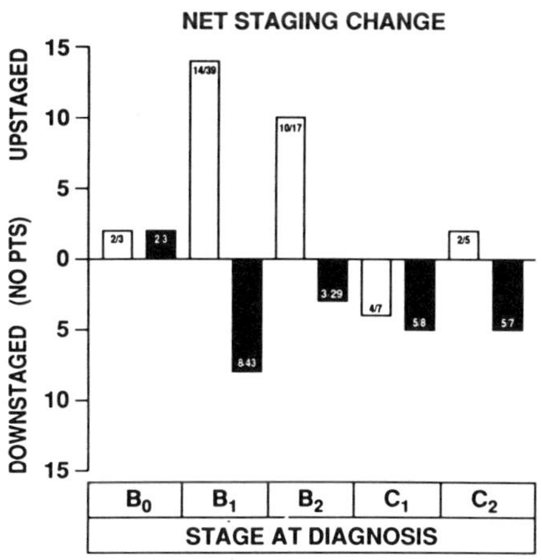

Fig. 1. Effect of 3 month combination therapy with flutamide and an LHRH agonist on the final histopathological stage at surgery v. the clinical staging at diagnosis. Data are expressed as number of patients showing upstaging or downstaging in each group (Labrie *et al*, in press)

men who received neoadjuvant combination therapy. In fact, organ confined disease increased from 61.5% (24 of 39) to 88.4% (38 of 43) in stage B_1 disease, from 23.5% (4 of 17) to 65.5% (19 of 29) in stage B_2 disease, from 57.1% (4 of 7) to 87.5% (7 of 8) in stage C_1 disease and from 20% (1 of 5) to 71.4% (5 of 7) in stage C_2 disease. On the other hand, specimen confined disease or cancer negative margins increased from 66.2% (47 of 71) in men who had radical prostatectomy alone to 92.2% (83 of 90) ($p<0.001$) in those who received neoadjuvant combination therapy before radical prostatectomy (Fig. 3B).

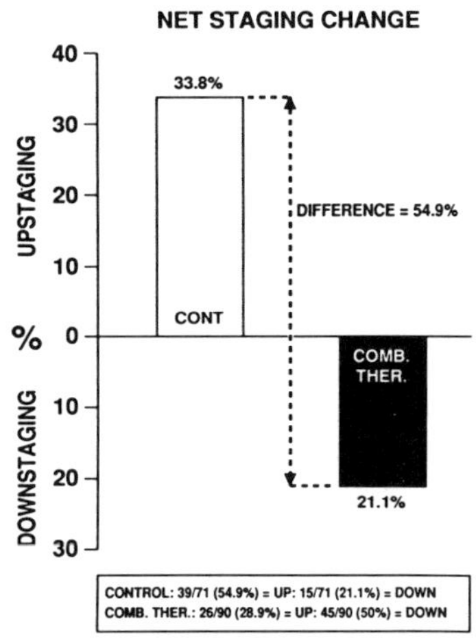

Fig. 2. Net change of stage between initial staging at diagnosis and final staging at radical prostatectomy in patients who had radical prostatectomy alone and those who received combination therapy for 3 months before radical prostatectomy. Data are expressed as percentage of patients in each group (Labrie *et al*, in press)

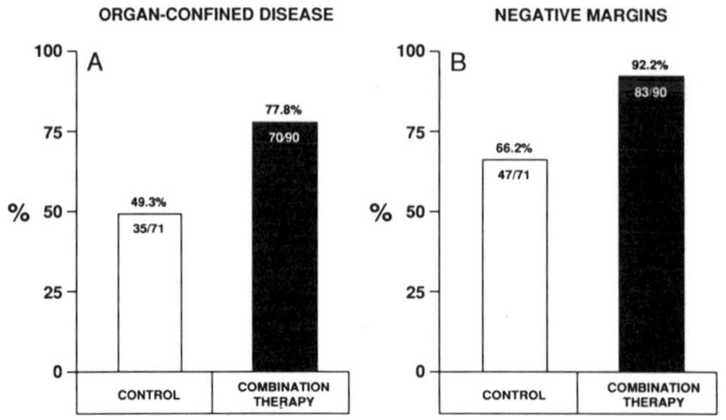

Fig. 3. Effect of 3 month neoadjuvant combination therapy with flutamide and an LHRH agonist on organ confined disease (A) and specimen confined disease (B) in stages B and C prostate cancer (Labrie *et al*, in press)

Thus, there is a 57.8% increase in the incidence of organ confined disease after 3 months of neoadjuvant combination endocrine therapy compared to control untreated men (Fig. 3A) while the incidence of cancer positive margins is 4.3-fold higher in the group of control untreated men (33.8% v. 7.8%) (Fig. 3B).

DISCUSSION

The essential objective of treatment of early stage prostate cancer is complete removal or elimination of cancer tissue. Although the long term effects of androgen deprivation achieved by neoadjuvant combination therapy on survival remain to be assessed by long term follow-up of the patients, the present data show that prostate cancer cell death or apoptosis occurs at a relatively high rate in the prostate area, under the influence of combination therapy: such cancer cell death leads to a relatively rapid downstaging of the disease. In fact, after only 3 months of neoadjuvant combination therapy with flutamide and an LHRH agonist, cancer positive surgical margins decreased from 33.8% to only 7.8% while organ confined disease increased from 49.3% to 77.8%.

The present data show that neoadjuvant combination therapy eliminates the previous serious limitation that 50% of men had a disease more advanced than expected at diagnosis when the final and true staging was obtained by histopathological examination of the surgical specimen. After 3 months of combination endocrine therapy, on average, the stage of the disease was decreased by 23% compared to the initial staging at diagnosis. Such histopathological findings, which remain to be supported by long term follow-up of the patients, offer the hope of a major improvement in the morbidity and mortality from prostate cancer.

SUMMARY

A total of 161 patients diagnosed as having stage B (134 patients) or C (27 patients) prostate cancer were randomly assigned to radical prostatectomy alone or to 3 months of neoadjuvant combination therapy with the antiandrogen flutamide and an LHRH agonist before radical prostatectomy. Neoadjuvant combination therapy before radical prostatectomy decreased cancer positive surgical margins from 33.8% in the control group to only 7.8%, thus leaving 92.2% of patients with negative margins at surgery for a 39.2% increase in specimen confined disease. Although on average the final stage determined at histopathological examination of the surgical specimen was more advanced than predicted at initial diagnosis in 33.8% of control patients, an opposite observation was made in the group of men who received the 3 month neoadjuvant combination therapy where the final stage, instead of being more advanced, was less advanced than at diagnosis in an average of 21.1% of men for a net 54.9% improvement of staging in favour of combination therapy. On the other hand, organ confined disease increased from 49.3% to 77.8% of patients after 3 months of combination therapy, for a 57.9% increase in the incidence of organ confined disease. Although long term follow up of these patients is required to determine the impact on survival, the marked influence of neoadjuvant combination therapy on the stage of the disease suggests the possibility of a major improvement in the morbidity and mortality from prostate cancer.

References

Boxer RJ, Kaufman JJ and Goodwin WE (1977) Radical prostatectomy for carcinoma of the prostate: 1951-1976: a review of 329 patients. *Journal of Urology* **117** 208–213

Brawer MK and Lange PH (1990) Adjuvant therapy after radical prostatectomy. *Problems in Urology* **4** 461–472

Catalona WJ and Stein AJ (1982) Staging errors in clinically localized prostatic cancer. *Journal of Urology* **127** 452–456

Elder JS, Jewett HJ and Walsh PC (1982) Radical perineal prostatectomy for clinical stage B2 carcinoma of the prostate. *Journal of Urology* **127** 704–706

Gibbons RP, Correar RJ Jr, Brannen GE and Weissman RM (1989) Total prostatectomy for clinically localized prostate cancer: long-term results. *Journal of Urology* **141** 564–566

Gomez JL, Dupont A, Cusan L *et al* (1992) Incidence of liver toxicity with the use of flutamide in prostate cancer patients. *American Journal of Medicine* **5** 465–470

Jewett HJ, Bridge RW, Gray Jr GF and Shelley WM (1968) The palpable nodule of prostatic cancer: results 15 years after radical excision. *Journal of the American Medical Association* **203** 403–406

Kolata G (1987) Prostate cancer consensus hampered by lack of data. *Science* **236** 1626–1627

Labrie F, Dupont A, Bélanger A *et al* (1982) New hormonal therapy in prostatic carcinoma: combined treatment with an LHRH agonist and an antiandrogen. *Journal of Clinical and Investigative Medicine* **5** 267–275

Labrie F, Dupont A and Bélanger A (1985) Complete androgen blockade for the treatment of prostate cancer, In: de Vita VT, Hellman S and Rosenberg SA (eds). *Important Advances in Oncology*, pp 193–217, JB Lippincott, Philadelphia

Labrie F, Bélanger A, Dupont A *et al* (1993a) Science behind total androgen blockade: from

gene to combination therapy. *Clinical and Investigative Medicine* **16** 487–504
Labrie F, Dupont A, Cusan L *et al* (1993b) Downstaging of localized prostate cancer by neoadjuvant therapy with flutamide and lupron: the first controlled and randomized trial. *Clinical and Investigative Medicine* **16** 511–521
Labrie F, Dupont A, Suburu R *et al* (1992) Serum prostatic specific antigen (PSA) as prescreening test for prostate cancer. *Journal of Urology* **147** 846–852
Labrie F, Cusan L, Gomez JL, Diamond P, Candas B Combination of screening and preoperative endocrine therapy: the potential for an important decrease in prostate cancer death. *Urology* (in press)
Lange PH and Narayan P (1983) Understaging and undergrading of prostate cancer: argument for postoperative radiation as adjuvant therapy. *Urology* **21** 113–118
Monfette G, Dupont A and Labrie F (1989) Temporary combination therapy with flutamide and Tryptex as adjuvant to radical prostatectomy for the treatment of early stage prostate cancer, In: Labrie F, Lee F and Dupont A (eds). *Early Stage Prostate Cancer: Diagnosis and Choice of Therapy,* pp 41–51, Excerpta Medica, New York
Olschewski M, Schumacher M and Davis KB (1992) Analysis of randomized and non-randomized patients in clinical trials using the comprehensive cohort follow-up study design, controlled. *Clinical Trials* **13** 226–239
Veenema RJ, Gursel EO and Lattimer JK (1977) Radical retropubic prostatectomy for cancer: a 20-year experience. *Journal of Urology* **117** 330–331
Walsh PC and Jewett HJ (1980) Radical surgery for prostatic cancer. *Cancer* **45** 1906–1911

The authors are responsible for the accuracy of the references.

Tumour Markers in Patients on Deferred Treatment: Prostate Specific Antigen Doubling Times

HANS-PETER SCHMID
Division of Urology, University of Basel, Kantonsspital, CH-4031 Basel, Switzerland

INTRODUCTION

In prostate cancer, the discrepancy between histologically identifiable (40%) and clinically diagnosed (8%) carcinomas (Stamey *et al,* 1993) gave rise to a considerable diagnostic and therapeutic dilemma. Prostate cancer was said to have an unpredictable natural history, and the therapeutic spectrum ranges from a wait and watch policy (UK, Scandinavia) to aggressive surgical treatment (USA, Germany).

Recent studies from the Stanford group demonstrated that with exact knowledge of tumour volume and quantitated histological grade, the prognosis for the patient with cancer that is clinically confined to the prostate becomes predictable (McNeal *et al,* 1990). On the basis of indirect evidence from the volumes of incidental carcinomas in autopsy series (McNeal *et al,* 1986) and unsuspected carcinomas in cystoprostatectomy specimens for bladder cancer (Stamey *et al,* 1993), it has been proposed that prostate cancer follows a simple exponential growth curve with a constant long doubling time throughout its entire natural history. However, these determinations fail to reveal whether there is prognostic predictability in the histological evolution of cancer with time. They are based on morphological evaluation at a single point in time.

The estimation of approximate prostate cancer volume by non-invasive means in the individual patient with clinical carcinoma has become possible. A linear relationship has been demonstrated between serum prostate specific antigen (PSA) level and cancer volume. On average, a rise in PSA of 3.5 ng/ml

Cancer Surveys Volume 23: *Preventing Prostate Cancer: Screening versus Chemoprevention*

reflects 1 cc (or 1 ml) of cancer, whether the cancer is within the prostate or extracapsular (Stamey *et al,* 1989). Because serum PSA is proportional to prostate cancer volume, serial PSA determinations in the absence of any therapy to the prostate should reflect tumour growth rate (doubling time) and the shape of the growth curve.

MATERIALS AND METHODS

Forty three patients with histologically proven prostate cancer who were referred to Stanford University Medical Center between February 1985 and April 1989 were followed up with serial serum PSA determinations. Only patients with two or more PSA determinations at least 12 months apart were included in this study. Between the initial and final PSA determinations, no specific treatment for prostate cancer (radical prostatectomy, radiation therapy, hormonal therapy, chemotherapy) was given nor was any manipulation, for example, transurethral resection of the prostate or prostate biopsy, performed.

The mean age of the patients at time of initial PSA determination was 71 years (range 51–83 years). The mean follow-up from initial to final PSA determination was 30 months; the median follow-up was 26 months (range 12–63 months).

The clinical stages at the time of initial PSA determination are shown in Table 1. Among the patients for whom treatment was deferred, eight refused therapy; ten were thought to have too small a cancer to warrant treatment (most patients with clinical stage A disease); ten had no symptoms with advanced disease (clinical stages C, D1 and D2); nine were too old or in poor health; five had stable PSA levels and wanted to wait; and one insisted on a radical prostatectomy after being followed up for 24 months, having only a microscopic focus of cancer.

For 22 patients, three or more PSA determinations obtained between the initial and final PSA determination were available—that is, five or more values overall (mean 6.8 determinations; range 5–12 determinations). The distribution of clinical stages in these patients is similar to that of the 21 patients for whom we have only initial and final serum PSA determinations during the period of observation.

The PSA was determined by the Yang assay, a polyclonal radioimmunoassay (Pros-check PSA, Yang Laboratories, Bellevue, WA). All blood was drawn on an ambulatory basis before rectal examination.

PSA doubling time (T′) was calculated according to the formula $T' = (\log 2 \times t)/(\log [\text{final PSA}] - \log [\text{initial PSA}])$, where t is the time from initial to final PSA determination in months.

Slides of the transurethral resection chips or needle biopsy cores obtained at outside facilities were reviewed at Stanford. The Gleason grading system

TABLE 1. All 43 patients stratified according to doubling times and clinical stages

	Stage	Group and PSA doubling time (months)					Total in each clinical stage
		5 stable	4 >48	3 24–48	2 12–24	1 <12	
Clinical disease confined to the prostate (n=28)	PSA-Ca		1				1
	TRUS-Ca	2	2		1		5
	A 1	1	2	1	1		5
	A 2		5				5
	B 1	1	2	1			4
	B 2		3	4			7
	B 3	1					1
Clinical disease not confined to the prostate (n=15)	C		4			1	5
	D 1	1	1	1	3		6
	D 2			1		3	4
Total in each group		6	20	8	5	4	43

PSA-Ca = cancer detected by PSA level
TRUS-Ca = cancer detected by transrectal ultrasound

was used for histological assessment and the sum of the primary and secondary Gleason grades (Gleason score) is reported.

RESULTS

Growth Curve of Prostate Cancer

Twenty two patients had a total of five or more PSA determinations over more than 12 months; 5 of 12 patients whose cancer was clinically confined to the prostate at initial PSA determination are represented in Fig. 1. Five of the ten patients who had non-organ confined disease at initial PSA determination are represented in Fig. 2. For both subgroups, the intermediate PSA values closely followed a straight line connecting initial and final values on a log-PSA versus time scale (Figs. 1 and 2). Thus, the increase in serum PSA was judged to trace an exponential (log-linear) curve throughout the measured interval for all stages. On the basis of these findings, we included in our analysis 21 additional patients in whom only initial and final PSA determinations were known. Data for the entire group were evaluated in terms of a single number, the tumour doubling time.

Doubling Time of Prostate Cancer

Among the total of 43 patients, 37 (86%) had an increase in PSA during the follow-up period, whereas in 6 (14%), PSA levels remained stable. This distribution is similar to that in the initial group of 22 patients for whom multiple PSA values were available.

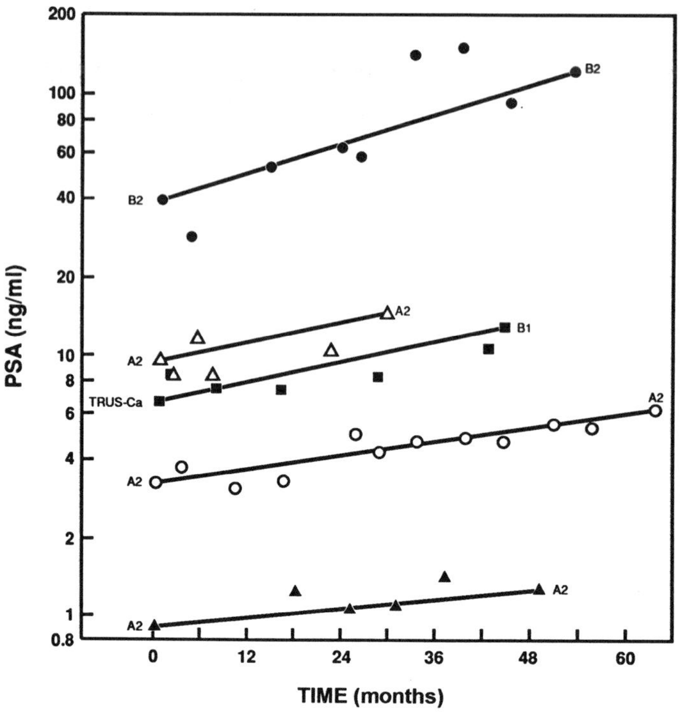

Fig. 1. Follow-up with multiple PSA determinations in five patients with cancers that are clinically confined to the prostate (stages B3 or less). Values for PSA between the initial and final PSA determinations follow the connecting line on the log-PSA versus time scale. The symbols are used only to distinguish PSA points for individual patients (from Schmid *et al*, 1993). TRUS-Ca = cancer detected by transrectal ultrasound

Among the patients with stable disease, the final PSA determination averaged 92% of the initial PSA determination, within the range of test accuracy on repeat determinations (Stamey *et al*, 1987). Local progression by digital rectal examination was undetectable in five of these six patients and may have been artefactual in the sixth patient (biopsy may have masked the nodule at initial examination). Bone scans remained consistently normal.

Table 1 shows that in the category of clinical disease confined to the prostate, 26 of 28 patients (93%) had a doubling time of more than 24 months; a doubling time of more than 24 months was found in 8 of 15 patients (53%) with cancer not confined to the prostate. This difference was statistically significant using a chi square test (p=0.01).

It should be noted that seven of nine patients with doubling times of less than 24 months had clinical disease not confined to the prostate (Table 1). Among this group, all three patients who had distant metastases had doubling times of less than 12 months. Only one of four patients who had distant metastases (stage D2) had a doubling time of more than 24 months. Conversely, five of six patients with stable PSA values and 15 of 20 with doubling times

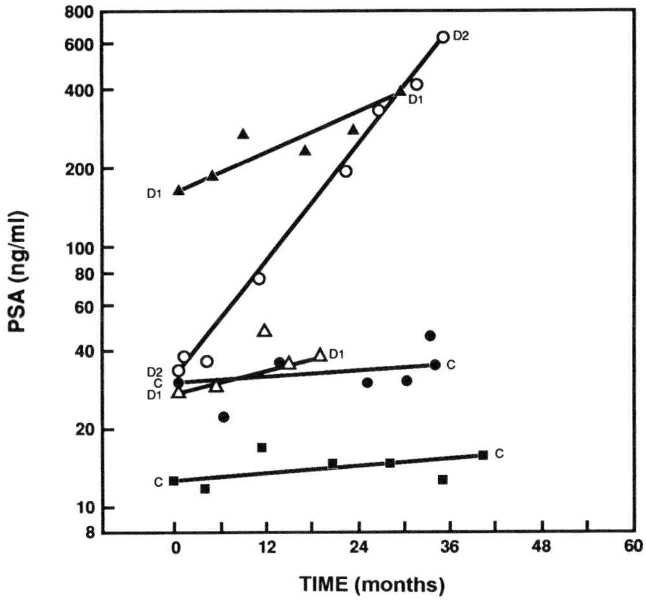

Fig. 2. Follow-up with multiple PSA determinations in five patients with cancers that were not confined to the prostate (stages C and greater). Values for PSA between the initial and final PSA determinations follow the connecting line on the log-PSA versus time scale. Symbols are the same as those in Fig. 1 (from Schmid *et al*, 1993).

longer than 48 months had organ confined disease (Table 1). These two groups probably represent cancers of smaller volumes, as indicated in Table 2, by median initial PSA values of 5.7 and 10.7 ng/ml, respectively. By contrast, the initial median PSA value was 27.3 ng/ml in patients with doubling times of 12–24 months, and it was 26.9 ng/ml in those with doubling times of less than 12 months, which is consistent with much larger tumour volume.

Data for the two groups are combined in Fig. 3; the 27 patients with clinically localized cancer throughout the follow-up period had a median initial PSA value of 6.7 ng/ml and doubling time of 69.3 months. For the 15 patients with cancer that was not localized, the median initial PSA value was 30.8 ng/ml and median doubling time 43.0 months. If the doubling times of the six patients who had stable PSA levels and those of the five patients whose increase in PSA was less than or equal to 1 ng/ml are excluded, the median doubling timc for organ confined cancers decreases from 69 to 50 months and that for cancers not localized decreases from 43 to 24 months.

Higher histological grades also were associated with faster doubling times (Table 2). There was a statistically significant relationship (p=0.05, using chi square analysis) between a Gleason score of 6 or lower versus a Gleason score of 7 or higher and a doubling time of more than 24 months versus one of less than 24 months.

TABLE 2. Relationship of doubling time with median PSA, medical clinical stage and Gleason score

Group	Doubling time (months)	No of patients (n=43)	Median initial PSA (ng/ml)	Median final PSA (ng/mg)	Median initial stage	Median final stage	Median Gleason score	No of patients with Gleason score of	
								≤6 (n=29)	≥7 (n=14)
1	<12	4	26.9	470.5	D 2	D 2	7.5	1	3
2	12–24	5	27.3	112.8	D 1	D 1	7.0	2	3
3	24–48	8	13.0	29.1	B 2	B 3	6.5	4	4
4	>48	20	10.7	13.5	A 2/B 1	B 1	6.0	18	2
5	stable	6	5.7	5.5	A 1/B 1	B 1/B 2	6.0	4	2

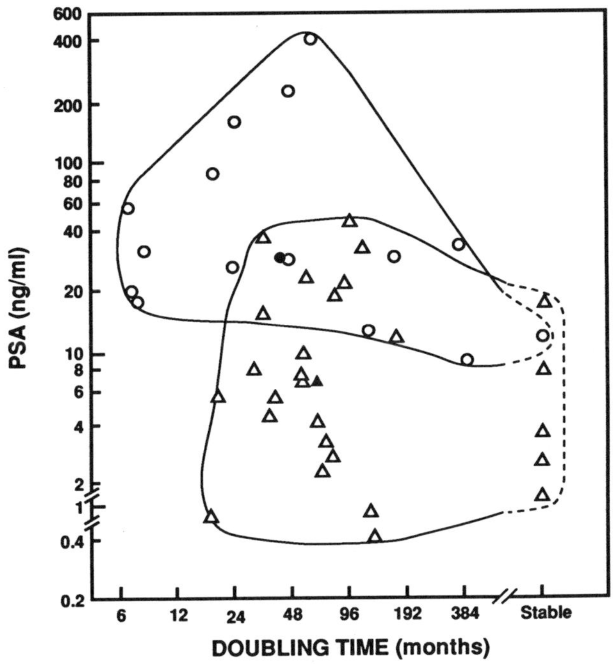

Fig. 3. Log (initial PSA level) versus log (PSA doubling time). (*Open triangle*) 27 patients with clinically localized cancers throughout the follow-up period (excludes one patient whose tumour progressed from stage B2 to stage D2). (*Closed triangle*) Median initial PSA value for this group was 6.7 ng/ml and median doubling time was 69 months. (*Open circle*) 15 patients with cancers not localized. (*Closed circle*) Median initial PSA value for this group was 30.8 ng/ml and median doubling time was 43 months (from Schmid *et al*, 1993)

Effect of BPH on Doubling Time Calculation

Benign prostatic hyperplasia (BPH) is known to raise serum PSA levels at an average of 0.3 ng/ml per cc (or gram) of BPH tissue (Stamey *et al*, 1987). Cancer raises PSA, on average, 3.5 ng/ml per cc of cancer (Stamey *et al*, 1989). Thus, any given serum level is composed of PSA from normal prostatic tissue (as great as 2.5 ng/ml by the Yang assay), BPH and cancerous tissue.

It is clear that the presence of BPH contributes PSA to the serum in amounts that may produce erroneously long estimates of tumour doubling time. Figure 4 shows a diagram of the nature of the relationship. The greater the amount of BPH that accompanies prostate cancer, the more likely the doubling time of the cancer will be overestimated. The less the amount of BPH, the more accurate the rise in serum PSA will be in reflecting the doubling time of the cancer.

DISCUSSION

The present study on tumour markers in patients on deferred treatment adds strong support to the concept that prostate cancer is probably the most predic-

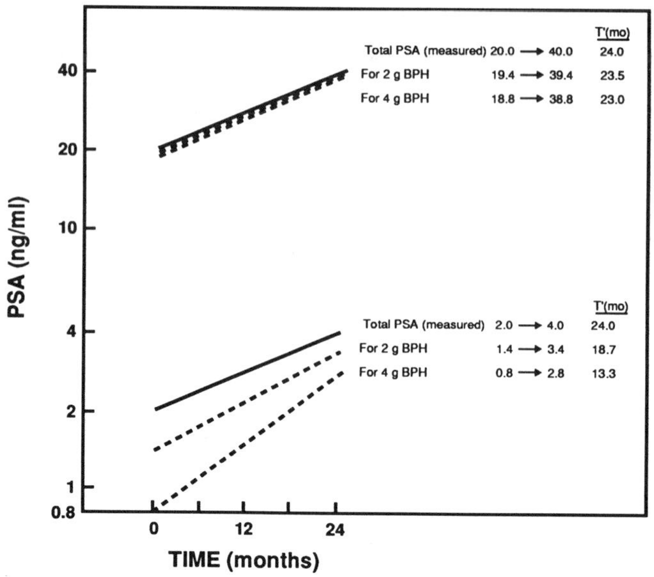

Fig. 4. Theoretical example of the influence of BPH and absolute PSA level on doubling times (T ′) of prostate cancer. Calculations are based on an average of 1 cc BPH equals 0.3 ng/ml PSA in the serum. The more BPH, the faster the doubling time, and the lower absolute PSA levels, the stronger the BPH influence on doubling time. See text for details (from Schmid *et al,* 1993)

table of all human solid tumours. The malignant potential (biological aggressiveness) of prostate cancer is directly related to tumour volume (McNeal *et al,* 1986, 1990) and tumour volume is proportional to serum PSA (Stamey *et al,* 1989). Therefore, changes in serum PSA with time in patients on deferred treatment should reflect the natural history of the disease.

Two important points must be stressed in our data on serial PSA determinations in untreated patients with prostate cancer. Firstly, the increase in PSA with time was exponential (log-linear) for all clinical stages (Figs. 1 and 2). This linearity allowed us to calculate a doubling time for PSA. Secondly, the vast majority of cancers that were clinically confined to the prostate doubled at rates exceeding 2 years (Table 1), and the median doubling time of this group was 4 years. These prolonged doubling times may explain the discrepancy between histologically identifiable (40%) and clinically diagnosed (8%) carcinomas (Stamey *et al,* 1993). The tumour volume distribution in the general population is such that 80% of all prostate cancers are less than 0.5 cc in volume (Stamey *et al,* 1993). The current study indicates that in most patients, it would require approximately 12 years for a 0.5 cc cancer to reach 4 cc in volume if its doubling time was 4 years. Thus, in view of the slow growth rate of prostate cancer, these small tumours will probably never become clinically significant.

Histological grade is also closely linked to tumour volume. Higher grades evolve from better grades with the passage of time and are found in overproportional frequency in cancers of larger volumes (McNeal *et al,* 1990). In

TABLE 3. Algorithm for early detection of prostate cancer

PSA (ng/ml) Yang assay (Hybritech assay)	Digital rectal examination	
	positive	negative
0.0–7.3 (0.0–4.0)	a	c
7.4–18.4 (4.1–10.0)	a	c
>18.4 (>10.0)	a	b

[a]Transrectal ultrasound (TRUS) guided biopsies
[b]TRUS guided systematic biopsies (Hodge *et al,* 1989)
[c]Follow-up (PSA and digital rectal examination)

other words, there is a progressive dedifferentiation of prostate cancer with time (ie tumour volume; Cumming *et al,* 1990). The data in Table 2 are in keeping with this concept; median Gleason score increases with higher clinical stages and increasing PSA values. Recently, Chodak *et al* (1994) pooled and analysed six non-randomized studies on patients with clinically localized prostate cancer whose disease was managed conservatively. The disease specific survival after 10 years was 87% for patients with histological grades 1 and 2 and dropped to 34% in untreated patients with grade 3. The favourable outcome of patients with grades 1 and 2 cancers may be explained by smaller tumour volumes and the long doubling time of these tumours.

Furthermore, our findings regarding serial PSA elevations may be important in making decisions about the group of patients identified as having PSA values in a borderline elevated range (Yang, Bellevue, WA, 7.4–18.4 ng/ml; Hybritech, San Diego, CA, 4.1–10.0 ng/ml) with a negative digital rectal examination (Table 3). These patients may currently require extensive and expensive additional studies. Following up such patients with serial PSA determinations on a yearly basis appears to be a prudent alternative (Schmid, 1994), given all the available information we now have about the natural history of prostate cancer.

Caution is warranted, however, for clinical judgment of prostate cancer that is accompanied by large amounts of BPH. Assuming the average rise in serum PSA caused by 1 cc of BPH to be 0.3 ng/ml (Stamey *et al,* 1987), it is determined that the greater the amount of BPH, the more likely the doubling time of the cancer will be overestimated (Fig. 4). This effect of BPH is critical primarily at lower PSA concentrations. The clinical importance of this observation is obvious. When following the doubling time of any prostate cancer by sequential measurement of serum PSA, the clinician should have an estimate of prostate size. The smaller the gland, the more accurately changes in PSA reflect the true doubling time of prostate cancer.

SUMMARY

Evidence is presented that cancer which is clinically confined to the prostate follows a predictable natural course. Biological aggressiveness of prostate cancer is directly related to tumour volume, and tumour volume is proportional to serum prostate specific antigen (PSA). Thus, the increase in PSA with time in patients on deferred treatment should reflect the growth rate (doubling time) of prostate cancer.

In 43 untreated patients with prostatic carcinomas, serum PSA was serially determined over an average time span of 30 months. Log-PSA values were plotted versus time, tested for linearity and compared between different clinical stages and histological grades.

The increase in serum PSA was exponential (log-linear) throughout the measured interval. This linearity allowed us to calculate a PSA doubling time. For clinically localized cancers, the median doubling time was 4 years. Doubling times were faster in patients with higher clinical stages and worse histological grades. Tumour doubling times were overestimated in patients with large volume benign prostatic hyperplasia, since hyperplasia also increases serum PSA, albeit 12 times less than cancer.

We conclude that prostate cancer follows a constant (log-linear) growth pattern with a doubling time that is very slow. This extraordinarily long doubling time may explain the favourable outcome of patients with low grade tumours on deferred treatment. Furthermore, this slow doubling time has important implications for early detection of prostate cancer.

References

Chodak GW, Thisted RA, Gerber GS *et al* (1994) Results of conservative management of clinically localized prostate cancer. *New England Journal of Medicine* **330** 242–248

Cumming JA, Ritchie AWS, Goodman CM, McIntyre MA and Chisholm GD (1990) De-differentiation with time in prostate cancer and the influence of treatment on the course of the disease. *British Journal of Urology* **65** 271–274

Hodge KK, McNeal JE, Terris MK and Stamey TA (1989) Random systematic versus directed ultrasound guided transrectal core biopsies of the prostate. *Journal of Urology* **142** 71–75

McNeal JE, Bostwick DG, Kindrachuk RA, Redwine EA, Freiha FS and Stamey TA (1986) Patterns of progression in prostate cancer. *Lancet* **i** 60–63

McNeal JE, Villers AA, Redwine EA, Freiha FS and Stamey TA (1990) Histologic differentiation, cancer volume, and pelvic lymph node metastasis in adenocarcinoma of the prostate. *Cancer* **66** 1225–1233

Schmid H-P (1994) *The Clinically Organ-confined Adenocarcinoma of the Prostate: Natural History, Selection Criteria for Radical Prostatectomy and Prognostic Factors Based on Long-term Follow up*, Steinkopff-Verlag, Darmstadt, Germany

Schmid H-P, McNeal JE and Stamey TA (1993) Observations on the doubling time of prostate cancer: the use of serial prostate-specific antigen in patients with untreated disease as a measure of increasing cancer volume. *Cancer* **71** 2031–2040

Stamey TA, Yang N, Hay AR, McNeal JE, Freiha FS and Redwine E (1987) Prostate-specific antigen as a serum marker for adenocarcinoma of the prostate. *New England Journal of Medicine* **317** 909–916

Stamey TA, Kabalin JN, McNeal JE *et al* (1989) Prostate specific antigen in the diagnosis and treatment of adenocarcinoma of the prostate: II radical prostatectomy treated patients. *Journal of Urology* **141** 1076–1083

Stamey TA, Freiha FS, McNeal JE, Redwine EA, Whittemore AS and Schmid H-P (1993) Localized prostate cancer: relationship of tumor volume to clinical significance for treatment of prostate cancer. *Cancer* **71** 933–938

The author is responsible for the accuracy of the references.

Endocrine Treatment of Metastatic Disease

Hormone Therapy: An Overview

P H SMITH
Department of Urology, St James's Hospital, Leeds LS9 7TF

INTRODUCTION

After the introduction of hormonal therapy for carcinoma of the prostate in the early 1940s (Coltham, 1941; Huggins and Hodges, 1941), the outlook for the patient with prostate cancer was greatly improved. His bone pain was relieved, at least for a time, and his urinary symptoms decreased. However, it was quickly recognized that up to 20% of tumours were are not responsive to hormone therapy and that treatment of patients with hormone responsive tumours was palliative rather than curative. For an elderly patient, this meant that the probability of dying from another cause during a period of remission was increased; for the young patient, it merely meant that his inevitable death from his disease process was postponed.

In patients who did not respond and in those in whom relapse occurred, increasing doses of oestrogens were used, often combined with orchidectomy. Doses of stilboestrol up to 100 mg daily were recommended (Ferguson, 1970).

In 1960, the Veterans Administration Cooperative Urological Research Group (VACURG) decided to evaluate oestrogen therapy and orchidectomy in a scientific way. In their first trial, which compared placebo (as initial therapy) + stilboestrol 5 mg daily, orchidectomy and orchidectomy plus stilboestrol 5 mg daily, no survival advantage was seen for immediate treatment (Veterans Administration Cooperative Urological Research Group, 1967). This disturbing finding was compounded by the discovery that stilboestrol 5 mg daily was associated with a significant risk of cardiovascular complications, including death from cardiovascular disease. This risk was seen especially in patients who did not have metastases at the time of first diagnosis. The cardiovascular death rate in these patients was 42% compared with 35% in those who did not receive oestrogen—a 20% difference.

These findings immediately led to other VACURG studies and to the development of other groups that investigated alternative approaches to therapy. Major contributions came from the Urological Group of the European Organisation for Research on the Treatment of Cancer (EORTC) and from the National Prostate cancer Project (NPCP) (see below).

EVALUATION OF ALTERNATIVE TREATMENTS

In the early 1970s, the treatment options included various doses of oestrogens, orchidectomy, estramustine phosphate, the first anti-androgen (cyproterone acetate) and medroxyprogesterone acetate (MPA). The VACURG investigated the effect of different oestrogens and MPA, the EORTC Urological Group committed itself to an evaluation of all the alternative hormonal agents and the NPCP chose to evaluate the role of cytotoxic agents in cancer of the prostate.

VACURG

The second and third studies of the VACURG compared different doses of stilboestrol and evaluated conjugated oestrogens. In the second VACURG study, patients were treated with placebo or with stilboestrol at doses of 0.2, 1 and 5 mg daily, whereas in the third VACURG study, patients were randomized to receive conjugated oestrogens 2.5 mg, MPA 30 mg, stilboestrol 1 mg or MPA 30 mg + stilboestrol 1 mg (Table 1).

The second VACURG study showed that stilboestrol 1 mg daily was as effective as 5 mg daily, but with fewer cardiovascular side effects. In the third study, conjugated oestrogens were found to be less effective than stilboestrol (Byar, 1973, 1978).

NPCP

In the early 1970s pressure from the then President Nixon led to the funding of national research programmes designed to cure certain cancers. One of these programmes was devoted to prostate cancer. As the NPCP developed, so the work of the VACURG came to an end. The NPCP evaluated the place of chemotherapy in patients with advanced disease and in those with newly diagnosed prostate cancer. The group undertook a large number of trials. The results of some of these trials for advanced disease are shown in Table 2 and those for newly diagnosed patients are shown in Table 3 (Smith, 1986).

High response rates were initially reported in patients with advanced dis-

TABLE 1. Entry into VACURG clinical trials for patients with extracapsular local disease or metastases

	Study 1a		Study 2b		Study 3c	
Stage	No	Treatment	No	Treatment	No	Treatment
III	216	Pcb	75	Pcb	140	Conj oestr (2.5 mg)
	264	DES (5 mg)	73	DES (0.2 mg)	136	MPA (30 mg)
	55	Orch	73	DES (1 mg)	134	MPA + DES (1 mg)
	266	Orch + Pcb	73	DES (5 mg)	135	DES (1 mg)
	258	Orch + DES (5 mg)				
IV	223	Pcb	53	Pcb	123	Conj oestr (2.5 mg)
	211	DES (5 mg)	52	DES (0.2 mg)	119	MPA (30 mg)
	57	Orch	55	DES (1 mg)	117	MPA + DES (1 mg)
	203	Orch + Pcb	54	DES (5 mg)	119	DES (1 mg)
	216	Orch + DES (5 mg)				

Conj oestr = conjugated oestrogens; DES = diethylstilboestrol; MPA = medoxyprogesterone acetate; Orch = bilateral orchidectomy; Pcb = placebo
[a]Patients admitted from March 1960 to March 1967
[b]Patients admitted from April 1967 to May 1969
[c]Patients admitted from June 1969 to September 1975

ease. Unfortunately, however, these good results stemmed from a decision to group complete response, partial response and stable disease as "objective response". This fallacy led to considerable confusion and eventually to the recognition that chemotherapy as used by the NPCP had contributed little if anything to the management of patients with prostate cancer. Once the essentially negative outcome of these trials was apparent to all, no further studies were commissioned.

EORTC Urological Group

This group has undertaken a number of clinical trials (Table 4). In the first two studies (protocols 30761 and 30762), stilboestrol 1 mg three times daily, which produced castration levels of testosterone (Robinson and Thomas, 1991), was evaluated against estramustine phosphate, cyproterone acetate and MPA. None of the alternative agents showed any survival advantage over stilboestrol; in fact, MPA was worse than the other agents. It was also clear that even 3 mg of stilboestrol daily was associated with cardiovascular hazard (de Voogt *et al,* 1986; Pavone-Macaluso *et al,* 1986; Smith *et al,* 1986; de Voogt *et al,* 1986).

The incidence of cardiovascular complications in patients given stilboestrol was 30% in the patients in protocol 30762 but only 2.7% in protocol 30761, in which study the incidence of cardiovascular side effects of cyproterone acetate was 4%. The reason for this enormous discrepancy has never been explained.

TABLE 2. Results of some NPCP trials using chemotherapy for patients with advanced disease

Protocol no	Evaluable patients	Randomized to treatment	% Response CR + PR	% Response ("objective response")
Without prior irradiation				
100	110	Standard	19	19
		CTX 1 g/m^2 every 3 weeks	7	46
		5FU 600 mg/m^2 weekly	12	36
300	129	CTX 1 g/m^2 every 3 weeks	–	26
		DTIC 200 mg/m^2 daily x 5 every 3 weeks	4	28
		PCB 100 mg/m^2 daily x 21 every 6 weeks	–	13
700	98	CTX 1 g/m^2 every 3 weeks	7[a]	35
		MeCCNU 175 mg/m^2 every 6 weeks	4	30
		HU 3 g/m^2 every 3 days	8[a]	15
With prior irradiation				
200	105	CTX	–	19
		EST	2	31
		Streptozotocin 500 mg/m^2 daily x 5 every 6 weeks	–	32
400	116	EST + prednimustine 300 mg daily	2	13
		Prednimustine 300 mg daily	–	13
800	90	EST	4	26
		VCR 1 mg/m^2 every 2 weeks	3	15
		EST + VCR	–	24
1200	115	EST	–	18
		CDDP 60 mg/m^2 every 4 weeks	–	21
		EST + CDDP	–	33

CDDP = cisplatinum; CTX = cyclophosphamide; DTIC = imidazole carboxamide dimethyl triazone; EST = estramustine phosphate; 5FU = 5 fluorouracil; HU = hydroxurea; MeCCN = methylchloroethylcyclohexynitrosourea; PCB = procarbazine; Standard = varying forms of palliative therapy; VCR = vincristine

[a]Includes one patient with complete response

In protocol 30761, most patients came from Italy, France, Holland and Belgium, whereas in protocol 30762, the vast majority came from the UK. Since the publication of these studies, the emphasis has always been on the high incidence of complications in the one study, rather than on any reason why there should have been a difference between the two studies.

In the next group of studies, total androgen ablation in one form or another was tested against monotherapy with stilboestrol 1 mg daily (in one study) and orchidectomy (in two studies). In the first two studies (protocols 30805 and 30843), no survival advantage was seen for any treatment arm (Klijn *et al*, 1993; Robinson, 1993), but cardiovascular side effects were still seen in some patients receiving stilboestrol therapy.

TABLE 3. Results of some NPCP trials using chemotherapy for patients with newly diagnosed metastatic disease

Protocol no	Evaluable patients	Randomized to treatment	% Response CR + PR	% Response ("objective response")
500	246	DES/orch	38	81
		DES + CTX 1 g/m^2 every 2 weeks	34	89
		CTX + EST 600 mg/m^2 daily	27	83
1300	286	DES/orch	15	79
		EST 600 mg/m^2 daily	14	76
		DES/orch + CTX 650 mg/m^2 every 3 weeks + 5FU 350 mg/m^2 weekly	15	79

CTX = standard chemotherapy; DES = diethylstilboestrol 1 mg tds; EST = estra-mustine phosphate; 5FU = 5-fluorouracil; orch = orchidectomy

The gradually increasing focus on the cardiovascular side effects of stilboestrol led to the notion that orchidectomy is the gold standard of therapy. This notion was completely illogical but nevertheless reassured every urologist at the time. We had no sooner come to repeat this mantra on a daily basis than Labrie introduced "total androgen ablation" with the combination of an anti-gonadotropin agent and an anti-androgen. This concept was initially decried, was later resisted with vigour and is now regarded as "the best treatment" by many.

TABLE 4. Randomized trials of the EORTC Urological Group for patients with advanced prostatic cancer for which results are available

Patients	Treatment	Survival difference
Monotherapy:		
Protocol 30761	CPA 250 mg daily	NS
T2-4 MO, TX M1	MPA	
Protocol 30762	estramustine phosphate	NS
T2-4 MO, TX M1	DES 1 mg tds	
Androgen Ablation:		
Protocol 30805	orchidectomy	NS
TX, NX, M1	DES 1 mg daily	
	orchidectomy + CPA 60 mg tds	
Protocol 30843	orchidectomy	NS
TX, NX, M1	buserelin (+ CPA for 2 weeks only)	
	buserelin + CPA 50 mg tds	
Protocol 30853	orchidectomy	7 month survival advantage for goserelin, flutamide
TX, NX, M1	goserelin 36 mg every 28 days + flutamide 250 mg tds	

CPA = cyproterone acetate; DES = diethylstilboestrol; MPA = medroxyprogesterone acetate; NS = no significant difference

The last major study of the EORTC group compared total androgen ablation (goserelin and flutamide) against orchidectomy (protocol 30853) (Denis *et al,* 1993). This study showed a survival advantage of approximately 7 months for the combined therapy, but in my view at least, it is somewhat marred by the fact that, on progression following orchidectomy, only 19% of patients received the next logical therapy—that is, an anti-androgen. This study therefore compared monotherapy versus total androgen ablation in the vast majority of patients, rather than total androgen ablation at diagnosis versus monotherapy followed by total androgen ablation on progression.

National Cancer Institute Intergroup Study

As the NPCP evolved from the VACURG, so the National Cancer Institute (NCI) grouping has evolved from the NPCP. Its first contribution had a major impact. In this study, patients were randomized to receive leuprolide (leuprorelin) (a luteinizing hormone releasing hormone [LHRH] analogue) or leuprolide + flutamide. The combined treatment showed a survival advantage of 7.3 months, this being limited to patients with minimal disease (metastases confined to the axial skeleton and pelvis) and to those with more extensive disease but with a good performance status (Crawford *et al,* 1989).

Unfortunately, an unexpectedly large number of deaths occurred in the first 3–6 months. A similar "shoulder", demonstrating early progression in the LHRH arm, had been seen in protocol 1700 of the NPCP study (Hubon *et al,* 1988), and as Crawford observed in an analysis of the NCI study (Crawford *et al,* 1989), it remains to be seen whether the survival advantage in this study was due to the combined therapy or was a consequence of an increase in the early death rate following LHRH therapy alone, which is known to stimulate the tumour by increasing the plasma testosterone during the first 2–3 weeks (known as the "flare phenomenon"). The same group is now recruiting 1200 patients to a study in which orchidectomy will be compared with orchidectomy + flutamide; this should clarify the issue.

As might be expected, urologists who have given up stilboestrol because of its cardiovascular side effects and who have clung (illogically) to orchidectomy as the "gold standard" have been quick to seek salvation in the potential bene-

TABLE 5. Approximate costs of hormonal therapy in the UK (Parmar et al, 1994)

Weekly costs (assuming median survival 2 years)	
Aspirin 75 mg (£0.02)	
Stilboestrol 1 mg (£0.95)	£1
Orchidectomy	£20
LHRH	£30
Anti-androgen	£30
Androgen ablation	£60

fits offered by total androgen ablation. The possibility of improved survival does, however, involve considerable financial cost and impairment of quality of life from the side effects of flutamide, the anti-androgen now increasingly used. Nevertheless, no pharmaceutical company is likely to wish to reverse this trend, and no lawyer can make a reasonable claim that his client's treatment was inadequate if both forms of treatment have been given.

THE PRESENT SITUATION

Urologists can now offer the patient treatment with:

- An anti-androgen, either the steroidal anti-androgen cyproterone acetate (which has some anti-gonadotropic function) or a non-steroidal anti-androgen (flutamide or nilutamide). Other non-steroidal anti-androgens including casodex may become available.
- Total androgen ablation, in which an anti-gonadotropic agent is combined with an anti-androgen. If this treatment is chosen, it is almost certainly safer to give the anti-androgen for at least 7 days before the first injection of the LHRH analogue to minimize disease flare.
- Follow-up with treatment on progression, that is, deferred therapy. This approach has yet to be proved inferior to immediate treatment for patients without symptoms.
- An anti-gonadotropic agent (stilboestrol, orchidectomy, other oestrogenic agents).

Anti-androgens as Monotherapy

A case can be made for the use of an anti-androgen as initial treatment, especially for patients with asymptomatic metastatic disease with good prognostic factors. Such a trial is already under way within the EORTC group (protocol 30892) and compares cyproterone acetate with flutamide. This protocol has recruited more than 200 patients, but no information is yet available. Such a study might lead to the choice of a preferred anti-androgen and to a clearer recognition of the concept of sequential combination therapy. The implications for both cost and quality of life would be considerable.

Meta-analysis of Total Androgen Ablation

A meta-analysis of total anti-androgen ablation has now been published (Denis and Murphy, 1993). This clearly shows that in trials in which the comparisons were LHRH versus LHRH + anti-androgen, orchidectomy versus orchidectomy + anti-androgen or orchidectomy versus LHRH analogue + anti-androgen, there was no significant difference in overall survival for any of these groups. The impairment of quality of life with such therapy is considerable and the financial cost high (Table 5).

Deferred Therapy

Most patients with prostate cancer are elderly, and of those presenting with clinical symptoms, fewer than one third die from their tumour. The recognition that most deaths in elderly patients with prostate cancer are from other causes and that treatment inevitably impairs quality of life without offering a cure has led many urologists to question whether treatment at diagnosis is mandatory. The VACURG study did not show any advantage for immediate rather than deferred treatment, and this concept is now being investigated again both by the EORTC and by the UK's Medical Research Council (MRC). The EORTC's trial of immediate or delayed orchidectomy or LHRH therapy (with 2 weeks of cyproterone acetate) is restricted to patients with asymptomatic non-metastatic prostate cancer (EORTC protocol 30891); the MRC study also compares immediate or delayed orchidectomy or LHRH but includes patients with asymptomatic metastases and those with non-metastatic disease.

The EORTC study has now recruited more than 300 patients and the MRC study has recruited more than 800 patients. An answer to this basic question should emerge by the end of this decade. If immediate therapy is not associated with any survival advantage, the implications for the patient, the community and the medical profession are clear.

Oestrogens Today

Although oestrogens are unpopular, there is no doubt that stilboestrol is more effective in lowering testosterone and in postponing death from cancer than is orchidectomy or any other treatment so far tested. Because of this, urologists have suggested the possibility of systemic oestrogen therapy, which is thought to be less cardiotoxic. This is being investigated, especially in Finland and Sweden, where the recommended treatment is polyestradiol phosphate estradurin 240 mg per month (a 6 ml intramuscular injection). In addition, intermittent therapy has been postulated as an alternative, this being introduced initially in 1974 (Eisen *et al,* 1974). Studies in animals suggest that intermittent anti-gonadotropic therapy may be of value for a time in that tumour suppression will occur following tumour implantation on three or four successive occasions if the animal is castrated after the tumour has been transplanted and allowed to grow. After four transplants, however, the tumour tends to become independent (Akakura *et al,* 1993).

It is also of interest to review the degree of cardiovascular toxicity found in patients treated with oestrogen. The excess mortality in the first VACURG study was approximately 20% and was largely confined to patients with non-metastatic disease (Veterans Administration Cooperative Urological Research Group, 1967). In three relevant protocols of the EORTC (protocols 30761, 30762 and 30805), the information is also interesting. In the first place, we have never explained the enormous difference (2.7% v. 30% complications) between protocols 30761 and 30762. Secondly, in protocol 30762, the recog-

TABLE 6. Incidence (%) of pre-existing cardiovascular disease according to treatment group in EORTC protocol 30805

	Orchidectomy	Orchidectomy + cyproterone acetate	Stilboestrol
Total	21.8	21.6	30.8
Hypertension	12.7	9.9	17.8
Ischaemic heart disease	5.5	6.3	10.3
Angina	2.7	6.3	7.5
Infarction	4.5	2.7	7.5
Deep vein thrombosis	0.9	1.8	2.8
Cerebrovascular accident	0.9	1.8	1.9

nized increase in death from cardiovascular disease was neither exclusive to nor dominant in those with the existing cardiovascular disease at entry. There was no difference between the two treatment arms, and no cardiovascular deaths occurred in the 29 patients aged under 60 years or in the 28 aged over 80.

In addition, in protocol 30805, in which a dose of 1 mg of stilboestrol daily was used, there was a 50% excess of pre-existing cardiovascular disease in the patients receiving stilboestrol (Table 6). Analysis of the cardiovascular deaths showed that the excess cardiovascular mortality was seen not in the patients with pre-existing cardiovascular disease but in those without it.

If the death rate from cardiovascular disease in patients receiving stilboestrol could be reduced, a survival benefit of 20% might emerge. Such an improvement is equivalent to that seen in the recent NCI and EORTC trials from total androgen ablation.

Reduction of Cardiovascular Side Effects following Treatment with Stilboestrol

The VACURG showed that oral treatment with 1 mg stilboestrol daily was as effective as 5 mg but less toxic, whereas 0.2 mg was ineffective. We also know from protocol 30805 that there is cardiovascular toxicity with 1 mg daily, mainly in patients without cardiovascular disease at entry to the study. The possible use of intermittent therapy or systemic treatment has been referred to above, and other possibilities to reduce cardiovascular complications must also be considered.

Aspirin is increasingly used in patients who are liable to vascular thrombosis. It is simple, cheap and safe in those not subject to peptic ulceration or other diseases likely to lead to bleeding. In the past, it has always been suggested that although this drug might be suitable for those with arterial stenoses (whether leading to transient ischaemic attacks, in those following coronary thrombosis or following coronary artery surgery), the drug was not of general value because it did not reduce the incidence of deep vein thrombosis or pulmonary embolism.

Such conventional views were widely held by surgeons, physicians and clinical haematologists. They have been shaken, however, by three papers (Antiplatelet Trialists' Collaboration, 1994a,b,c) that have shown clearly a 30% reduction in incidence of heart attack and stroke and a 15% reduction in the death rate in patients treated with aspirin, together with a 25% reduction in incidence of venous thrombosis and a 40% reduction in incidence of pulmonary embolism. These studies were carried out in many thousands of patients and offer the opportunity for a re-evaluation of oral oestrogen therapy, now combined with aspirin. This is just the project that the VACURG wished to undertake 20 years ago as their fourth and fifth studies at the time that their funding was withdrawn and the NPCP developed.

The logic for further assessment of oral oestrogens with aspirin appears inescapable, since oestrogens are the most effective agents and, in the absence of cardiovascular toxicity, should demonstrate a 20% increase in survival.

SUMMARY

Hormonal treatment of prostate cancer has advanced little in the past 20 years. Total androgen ablation may offer a 20% survival advantage when compared with monotherapy, as might the use of stilboestrol if its cardiovascular side-effects could be abolished with aspirin or some other agent. Neither approach, however, is likely to lead to a cure. Currently available cytotoxic chemotherapy appears to offer little survival advantage. There is an urgent need for the development of other treatments.

Acknowledgement

I should like to thank Miss Diane Roberts for her help with preparing the manuscript.

References

Akakura K, Bruchovsky N, Goldenberg SL *et al* (1993) Effects of intermittent androgen suppression on androgen-dependent tumours. *Cancer* **71** 2782–2790

Antiplatelet Trialists' Collaboration (1994a) Collaborative overview of randomised trials of antiplatelet therapy, I, Prevention of death, myocardial infarction and stroke by prolonged antiplatelet therapy in various categories of patients. *British Medical Journal* **308** 81–106

Antiplatelet Trialists' Collaboration (1994b) Collaborative overview of randomised trials of antiplatelet therapy, II, Maintenance of vascular graft or arterial patency by antiplatelet therapy. *British Medical Journal* **308** 159–168

Antiplatelet Trialists' Collaboration (1994c) Collaborative overview of randomised trials of antiplatelet therapy, III, Reduction in versus thrombosis and pulmonary embolism by antiplatelet prophylaxis among surgical and medical patients. *British Medical Journal* **308** 235–246

Byar DP (1973) The Veterans Administration Cooperation Urological Research Group's studies of cancer of the prostate. *Cancer* **32** 1126–1130

Byar DP (1978) Review of the Veterans Administration studies of cancer of the prostate and new results concerning treatment of stage I and II tumours, In: Pavone-Macaluso M, Smith PH and Esdmyr F (eds). *Bladder Tumours and Other Topics in Urological Oncology*, p

475, Plenum Press, New York

Coltham S (1941) Studies on prostate cancer, III, The effects of fever, of desoxhycorticosterone and of estrogen on clinical patients with metastatic carcinoma of the prostate. *Journal of Urology* **46** 997–1006

Crawford ED, Eisenberger MA, McLeod DG *et al* (1989) A comparison of leuprolide with and without flutamide in previously untreated patients with disseminated prostate carcinoma: a placebo controlled study. *New England Journal of Medicine* **321** 419–424

Denis L and Murphy GP (1993) Overview of phase III trials on combined androgen treatment in patients with metastatic prostatic cancer. *Cancer* **72 (Supplement 12)** 3888–3895

Denis LJ, Whelan P and Carneiro de Moura JL (1993) Goserelin acetate and flutamide versus bilateral orchidectomy: a phase III EORTC trial (30853). *Urology* **42** 119–129

de Voogt HJ, Smith PH, and Pavone-Macaluso M (1956) Cardiovascular side effects of diethylstilboestrol, cyproterone acetate, medroxyprogesterone acetate and estramustine phosphate used for the treatment of advanced prostatic cancer: results from European Organization for Research on Treatment of Cancer trials 30761 and 30762. *Journal of Urology* **135** 303–307

Eisen M, Napp HE, and Vock R (1974) Thrombocytere-aggregationshemming bei oestrogenbehandelten prostata-carcinoma-patients. *Urologe* **A14** 132–136

Ferguson JD (1970) Cancer of the prostate II. *British Medical Journal* **4** 512–514

Hubon RP, Murphy GP and National Prostate Cancer Project (1988) A comparison of diethylstilboestrol or orchidectomy with buserelin and methotrexate plus diethylstilbestrol or orchidectomy in newly diagnosed patients with clinical stage D2 cancer of the prostate. *Cancer* **62** 1881–1887

Huggins C and Hodges CV (1941) Studies on prostatic cancer, I, The effect of castration of estrogen and the androgen injection on serum phosphatases in metastatic carcinoma of the prostate. *Cancer Research* **1** 293–297

Klijn JGM, de Voogt HJ, Studer E *et al* (1993) Short term versus long term addition of cyproterone acetate to Buserelin therapy in comparison with orchidectomy in the treatment of metastatic prostatic cancer. *Cancer* **72 (Supplement)** 3858–3862

Parmar H, Bottomley D, Hanham IW *et al* (1994) Cost benefit analysis of the treatment options for advanced prostate cancer. *Urology Topics* **11** 124–126

Pavone-Macaluso M, de Voogt HJ, Viggiano G *et al* (1986) Comparison of diethylstilboestrol, cyproterone acetate and medroxyprogestrone acetate in the treatment of advanced prostate cancer: final analysis of a randomised phase III trial of the EORTC GU group. *Journal of Urology* **136** 624–631

Robinson MRG (1993) A further analysis of European Organisation for Research and Treatment of Cancer protocol 30805: orchidectomy versus orchidectomy plus cyproterone acetate versus low dose diethylstilboestrol. *Cancer* **72 (Supplement)** 3855–3857

Robinson MRG and Thomas BS (1991) Effect of hormonal therapy on plasma testosterone levels in prostatic carcinoma. *British Medical Journal* **4** 391–394

Smith PH (1986) Cancer of the prostate, In: Slevin MC and Staquet MJ (eds). *Randomised Trials in Cancer: A Critical Review by Sites*, pp 605–630 Raven Press, New York

Smith PH, Suciu S and Robinson MRG (1986) A comparison of the effect of diethylstilboestrol with low dose estramustine phosphate in the treatment of advanced prostate cancer: final analysis of a phase III trial of the European Organization for Research on Treatment of Cancer. *Journal of Urology* **136** 619–623

Veterans Administration Cooperative Urological Research Group (1967) Treatment and survival of patients with cancer of the prostate. *Surgery, Gynecology and Obstetrics* **124** 1011–1017

The author is responsible for the accuracy of the references.

Immediate versus Deferred Treatment for Advanced Disease

DAVID KIRK
Department of Urology, Western Infirmary, Glasgow G11 6NT

INTRODUCTION

Although it is over half a century since Huggins first recognized the hormonal dependence of prostate cancer (Huggins and Hodges, 1941), hormonal therapy still provides the only real chance of influencing the course of the disease once it is too advanced for local treatment (Resnick and Grayhack, 1965). Any response will be temporary, with relapse occurring usually within 2 years in patients with metastases. Although radiotherapy and other palliative measures may then be helpful in relieving symptoms, relapse after hormone therapy usually is fatal within a matter of months (Beynon and Chisholm, 1984). It seems sensible that the use of hormonal therapy be timed to achieve maximum benefit.

THE CONCEPT OF DEFERRED TREATMENT

Treatment of advanced prostate cancer at diagnosis will delay the onset of symptoms and may well prolong survival, although this is not inevitably so (Lepor *et al,* 1982). Alternatively, the patient may be treated when symptoms occur, and if he responds, a further symptom free period will follow, with possibly a similar survival. Any side effects resulting from treatment will occur for

Cancer Surveys Volume 23: *Preventing Prostate Cancer: Screening versus Chemoprevention*
 0-87969-466-1/95. $5.00 + .00

a shorter period of time, and an elderly patient might die from an unrelated cause before the development of symptoms requiring treatment. Thus, unless early treatment can be shown to have advantages, deferment until an indication arises might be preferable (Kirk, 1987). As new and more expensive methods of androgen deprivation are introduced, an economic aspect also enters the argument.

CHANGING VIEWS: THE HISTORICAL DEBATE

Which patients require treatment and when treatment should be started remain key issues. They have been discussed since the inception of hormonal therapy and have yet to be resolved. Initial tentative use of deferred treatment was swept away in 1950 for some 25 years by the confident belief that the use of hormonal therapy prolonged the patient's life and that the benefit was greater the earlier it was started (Nesbit and Baum, 1950). These apparent benefits of hormonal treatment came from comparing the survival of hormone treated patients with that of patients managed before hormonal therapy was available—that is, historical controls (Nesbit and Plumb, 1946). The Veterans Administration Cooperative Research Group (VACURG) studies included randomized control groups treated initially with a placebo but started on active treatment on progression, without apparent compromise to their survival (Byar, 1973). Reviewing the data, Byar stated: "These data support the concept that treatment can be delayed ...". Recently, there has been more doubt about the justification for deferring hormonal therapy. This results partly from Crawford and colleagues' (1989) observation that if total androgen ablation is more effective than monotherapy, the difference is most marked in those with least disease. The argument that to defer treatment is to allow the tumour to lose its hormone sensitivity is similar to that used by Nesbit and Baum in 1950. On the other hand, a review of the records of patients with prostate cancer treated at Johns Hopkins Hospital immediately before and immediately after the introduction of hormonal treatment could not demonstrate any increase in life expectancy attributable to its use (Lepor *et al,* 1982). This has led to the view that hormonal therapy has no effect on survival. However, some patients present with life threatening conditions such as ureteric obstruction response of which to treatment must save life. What is in doubt is whether a further prolongation of life would have resulted if treatment could have been started at an earlier stage of the disease (Kirk, 1991).

THE SYMPTOM FREE PATIENT

The indications for hormonal treatment in patients presenting with painful metastatic disease and other manifestations of advanced prostate cancer are fairly clear (Catalona and Scott, 1986). However, in many patients, no immediate benefit would seem to accrue from hormonal treatment. Examples are patients presenting with outflow obstruction readily managed by transurethral prostate resection, with no metastases or with metastases that are not a source of symptoms, and patients with confined disease in whom a positive pelvic lymph node biopsy has ruled out radical local treatment. Arguments can be advanced either for starting hormonal treatment immediately or for its deferment until unquestionable need arises. Paradoxically, although early treatment might seem to be most important in the younger patient, he is just the one who may be most upset by the resulting loss of sexual function. Thus, if no disadvantage could be found from delaying treatment, there would seem to be every reason for so doing.

THE CASE FOR EARLY TREATMENT

Cancer therapy is generally more effective the smaller the tumour bulk. Since deferring treatment will allow tumour growth to continue, it does seem sensible to start any treatment as soon as possible. Hormonal treatment is not quite the same as cytotoxic chemotherapy or radiotherapy, which are usually administered for a finite period with a view to destroying all or a significant portion of the tumour. Androgen deprivation requires continuous administration, during which it controls rather than eliminates the tumour and could be less dependent on tumour bulk. However, hormonal therapy differs in another respect: relapse results from loss of hormone sensitivity, some tumours are hormone insensitive at presentation and varying sensitivity will produce greater or lesser responses in others. Does a prostate tumour become less hormone sensitive as it progresses? This important question has once more been posed by Crawford *et al* (1989) in their study of total androgen ablation, in which better response rates occurred in patients presenting with less advanced disease—the "minimal disease group" defined as those with metastases confined to the axial skeleton. These are just the patients who might be considered most suitable for deferred treatment. If these results are correct, leaving such patients until their disease became more advanced might reduce their response to that of the more advanced patients in the trial—in other words, deferring treatment will reduce the response to treatment when eventually it is started. Alternatively, it could well be the nature of the most hormone sensitive tumour to present at an early stage, and allowing that tumour to progress might not compromise its hormone sensitivity. Trials ask and seek to answer questions. They can only satisfactorily answer the question they were designed to answer. Crawford's group set out to compare the responses to total androgen ablation and conventional treatment, a totally different problem from the timing of treatment.

The question of timing will be resolved largely on clinical evidence. Survival, the risk of complications such as spinal cord compression and subtle ill effects such as weight loss not recognized as "symptoms" are all possible factors favouring early treatment (Kirk, 1987). To resolve these issues requires a specifically designed clinical trial.

TABLE 1. MRC study of immediate versus deferred hormonal therapy. Interim data: principle indications for treatment in patients randomized to deferred treatment who subsequently have been treated

Treatment	No of patients[a]
Patients randomized to deferred treatment (with data available)	368
Patients treated (follow-up 1–6 yr)	222
Indications for deferred treatment	
Metastatic disease (pain in 91)	103
Local progression	101
Rising markers	22
General ill health	14
Bleeding	11
Patient's request	4

[a]In some patients, there was more than one reason for deferred treatment

MEDICAL RESEARCH COUNCIL STUDY

A study of deferred treatment conducted by the Medical Research Council (MRC) in Britain (Kirk, 1985) closed to recruitment at the end of 1993 with an entry of 938 patients. With advice from the Protocol Review Committee on the need for a further period of follow-up, its first report is expected during 1996, although longer follow-up may be needed to obtain a definitive result. Given the limited life expectation of most men with prostate cancer, many urologists now feel that treatment should be aimed as much at avoiding complications and symptoms as at prolonging survival, and this aspect is being monitored in the MRC study (Kirk, 1987). Although the immaturity of its data prevents any conclusion being drawn from the MRC trial about its main endpoints, some items of interest can be gleaned from the considerable amount of follow-up data already available. Table 1 gives the reasons for intervention in patients originally randomized to deferred treatment. It is interesting that local progression—usually the need to perform a (second) transurethral resection—is as common an indication for treatment as are symptoms or other problems from metastatic disease.

Patients entered into the study were stratified according to whether or not they had metastases (M_0 or M_1). Early follow-up returns indicated, not surprisingly, that M_1 patients allocated deferred treatment came to need treatment sooner than M_0 patients. However, interim analysis shows that 40% of M_1 patients remain untreated at 12 months, so that a substantial number of even those with metastases can be saved the undesirable effects of treatment for a useful period of time before an indication of treatment occurs. By comparison with the VACURG studies (Byar, 1973), where the patients were on average older, a much higher proportion of deaths are due to prostate cancer than to incidental causes (Table 2).

TABLE 2. Deaths in patients with advanced prostatic cancer: proportion of deaths due to carcinoma of prostate

	VACURG[a]	MRC[b]
Patients assessable	945	880
Patients dying	732	511
Deaths due to prostate cancer	283 (39%)	323–358[c] (63–70%)

[a]Data from Byar (1973): VACURG study 1, disease stages III and IV, non-oestrogen treated patients
[b]Interim data from MRC immediate versus deferred treatment study
[c]35 patients at present with cause of death unknown: range gives estimated minimum and maximum numbers of deaths due to carcinoma of prostate

TOTAL ANDROGEN ABLATION

If the final adjudication on total androgen ablation confirms its greater efficacy over conventional monotherapy, it could be argued that the MRC trial has become irrelevant because it has been investigating an "out of date treatment" (Crawford ED, personal communication). However, any benefit from total androgen ablation is unlikely to be of the order originally proposed by Labrie *et al* (1984), and although there may be quantitative benefits in terms of months to progression and survival, a qualitative therapeutic difference seems unlikely. Any beneficial effect or otherwise of immediate treatment emerging from the MRC study should apply equally to total androgen ablation, although a case might exist for a trial to confirm this.

If total androgen ablation does become the hormonal treatment of choice, it affects both the positive and the negative sides of the deferred versus immediate treatment argument. The use of anti-androgens introduces an additional range of potential side effects for the patient. There also is a considerable increase in expense, which will be substantial even if total androgen ablation is confined to those who are currently offered hormonal therapy. What would be the effects on drug bills if all the men at present managed by deferred treatment were suddenly to be started on both a luteinizing hormone releasing hormone analogue and a non-steroidal anti-androgen? Clearly, if this were the right management, this expense would have to be borne, but whether this is so is far from certain.

ROLE OF PROSTATE SPECIFIC ANTIGEN

As the use of prostate specific antigen (PSA) has become more widespread, rising tumour markers has become a commoner indication for abandoning deferred treatment in MRC trial patients (Table 1). A high PSA correlates with tumour progression (Armitage *et al,* 1988). In the author's own practice, the level of PSA, and more particularly its rate of change, is increasingly used in deciding if and when to treat a patient with prostate carcinoma. The use of PSA in assessing and monitoring patients in this way can reduce some of the concern about missing tumour progression in patients assigned to deferred treatment.

IMMEDIATE OR DEFERRED TREATMENT: THE CURRENT POSITION

The timing of treatment is unlikely to have a dramatic effect on survival, otherwise the current controversy would not exist. Indeed, immediate treatment is often advocated as much to avoid complications or catastrophes (such as paraplegia) or to improve the health of a patient with unrecognized non-specific effects from his tumour. These may be avoidable by careful assessment in selecting patients for deferred treatment and by subsequent close follow-up. This approach is now facilitated by the availability of PSA measurements. Any stated advantages of routine immediate treatment have to be balanced against the definite disadvantages. It is argued that the newer methods of hormonal therapy now available are more acceptable to the patient and the disadvantages less (Kozlowski *et al,* 1991). This is relative, with hot flushes and loss of potency still being significant problems for some men. It is true (Table 2) that as men live longer and are fitter, the chances of death from other causes occurring before treatment of their cancer is needed is much reduced, but equally as men live longer, there will be increasing numbers with carcinoma diagnosed at an age where deferred treatment may be desirable.

FUTURE RESEARCH

The MRC trial is unlikely to be the last word on this topic. The question of maximal androgen blockade, its timing and the timing of its individual components might merit future study. The role of PSA monitoring, which was not available when the MRC study began, needs closer scrutiny. If a method of androgen deprivation definitely devoid of significant side effects becomes available, its use as adjuvant treatment in all men with the disease, as with tamoxifen in breast cancer, would be worthy of a large scale trial.

DEFERRED TREATMENT IN CLINICAL PRACTICE

Deferring treatment restricts the period when the patient is prone to the undesirable effects of therapy and provides the satisfaction of seeing symptomatic benefit from treatment, but it must be emphasized that it is not the easy option. The risk that irreversible problems, even death, could occur before treatment is started is real but should be avoidable. Where treatment is deferred careful follow-up is essential; the patient and his general practitioner have to be fully aware of the situation, and the urologist willing and able to respond immediately to new developments. The situation is analogous to surveillance in men with stage 1 testicular teratoma, and when an appropriate level of supervision is not possible, deferred treatment should not be attempted. However, at least in selected patients, there do seem to be some advantages in this approach.

Suitable patients for deferred treatment are those with no immediate prospect of complication, and rigorous assessment must precede the decision. A large spinal metastasis that might lead to sudden paraplegia, mild anaemia, a recent history of weight loss and a large poorly differentiated tumour liable to reocclude the urethra or invade the rectum or ureters are all indications for treatment. However, all these situations could be covered by the term "symptom free disease". A man of 85 with a coincidental life threatening illness is clearly a different prospect from a fit 60 year old. The presenting level of PSA, and whether it is stable or rising, must also be taken into account. Once the patient has been fully assessed, in many instances, it is important to discuss the issue with the patient and his relatives. Patients increasingly wish to be involved in decisions about their own treatment, and this seems to be an area where that is particularly appropriate.

SUMMARY

The timing of hormonal treatment has been controversial for the last 50 years. The VACURG studies suggested that deferring treatment in symptom free patients might not compromise survival. Recent studies of maximal androgen blockade have revived an old observation that disease presenting earlier may be more hormone sensitive. The arguments in favour of immediate versus deferred treatment depend on the balance of advantages against side effects and costs, but a clear advantage in terms of survival from immediate treatment has yet to be demonstrated. An MRC study of this issue has recruited 1938 patients and should make its first report in 1996. Meanwhile, in many men, deferred treatment remains a valid management option, provided it is used with caution and careful follow-up.

References

Armitage TG, Cooper EH, Newling DWW, Robinson MRG and Appleyard I (1988) The value of measurements of serum prostate specific antigen in patients with benign prostatic hyperplasia and untreated prostate cancer. *British Journal of Urology* **62** 584–589

Beynon LL and Chisholm GD (1984) The stable state is not an objective response in hormone-escaped carcinoma of the prostate. *British Journal of Urology* **56** 702–705

Byar DP (1973) The Veterans Administration Cooperative Research Group's studies of cancer of the prostate. *Cancer* **32** 1126–1130

Catalona WJ and Scott WW (1986) Carcinoma of the prostate, In: Walsh PC, Gittes RE, Perlmutter AD and Stamey TA (eds). *Campbell's Urology*, pp 1463–1534, WB Saunders, Philadelphia

Crawford ED, Eisenberger MA, McLeod DG *et al* (1989) A controlled trial of leuprolide with and without flutamide in prostatic carcinoma. *New England Journal of Medicine* **321** 419–424

Huggins C and Hodges CV (1941) Studies in prostate cancer. 1. The effect of castration of oestrogen and of androgen injection on serum phosphatease in metastatic carcinoma of the prostate. *Cancer Research* **1** 293–297
Kirk D (1985) Prostatic carcinoma. *British Medical Journal* **290** 875–876
Kirk D (1987) Trials and tribulations in prostatic cancer. *British Journal of Urology* **59** 375–379
Kirk D (1991) Deferred treatment for advanced prostatic cancer, In: Waxman J and Williams G (eds). *Urological Oncology*, pp 117–125, Edward Arnold, Sevenoaks
Kozlowski JM, Ellis WJ and Grayhack JT (1991) Advanced prostatic carcinoma: early versus late endocrine therapy. *Urologic Clinics of North America* **15** 15–24
Labrie F, Belanger A, Dupont A, Emond J, Lacoursiere Y and Monfette G (1984) Combined treatment with LHRH agonist and pure antiandrogen in advanced carcinoma of prostate. *Lancet* **ii** 1090
Lepor Ross A and Walsh PC (1982) The influence of hormonal therapy on survival of men with advanced prostatic cancer. *Journal of Urology* **128** 335–340
Nesbit RM and Baum WC (1950) Endocrine control of prostatic cancer: clinical survey of 88 cases. *Journal of the American Medical Association* **143** 1317–1320
Nesbit RM and Plumb RT (1946) Prostatic carcinoma: a follow-up on 795 patients treated prior to the endocrine era and a comparison of survival rates between these and patients treated by endocrine therapy. *Surgery* **20** 263–272
Resnick MI and Grayhack JT (1965) Treatment of stage IV carcinoma of the prostate. *Urologic Clinics of North America* **2** 141–161

The author is responsible for the accuracy of the references.

Intermittent Endocrine Therapy and Its Potential for Chemoprevention of Prostate Cancer

R T D OLIVER • C J G GALLAGHER
Royal London Hospital Medical College, 1 Turner Street, London E1 2AD

INTRODUCTION

With society's increasing longevity, the excess of occult prostate cancer known to exist from autopsy studies (Breslow *et al,* 1977) is becoming a more significant cause of death as more people survive into old age. Most prostate cancer still presents to surgeons with symptoms of outflow obstruction, although occasional cases present to haematologists with a leucoerythroblastic anaemia, to rheumatologists with backache, to nephrologists with unexplained obstructive renal failure or to geriatricians with other problems of old age.

At the present time, there is no established place for either chemotherapy or immunotherapy in the routine management of these cases. As large numbers of patients have been entered into chemotherapy trials (Sher and Sternberg, 1985), the lack of value is clearly established; as virtually no work has been done on immunotherapy the question remains open. Hormone therapy is still accepted as first line medical treatment for metastatic disease. As experimental animals undergoing castration retain hormone sensitive stem cells, hormone therapy is considered to be a cytostatic rather than a cytotoxic treatment and continued indefinitely. Because of this and the associated problems of impotence, hormone therapy is conventionally considered unsuitable for

TABLE 1. Natural history of prostatic cancer

Primary treatment	MO (n = 326)	M+ (n = 263)
Surveillance	90%[a]	94%[a]
Stilboestrol	71%	90%
Orchidectomy	69%	80%
Orchidectomy + stilboestrol	56%	79%

Data from Nesbit and Baum (1950)
[a]Percentage dead after 5 years

early cases despite the considerable morbidity of surgery (Fowler and Wennberg, 1993; Talcott *et al,* 1994) and evidence from radiotherapy studies in prostate and breast cancer showing increased numbers of late deaths (Adolfsson *et al,* 1993; Houghton *et al,* 1994) possibly due in part to the long sustained T cell lymphopenia (Stjernswald *et al,* 1972; Rysscher *et al,* 1992). The recent observations from the meta-analysis of oophorectomy and tamoxifen trials in breast cancer have raised the possibility that hormone therapy may have a long term cure potential in that disease (EBCTCG, 1992a,b) and by implication a similar potential in prostate cancer. There is some support for this in the Nesbit and Baum (1950) studies of immediate versus deferred hormone treatment, which demonstrate that the survival advantages of immediate hormone therapy are only seen in patients without blood borne metastases (MO) (Table 1).

It is the aim of this chapter to review the limitations of chemotherapy compared to radiotherapy for hormone resistant metastatic disease, to assess new methods for differentiating hormone and chemotherapy sensitive patients to maximize benefit and finally to consider how to apply this knowledge and new data on the effect of sex hormones on thymus physiology to justify the use of intermittent hormone therapy as a form of chemoprevention for prostate cancer.

LIMITATIONS OF CHEMOTHERAPY COMPARED TO RADIATION HORMONE THERAPY

There can be little doubt that occasionally patients with prostate cancer can do extremely well with chemotherapy. My first such patient was moribund and confined to bed because lymphangiitis carcinomatosa caused severe dyspnoea. In addition, he had multiple painful bone metastases and pelvic lymph nodes and was taking high doses of morphine. Within 72 hours of treatment with carboplatin, he had been discharged off morphine and returned to work within 4 weeks. The lymphangiitis disappeared (Fig. 1), his acid phosphatase returned to normal and he remained well for 11 months before bone pain and lymphangiitis returned. He died 14 months after starting treatment.

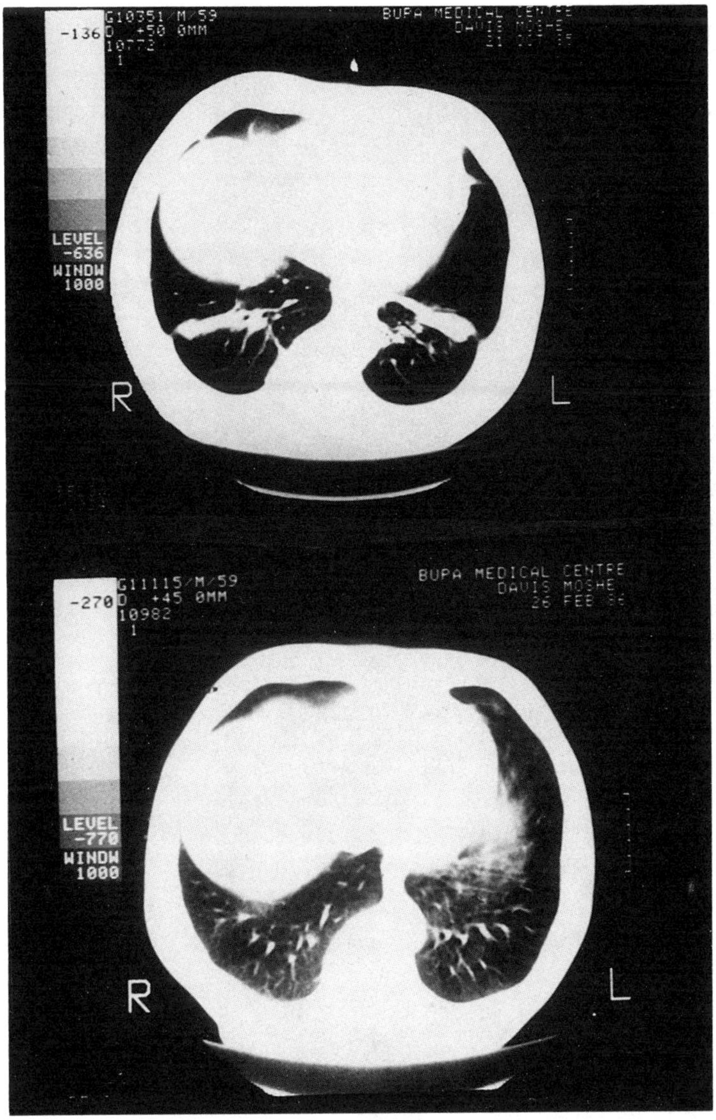

Fig. 1. Pre- (*top*) and postchemotherapy (*bottom*) (carboplatin) treatment for lymphangiitis carcinomatosa in a patient with carcinoma of the prostate

A second such patient had locally advanced metastatic (T_4 N0) disease that had returned after radiation and treatment with hormones. With treatment with 5-fluorouracil and mitomycin, he responded with a 60% reduction in tumour volume (Fig. 2) and was able to stop diamorphine for 6 months. Such cases, however, are the exception rather than the rule, and in general, there is better palliative benefit from radiation than from single agent chemotherapy (Oliver and Waxman, 1986). This is probably because the majority of patients have bone disease, which is difficult to measure as the sole site of disease, and in such patients, it is notoriously difficult to determine benefit from chemo-

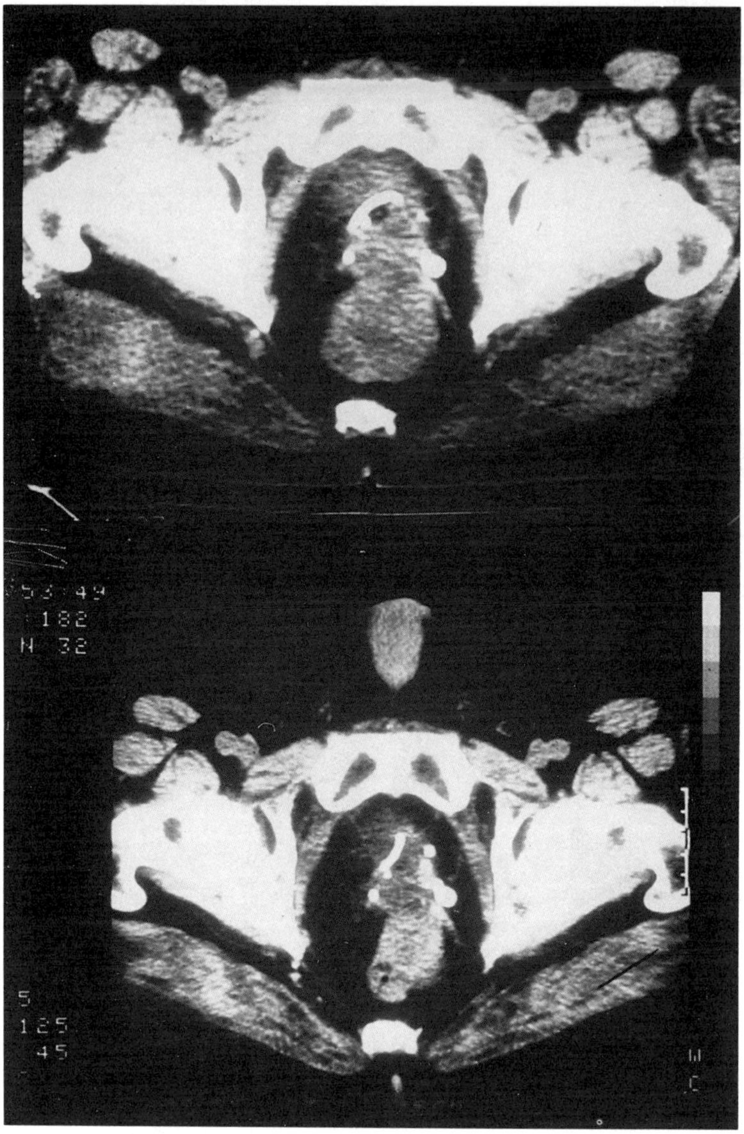

Fig. 2. Pre- (*top*) and postchemotherapy (*bottom*) (5-fluorouracil and mitomycin) for locally extensive recurrent primary carcinoma of the prostate

therapy whatever type of primary is responsible. Table 2 summarizes single agent chemotherapy data from the literature. It is not very impressive unless the large stable disease category is taken into consideration. Mitomycin appears to be the best agent, although this study was in a selected group of patients, all of whom had bidimensionally measurable soft tissue metastases. Despite this, the response rate of 29% is clearly equal to that in similarly selected cases for phase II studies of mitomycin in breast cancer where 26% of patients who failed first line treatment responded.

TABLE 2. Single agent studies in carcinoma of the prostate (for references see Oliver and Waxman, 1986)

	No of cases	Partial response (+ stable disease)
Mitozantrone	35	5(+20)%
Carboplatin	6	17%
Mitomycin	40	29%
Cisplatin	92	2(+27)%
Cyclophosphamide	119	6(+34)%
Methotrexate	58	5(+36)%
Interferon	35	11%

There have been only a few studies in prostate cancer that have suggested that combination chemotherapy produces a better response than single agent chemotherapy. The effect of selection on these studies is illustrated in the report from the MD Anderson Group. Although they achieved an initial response of 60% in the first patients (Logothetis *et al,* 1981), the response rate in their second cohort of patients was only 33% (Logothetis *et al,* 1983)—not much better than the single agent data at the cost of considerable toxicity.

Given the similarity that is often seen between prostate and breast cancer and the fact that two of the best agents for both are mitomycin and mitozantrone, and some activity is also detectable with methotrexate, there could be a case for studying methotrexate, mitomycin and mitozantrone in combination and compare this with mitomycin alone. This combination is increasingly being used as first line therapy in breast cancer because of its low toxicity (Powles *et al,* 1991).

SELECTION OF HORMONE AND CHEMOTHERAPY SENSITIVE PATIENTS PRIOR TO TREATMENT

In breast cancer, there has been more widespread use of chemotherapy both to treat metastases and for adjuvant treatment (Wood *et al,* 1994) despite the evidence that the response rates of metastatic disease to single agents are not substantially better than those in prostate cancer. There is increasing evidence from the studies in breast cancer that patients with endocrine sensitive tumours, defined on the basis of a high level of oestrogen receptor, are less sensitive to chemotherapy than to hormones and vice versa (Table 3). Comparison of response rates in breast cancer and prostate cancer to endocrine and single agent mitomycin treatment gives some encouragement that if there were methods of defining the primarily hormone resistant patients, it might be possible to improve the selection of prostate cancer patients who would benefit from chemotherapy. Although there are some reagents available to identify the androgen receptor in tissue sections, this approach has not been used extensively in prostate cancer and may not be of much value given data

TABLE 3. Opposing actions of endocrine therapy and chemotherapy on oestrogen receptive (ER) positive and negative breast cancer

5 year survival	Ovarian ablation (n = 167)	Cyclophosphamide, methotrexate, 5-fluorouracil (n = 165)
All cases (n = 332)	62%	63%
ER ≥ 20 (n = 132)	75%	61%
ER <20 (n = 100)	52%	68%

Data from Scottish and ICRF Breast Study (1993)

TABLE 4. Prostatic acid phosphatase (PAP) rate of decline and response duration of PAP producing metastases to leuprolide

PAP	No of cases	Progression free at 18 months
Normal at 16 weeks	10	80%
Persistent elevated PAP at 16 weeks	9	22%
	Fischer's exact test p <0.05	

TABLE 5. Breast cancer c-erbB2 production and prognosis

Histological grade + p <0.002
Mitotic index + p <0.0002
Progesterone receptor – p <0.0006
Oestrogen receptor – p <0.02
Serum level responders (n = 3) 9.3 units/ml
Non-responders (n = 33) 33 units/ml

Data from Watanabe *et al* (1994)

that some hormone resistant lines have mutated androgen receptors that can be stimulated by the anti-androgen flutamide (Chung, this volume) However, there is an even better approach possible in prostate cancer. Recently, it has become increasingly accepted that the rate of tumour marker normalization after starting endocrine treatment may give an in vivo functional measure of the hormone sensitivity of the patient's tumour and predict for chance of long term survival (Table 4).

Although the decline in prostate specific antigen may give a reasonable measure of hormone sensitivity as it is a marker of the differentiated component of prostate cancer, it has been less reliable in measuring chemosensitivity, presumably because the hormone resistant clones tend to lose markers of differentiation. In breast cancer, measurement of serum levels of c-erbB2 proto-oncogene protein is emerging as a good marker of the non-hormone sensitive clone (Table 5), and tissue expression may be a predictor of response to high dose chemotherapy (Muss *et al,* 1994). Although as yet there is considerably less evidence from prostate cancer that c-erbB2 is a marker of the hormone resistant clones, there have been reports demonstrating that, as in breast cancer, it is expressed in a similar minority population (Mellon *et al,* 1992). Clearly, more work is required to clarify this because if it were possible to select more easily the patients who might benefit, there would be a greater justification for the early use of chemotherapy. One other approach reported from the study of breast cancer and possibly relevant to the study of prostate cancer is the use of *Helix pomatia* lectin to demonstrate defects in tumour glycosylation, which predicts poor prognosis (Brooks and Leathem, 1991).

INFLUENCE OF SEX HORMONE MANIPULATION ON THE IMMUNE SYSTEM AND ITS RELEVANCE TO TREATMENT OF PROSTATE CANCER

An indication of the lack of interest in the use of biological therapy in prostate cancer is the small amount of data recorded on patients treated with interferon in the 17 years since it was first introduced into clinical trials in 1977 (Haelst-Pisani *et al,* 1992; Weiss, 1994). The 11% response is quite respectable compared with the other data on single agent chemotherapy, particularly as there is evidence that interferon, as part of its spectrum of actions on end cell differentiation functions, can increase the expression of hormone receptors (Berg *et al,* 1987). Even less has been published on the use of interleukin 2 (IL2), despite one complete remission of acid phosphatase tumour marker in the early phase I studies undertaken in the UK (Oliver *et al,* 1989a).

In the most recent trials of immunotherapy, IL2 has been studied alone and in combination with interferon in patients with renal cell cancer and melanoma where more than 5% of patients are achieving durable complete remission of metastatic disease for more than 2 years and in some cases continuing for more than 5 years (Oliver and Nouri, 1992). However, it is the studies of BCG in the treatment of superficial bladder cancer that provide the most clear-cut demonstration that biological treatments can induce rejection of tumour in humans (Oliver, 1991).

It is now nearly 20 years since the first reports appeared on the effectiveness of intravesical BCG and, most specifically, that the complete remission remained durable for longer than 12 months in more than 60% of patients (Lamm *et al,* 1980). That this response is mediated by an immune response comes from the demonstration that the degree of induction of HLA class II antigens on tumour cells (Prescott *et al,* 1989) and the amount of IL2 released into the urine (Fleishman *et al,* 1989) predict for the duration of the response. With increasing evidence that tumours lose normal expression of HLA and adhesion molecule expression as they become more malignant and more un-

TABLE 6. Influence of immunotherapy lentinan on progression free survival of breast cancer responders to hormone therapy

	No of cases	Progression free in primary tumour
Controls	16	13%
Lentinan polysaccharide	15	47%
$\chi^2 = 4.2$, $p < 0.05$		

Data from Kosaka *et al* (1985)

differentiated (Oliver *et al,* 1989a; Oliver and Nouri, 1992), it has become apparent that to gain the most from immunotherapy, it is necessary to focus on the early, more differentiated tumours.

As response to hormones is the normal function of the most differentiated component of these tumours, it might be expected that tumours with a high level of endocrine receptors would benefit most from immunotherapy. There have been few studies of immunotherapy in prostate cancer and none in tumours that have a high level of hormone response. Although there have been more studies of immunotherapy in breast cancer, the results have been very disappointing (EBCTCG, 1992b). However, only one of these has focused on specifically identifying the hormone responsive tumours and restricting immunotherapy use to the tumours that responded (Kosaka *et al,* 1985). Despite the small numbers of patients treated, the results (Table 6) were surprisingly good and clearly provide a strong justification for considering trials in prostate cancer patients showing endocrine sensitivity.

Given the failure of human papillomavirus screening to detect any involvement (reviewed in Cuzick, this volume), it is unlikely that a vaccine programme will be of value in preventing of this disease. However, screening for other infectious agents is clearly indicated, given the epidemiologist's evidence that prior history of a sexually transmitted disease is the strongest reported risk factor for prostate cancer (Key, this volume). The recent observations on the role of *Helicobacter* in the development of stomach cancer or gastric lymphoma (reviewed in Isaacson, 1994) provide a model of how a non-specific bacterial infection could be involved in promoting the development of prostate cancer.

There is one further justification for considering the use of combined hormones and immunotherapy. This is provided by observations from two recently completed unpublished studies investigating the effect of testosterone withdrawal on thymic physiology. The first demonstrated that 13 of 17 (75%) patients being treated with luteinizing hormone releasing hormone analogues had a lymphocytosis within 3–4 weeks of starting treatment (median increase 36%, range 4–115%) and that in these patients, survival was better than in those who failed to demonstrate lymphocytosis (Table 7). The second study in

TABLE 7. Impact of hormone therapy induced lymphocytosis on duration of first remission in prostate cancer

	No of cases	Mean remission (months)	Remission of over 12 months
Increased posthormone therapy lymphocytosis on day 28	13	13	31%
No posthormone therapy lymphocytosis on day 28	4	6.5	25%

Data from Joseph J and Oliver T (unpublished)

patients with cancer of the testis treated with chemotherapy demonstrated that the patients with evidence of testicular failure as measured by the presence of elevated levels of luteinizing hormones had the highest incidence of thymic hyperplasia (Table 8). These studies provide the first clinical evidence of something that has been previously well described in experimental animals (Grossman, 1985)—that is, that sex hormones are involved in involution of the thymus at puberty and that castration after puberty leads to thymic regeneration, which is reversed by sex hormone replacement. As yet, there are no studies in women to confirm these studies in men. However, reports from studies of red foxes demonstrate fluctuation in thymic size during the breeding cycle (Twigg and Harris, 1982), suggesting that it is highly likely that this is the case and may explain recent reports suggesting that breast cancer patients operated on during unopposed oestrogen stimulation have a higher incidence of lymph node metastases in the axilla (Fentiman and Gregory, 1993).

RELEVANCE OF THE NEW UNDERSTANDING OF INTERACTIONS BETWEEN ENDOCRINE AND IMMUNE SYSTEMS

Role of Surgery in Prostate Cancer

There is little doubt that although surgeons have made considerable progress in improving the technical results of surgery, there is no evidence yet that wide scale use of prostatectomy has reduced mortality from prostate cancer (Lu-Yao and Greenberg, 1994). It is equally clear in breast cancer that despite more and more complicated surgical attempts to remove the tumour, there is no improvement in survival (Urban and Castro, 1971).

Two non-cancer related factors have been put forward as possibly contributing to the failure of radical surgery to provide any benefit. The first relates to the immunosuppressive effects of the surgery and/or stress related to anaesthesia, which has long been known to be demonstrable both in experimental animal models and in the clinical setting (Cochran *et al*, 1972). Figure 3 shows an impressive demonstration in animal models that the degree of im-

TABLE 8. Correlation of luteinizing hormone levels in patients with cancer of the testis and thymic hyperplasia after chemotherapy

	Luteinizing hormone levels after chemotherapy	
	≥18 units/l	<18 units/l
Thymic hyperplasia (n = 16)	10	6
Normal thymus (n = 36)	11	25
$\chi^2 = 4.695$, $p \leq 0.025$		

Data from Sperandio P and Oliver T (unpublished)

munosuppression after surgery is proportional to the duration of anaesthesia. Although long known, there have been no clinical studies of this despite successful animal models where presurgery immunotherapy has prolonged survival (Weiss, 1994).

The second factor that has been postulated as diminishing the benefit of

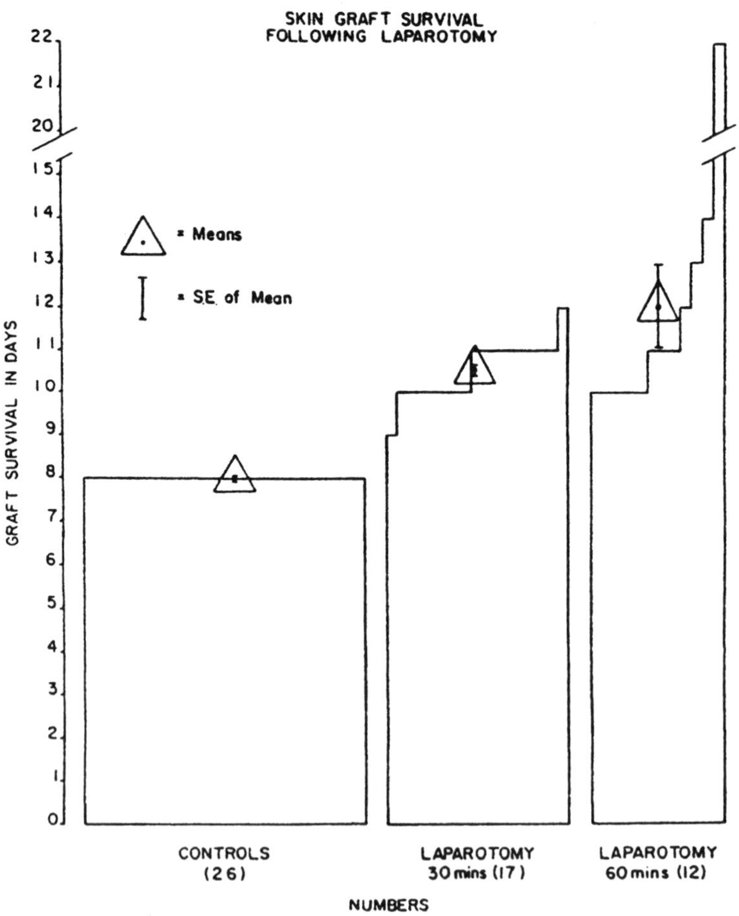

Fig. 3. Skin graft survival following laparotomy (Riddle, 1969)

radical surgery is post-trauma repair cytokine induction. It is now 80 years since Peyton Rous first observed that traumatic injury accelerated cancer growth (Joynes and Rous, 1914). Several researchers have subsequently confirmed this observation (Alexander *et al,* 1988), and recently new information from the study of induction of cytokine growth factors, such as epidermal growth factor, after trauma has provided a possible explanation of the mechanism involved (Skipper *et al,* 1989).

In breast cancer, there is one group of studies that has provided the most convincing evidence that there may be circumstances when the degree of surgical trauma does accelerate tumour recurrence. These data come from two studies of 249 and 155 patients reported by Badwe *et al* (1991a,b). They demonstrated that surgical treatment in premenopausal patients undertaken during the unopposed oestrogenic phase of the menstrual cycle (days 3–12) was associated with a 23–30% worse survival at 5 years when compared to patients operated on during other phases of the cycle. Support for the view that this may relate to the degree of surgical trauma when the cells are most metabolically active under the influence of oestrogens comes from their observations (Table 9) that the deleterious effect was more marked in patients who underwent mastectomy rather than lumpectomy and in patients with positive lymph nodes, but was very little influenced by oestrogen receptor status or size of tumour mass. Evidence suggesting that under the influence of unopposed oestrogens even needle biopsy might represent significant surgical disruption comes from the second study by Badwe *et al* (1991b), which demonstrated that none of six patients biopsied during the oestrogenic phase survived compared to five of five biopsied during the remaining part of the cycle. For unbiopsied patients, 5 year survival of patients who were operated on outside the oestrogenic phase was 67% versus 35% for those operated on during the oestrogenic phase.

Although 17 other studies have attempted to repeat this observation, only 7 were positive (Fentiman, 1994). It is not clear what causes this marked heterogeneity, although Fentiman and Gregory's analysis demonstrates that in their data the difference is weakest in patients undergoing lumpectomy and adjuvant chemotherapy; in addition, as well as paying attention to menstrual cycle timing of biopsy (Badwe *et al,* 1991b), they demonstrated that it may be necessary to pay attention to time of mammography, as in their study, mammography during the unopposed oestrogenic phase had a deleterious effect in univariate but not multivariate analysis (Fentiman and Gregory, 1993). In addition, they have taken particular care to verify menstrual histories, excluding 17% of their cases because their patient's periods were so irregular that their oestrogenic phase could not be calculated. On this basis, it is possible that the observation may still be genuine despite the large number of negative studies reported from other units. Biochemical support for the view that unopposed oestrogen at the time of surgical trauma is a significant factor accelerating recurrence and diminishing survival comes from a third study recently reported by Badwe *et al* (1994) demonstrating that there was no influence of

TABLE 9. Influence of surgery and menstrual cycle status on breast cancer survival

	Unopposed oestrogenic phase (days 3-12)		Rest of cycle	
	No	% 10 year	No	% 10 year
Breast conservation	15	70	39	84
Mastectomy	60	52	135	85
≤4 cm tumour	65	57	155	87
>4 cm tumour	10	44	19	63
Oestrogen receptor +ve tumours	43	57	102	81
Oestrogen receptor −ve tumours	19	42	46	83
Lymph node negative	33	82	91	89
Lymph node positive	42	36	83	78

Data from Fentiman and Gregory (1993, p. 154)

preoperative oestrogen level on survival but that the higher the preoperative progesterone, the better the survival of node positive patients.

If these observations from breast cancer are relevant to the use of surgery in prostate cancer, they suggest that there may be a case for a more circumspect approach to all surgery, including biopsy of the prostate in the diagnosis of these tumours. Support for this comes from a report demonstrating that tumours can grow out along the track made by needle biopsy (Bastacky *et al,* 1991); a report of poor survival of patients diagnosed after initial prostate screening associated with an aggressive approach to biopsy (Gerber *et al,* 1993); and evidence that an aggressive approach to needle biopsy produces sustained elevation of prostate specific antigen lasting more than a month. Use of prebiopsy hormone treatment as a form of neo-adjuvant immunotherapy might be a way to avoid this problem. Alternatively, use of polymerase chain reaction (Ghossein *et al,* 1994) on prostatic massage (Fergusson and Gibson, 1956) or ejaculate samples might be a less traumatic approach than biopsy for establishing the diagnosis before staring endocrine therapy.

Use of Intermittent Hormone Therapy for Chemoprevention of Prostate Cancer

Until recently, it had been assumed that once started, hormone therapy had to be continued indefinitely as the effect of the treatment only reduced the stem cells to the state that had existed prior to puberty. Recent unpublished evidence that hormone therapy through an indirect effect on the thymus (Tables 7 and 8) might produce improved immune response and could therefore produce tumour rejection has provided a scientific rationale to justify increasing interest in using hormone therapy intermittently. With a recent report

TABLE 10. Prostate specific antigen (PSA) doubling times and progression free survival

PSA doubling time	No of cases	Proportion with metastases at diagnosis
<24 months	9 (21%)	78%
24–48 months	8 (19%)	75%
>48 months	20 (47%)	25%
Stable disease	6 (14%)	0

Data from Schmid *et al* (1993)

(Akakura *et al,* 1993) demonstrating that at least four consecutive responses can be achieved by using short term hormone therapy, there is clearly a case for investigation of this approach, particularly in light of reports that patients can also demonstrate response after withdrawal of flutamide (Sher and Kelly, 1993).

During the last 5 years, we have begun to explore the concept of intermittent hormone therapy. We have stopped treatment in six patients with normal acid phosphatase on prostate specific antigen after 3 to 6 months of treatment. Three of these patients with early tumours remain progression free at 16, 18 and 24 months.

From this experience, we believe that greater confidence in the use of intermittent hormone therapy would open up a completely new approach to management of early small tumours in patients in whom treatment with hormones for 3 months only might be justified. Even more radical a departure from conventional approaches would be to consider intermittent hormone therapy as chemoprevention for prostate cancer as given its slow growth rate in the early stages with nearly 80% of patients not showing a prostate specific antigen doubling by 2 years (Schmid *et al,* 1993; Table 10), it might be possible to treat for only 1–3 months every 5–10 years.

CONCLUSIONS AND PROPOSALS FOR NEW STUDIES

This review has attempted to highlight new aspects of prostate cancer management that could revolutionize the treatment of this disease. The first is the possibility that the identification of patients with hormone responsive tumours on the basis of the rate of decline of prostate specific antigen could enable more focused exploration of immunotherapy. The second is that new-found confidence in the use of intermittent hormone therapy, as well as lessening the more distressing side effects of hormone therapy on sexual function, might encourage the use of such therapy as an alternative to surgery as primary therapy and in chemoprevention in individuals at high risk. Table 11 summarizes a series of trials that have been proposed to investigate these ideas.

TABLE 11. Proposals for future studies in prostate cancer

Metastases
  Hormone treatment for 4 weeks then stratify by PSA response
  (a) Good responders continued hormones ± immunotherapy
  (b) Poor responders continued hormones ± chemotherapy

Advanced Local Disease
  Short term (3 months) hormone treatment ± surgery/radiotherapy

Early Local Disease
  Surveillance v. 3 months' endocrine treatment. Advanced local disease protocol if localized at relapse

Chemoprevention
  One to three months' treatment at age of 55 with GNRHA + antiandrogen

SUMMARY

This chapter has reviewed the limitations of the use of chemotherapy in patients with hormone resistant prostate cancer. Although demonstrating that there is a small number of patients with very chemosensitive tumours, the age profile and intolerance to chemotherapy make it highly unlikely that this modality of treatment will be used more routinely despite the increasing evidence that the slow decline of prostate specific antigen with endocrine treatment can be used early to select patients who might respond to chemotherapy. Equally certain is that it will not be of use for chemoprevention of the early stages of this disease.

Although some data suggest that tumours that respond rapidly and completely to endocrine therapy may benefit from the use of non-specific immunotherapy, there is no evidence that any form of vaccination therapy would be of value in preventing the disease in the main because all attempts to find evidence of a virus, particularly a human papillomavirus subtype, involved in its aetiology have proved negative.

The discovery that standard endocrine therapy induces thymic regeneration and peripheral blood lymphocytosis, taken together with the demonstration that surgical trauma induced by a needle biopsy could accelerate tumour dissemination because of tumour activation by trauma induced release of tissue repair cytokines, has led to the proposal that short term endocrine treatment should be given to all prostate specific antigen positive patients prior to needle biopsy. New information on the slow kinetics of prostate cancer growth, with cancers detected by screening being found up to 20 years before clinical presentation and more than 80% of early tumours failing to double the prostate specific antigen level within 2 years, has led to proposals for a new strategy for endocrine chemoprevention of prostate cancer. This has in part been encouraged by greater confidence in the use of intermittent hormone therapy to treat patients with metastatic disease. These observations have led to the suggestion that it might be possible to prevent deaths by treating early cases detected from prostate specific antigen screening with short term (1–3 months) endocrine treatment every 5 to 10 years.

References

Adolfsson J, Steineck G and Whitmore WF (1993) Recent results of management of palpable clinically localized prostate cancer. *Cancer* **72** 310–322

Akakura K, Bruchovsky N, Goldenbery SL *et al* (1993) Effects of intermittent androgen suppression on androgen dependent tumors. *Cancer* **71** 2782–2790

Alexander P, Murphy P and Skipper D (1988) Preferential growth of blood borne cancer cells at site of trauma—a growth promoting role of macrophages. *Advances in Experimental Medicine and Biology* **233** 245–251

Badwe RA, Gregory WM, Chaudary MA *et al* (1991a) Timing of surgery during menstrual cycle and survival of premenopausal women with operable breast cancer. *Lancet* **337** 1261

Badwe RA, Richards MA and Fentiman IS (1991b) Surgical procedures, menstrual cycle phase and prognosis in operable breast cancer. *Lancet* **338** 815–816

Badwe RA, Wang DY, Gregory WM *et al* (1994) Serum progesterone at the time of surgery and survival in women with premenopausal operable breast cancer. *European Journal of Cancer* **30** 445–448

Bastacky SS, Walsh PC and Epstein JI (1991) Needle biopsy associated tumor tracking of adenocarcinoma of the prostate. *Journal of Urology* **145** 1003–1007

Breslow N, Chan CW, Dhom G *et al* (1977) Latent carcinoma of prostate at autopsy in seven areas. *International Journal of Cancer* **20** 680–688

Brooks SA and Leathem AJC (1991) Prediction of lymph node involvement in breast cancer by detection of altered glycosylation in the primary tumour. *Lancet* **338** 71–74

Cochran AJ, Spilg WG, Mackie RM and Thomas CE (1972) Post-operative depression of tumour-directed cell-mediated immunity in patients with malignant disease. *British Medical Journal* **4** 67–70

EBCTCG (1992a) Systemic treatment of early breast cancer by hormonal, cytotoxic or immune therapy. *Lancet* **339** 1–15

EBCTCG (1992b) Systemic treatment of early breast cancer by hormonal, cytotoxic or immune therapy. *Lancet* **339** 71–85

Fentiman AS and Gregory WM (1993) The hormonal milieu and prognosis in operable breast cancer. *Cancer Surveys* **18** 149–163

Fergusson JD and Gibson EC (1956) Prostatic smear diagnosis. *British Medical Journal* **1** 822–825

Fleishman JD, Toosi Z, Ellner DB *et al* (1989) Urinary interleukins in patients receiving intravesical bacillus Calmette-Guerin therapy for superficial bladder cancer. Cancer **64** 1447–1454

Fowler PJ and Wennberg JE (1993) Patient treated complications and follow up treatment after radical prostatectomy—national medicare experiment 1988-1990. *Urology* **42** 622–629

Gerber GS, Thompson IM, Thisted R and Chodak GW (1993) Disease-specific survival following routine prostate cancer screening by digital rectal examination. *Journal of the American Medical Association* **269** 61–64

Ghossein R, Scher H, Gerald W *et al* (1994) Detection of circulating tumour cells in peripheral blood of patients with advanced prostatic carcinoma. *Proceedings of the American Society of Clinical Oncology* **13** 735A

Grossman CJ (1985) Interactions between the gonadal-steroids and the immune system. *Science* **227** 257–261

Haelst-Pisani CMV, Richardson RL, Su J *et al* (1992) A phase II study of recombinant human alpha-interferon in advanced hormone-refractory prostate cancer. *Cancer* **60** 2310–2312

Houghton J, Baum M and Haybittle J (1994) Role of radiotherapy following total mastectomy in

patients with early breast cancer. *World Journal of Surgery* **18** 117–122
Isaacson PG (1994) Gastric lymphoma and *Helicobacter pylori*. *New England Journal of Medicine* **330** 1310–1311
Joynes F and Rous P (1914) On the cause of localization of secondary tumour at points of injury. *Journal of Experimental Medicine* **20** 404–412
Kosaka A, Hattori Y, Imaizumi A and Yamashita A (1985) Synergistic effect of lentinan and surgical endocrine therapy of the growth of DMBA-induced mammary tumours of rats and of recurrent human breast cancer. *Excerpta Medica International Conference*, pp 138–199, Excerpta Medica, Amsterdam
Lamm DL, Thor DE, Harris SC *et al* (1980) Bacillus calmette-guerin immunotherapy of superficial bladder cancer. *Journal of Urology* **124** 28
Logothetis C, Eschenbach AV, Samuels A and Haynie M (1981) Doxorubicin, mitomycin-C and 5-fluorouracil (DMF) in the therapy of hormonal resistant adenocarcinoma. *Proceedings of the American Society of Clinical Oncology* **18** 333A
Logothetis C, Samuels ML, Eschenbach AV *et al* (1983) Doxorubicin, mitomycin-C and 5-flurouracil (DMF) in the treatment of metastatic prostate cancer. *Journal of Clinical Oncology* **1** 368–379
Lu-Yao GL and Greenberg ER (1994) Changes in prostate cancer incidence and treatment in USA. *Lancet* **343** 251–254
Mellon K, Thompson S, Charlton R *et al* (1992) c-erbB-2 and the epidermal growth factor receptor in the benign and malignant prostate. *Journal of Urology* **147** 496–499
Muss HB, Thor AD, Berry DA and Kute A (1994) c-erbB-2 expression and response to adjuvant therapy in women with node-positive early breast cancer. *New England Journal of Medicine* **330** 1260–1266
Nesbit RM and Baum WC (1950) Endocrine control of prostatic carcinoma: clinical and statistical survey of 1818 cases. *Journal of the American Medical Association* **143** 1317–1320
Oliver RTD (1991) Topical BCG for recurrent superficial bladder cancer. *Lancet* **337** 821–822
Oliver RTD and Nouri AME (1992) T cell immune response to cancer in humans and its relevance for immunodiagnosis and therapy. Cancer Surveys **13** 173–204
Oliver RTD and Waxman JH (eds) (1986) *Cytotoxic Chemotherapy in Treatment of Endocrine Unresponsive Carcinoma of the Prostate*, pp 208–215, Blackwell, Oxford
Oliver RTD, Crosby D, Nouri A, Scott E and Galazka A (1989a) Evaluation of the effect of continuous infusion recombinant interleukin-2 (bioleukin) on peripheral blood leucocytes of patients with terminal malignancy. *British Journal of Cancer* **64** 934–937
Oliver RTD, Nouri AME, Crosby D *et al* (1989b) Biological significance of beta hCG, HLA and other membrane antigen expression on bladder tumours and their relationship to tumour infiltrating lymphocytes (TIL). *Journal of Immunogenetics* **16** 381–390
Powles T, Jones A, Judson I *et al* (1991) Randomised trial comparing combination chemotherapy using mitomycin C, mitozantrone and methotrexate with vincristine, anthracycline and cyclophosphamide in advanced breast cancer. *British Journal of Cancer* **64** 406–410
Prescott S, James K, Busuttil J *et al* (1989) HLA DR expression by high grade superficial bladder cancer treated with BCG. *British Journal of Urology* **63** 264–269
Riddle PR (1969) "Immunosuppressive effects of surgery." MS thesis, University of London
Rysscher D (1992) Irradiation induced T cell lymphopenia after breast cancer radiation treatment. *European Journal of Cancer* **28** 1729
Schmid McNeal JE and Stamey TA (1993) Observations on the doubling time of prostate cancer. *Cancer* **71** 2031–2040
Scottish and ICRF Breast Unit (1993) Adjuvant ovarian ablation vs CMF chemotherapy in premenopausal women with pathological stage II breast carcinoma: the Scottish trial. *Lancet* **341** 1293–1298
Sher HI and Kelly WK (1993) Flutamide withdrawal syndrome: its impact on clinical trials in hormone-refractory prostate cancer. *Journal of Clinical Oncology* **11** 1566–1572
Sher HI and Sternberg C (1985) Chemotherapy of urologic malignancies. *Seminars in Oncology*

3 239–280

Skipper D, Jeffrey M, Cooper A and Alexander P (1989) Enhanced growth of tumour cells in healing colonic anastomoses and laparotomy wounds. *International Journal of Colorectal Disease* **4** 172–177

Stjernswald J (1972) Irradiation induced T cell lymphopenia after breast cancer radiation treatment. *Lancet* **i** 1352

Talcott JA, Rieker P, Propert K and Kalish L(1994) Complications of treatment for early prostate cancer: a prospective multi-institutional outcomes study. *Proceedings of the American Society of Clinical Oncology* **13** 711A

Twigg G and Harris S (1982) Seasonal and age changes in the thymus gland of the red fox. *Journal of Zoology* **196** 355–370

Urban J and Castro E (1971) Selecting variations in extent of surgical procedure for breast cancer. *Cancer* **28** 1615–1623

van den Berg HW, Leahy WJ, Lynch M *et al* (1987) Recombinant human interferon alpha increases oestrogen receptor expression in human breast cancer cells (zr-75-1) and sensitises them to anti-proliferative effects of tamoxifen. *British Journal of Cancer* **55** 255–257

Watanabe T, Adachi J and Abe K (1994) Overexpression of C-erbB2 protein and response to endocrine therapy in breast cancer. Conference—The Challenge of Breast Cancer, Brugge. *Lancet* p 85 [Abstract 51]

Weiss KS (1994) A phase II study of recombinant leukocyte a human interferon intron a (int-a) in patients with hormone-refractory metastatic prostate cancer. *Proceedings of the American Society of Clinical Oncology* **13** 738A

Wood WC, Daniel MD, Budman R and Korzun AH (1994) Dose and dose intensity of adjuvant chemotherapy for stage II, node-positive breast carcinoma. *New England Journal of Medicine* **330** 1253–1259

The authors are responsible for the accuracy of the references.

Experimental Therapy and Other Aspects

Strontium-89 in the Management of Metastatic Prostate Cancer

DAVID KIRK
Department of Urology, Western Infirmary, Glasgow G11 6NT

INTRODUCTION

Strontium is named after the town of Strontian on the west coast of Scotland close to where the element was discovered at the end of the eighteenth century. Its significance as a chemical element lies in its various radioactive isotopes. Strontium-90, an alpha emitter, was a notorious component of the radioactive fallout from nuclear explosions. The research into the metabolism of strontium in the human skeleton stimulated by this remains useful (International Commission on Radiological Protection, 1972). It is important that patients receiving strontium-89 be made aware that this is a different isotope. Strontium-85 is a gamma emitter and can be used as an alternative to technetium-99 for radioisotope bone scans, confirming the uptake of strontium by metastatic "hot spots". Strontium-89 (Metastron) is a beta emitter, producing low penetration radiation. Its avid uptake into the osteoblastic metastases typical of carcinoma of the prostate delivers intense local irradiation. Compared with normal bone, the uptake and retention of strontium in metastatic disease is considerably enhanced and its biological half life in metastases approaches that of its radiation decay (Ackery and Yardley, 1993). It is administered by a single intravenous injection, with advantages in convenience and acceptability compared with conventional external beam radiotherapy.

THERAPEUTIC AND RESEARCH STRATEGIES

The development of strontium-89 as a therapy has progressed in a logical sequence. It was first used in patients in whom conventional radiotherapy had

Cancer Surveys Volume 23: *Preventing Prostate Cancer: Screening versus Chemoprevention*

failed. Once both open usage and a double blind placebo crossover study had confirmed its efficacy in this situation, its role in first line radiotherapy was explored, both as an adjunct and as an alternative to conventional irradiation. Studies in this area continue, and there is interest in investigating its use in earlier stages of the disease.

STRONTIUM-89 AFTER FAILURE OF CONVENTIONAL RADIOTHERAPY

Robinson (1986) in Kansas City initiated the current interest in strontium-89 as therapy for metastatic carcinoma of the prostate. The UK open study (Laing *et al,* 1991) confirmed Robinson's extensive experience with patients who had developed recurrent symptoms (or had failed to respond) after conventional external beam radiotherapy. Of 83 patients, 22% became pain free after a single injection of strontium-89, and only a quarter failed to achieve any benefit from this treatment. To exclude a placebo response and also to confirm that the therapeutic effect was due to irradiation and not to some chemical effect of elemental strontium, a double blind crossover trial against non-radioactive strontium was set up (Lewington *et al,* 1991). No patients receiving placebo achieved complete pain relief, which occurred in 15% of those treated with active strontium-89, any placebo responses being confined to the mildest category.

STRONTIUM-89 AT TIME OF PRIMARY RADIOTHERAPY

The effectiveness of strontium-89 after failure of radiotherapy led to its exploration as an alternative to conventional radiotherapy (Robinson *et al,* 1989). Strontium-89 administered as a single intravenous injection as an outpatient treatment has considerable advantages in convenience compared with external beam treatment. In addition, after local treatment of painful sites, all too often new sites of pain develop elsewhere, and although the use of hemibody (wide field) radiotherapy can reduce this, it seemed possible that a systemic treatment taken up by all metastases might prevent new sites of pain. Two comparative trials have been reported, one in Canada, where strontium-89 was used in an adjunctive role (Porter *et al,* 1993), and one in the UK, where strontium was compared directly as an alternative to radiotherapy (Quilty *et al,* 1994).

The double blind Canadian trial was designed to assess whether strontium-89 in a dose of 400 MBq (chosen as the maximum considered safe for use) given at the time of treatment would improve the results of conventional fractionated external beam radiotherapy in patients with one or two sites of metastatic pain (Porter *et al,* 1993). The control patients received a placebo "spiked" with a small non-therapeutic dose of radioactive strontium-85. At most intervals after treatment, an increased response was apparent in the patients receiving strontium-89. Perhaps of greater note was the slower development of further sites of pain in patients receiving adjunctive strontium-89, this difference in pain progression achieving a high level of statistical significance. However, this dose (400 MBq compared with the current standard dose of 150 MBq) produced unacceptable bone marrow toxicity with considerable depression of both white cell and platelet counts.

The UK study compared on a randomized but non-blinded basis strontium-89 alone versus conventional radiotherapy (Quilty *et al,* 1994). Patients were eligible if they were referred for radiotherapy treatment, having relapsed following hormonal therapy. Before randomization, patients were stratified according to whether their metastatic disease was more suitable for local radiotherapy or hemibody treatment (for diffuse or multiple sites of pain). Following stratification, the patients within each of the two groups were randomized to receive either strontium-89 200 MBq or the assigned radiotherapy. Patients were followed in the first instance for 3 months during which pain response, use of analgesic drugs etc were assessed at monthly intervals.

In both parts of the study, the therapeutic response to strontium-89 was equivalent to that of radiotherapy. However, as in the Canadian study, new sites of pain developed more rapidly in patients receiving conventional radiotherapy than in those who received strontium-89. This difference was apparent in both stratified groups, and in the local radiotherapy arm, it was associated with a highly significant reduction in the need for further radiotherapy in the patients receiving strontium-89. Although there was some bone marrow depression as measured by peripheral blood counts in the strontium-89 treated patients, this did not cause clinical problems. There was a significantly higher incidence of gastrointestinal side effects in patients receiving external beam radiotherapy, particularly hemibody treatment. Although this study was not double blind, the observation concerning slower pain progression is consistent with the similar observation in the double-blind Canadian study (Porter *et al,*1993) and is the major therapeutic benefit over external beam radiotherapy.

THE THERAPEUTIC ROLE OF STRONTIUM-89

As a method of pain palliation, strontium-89 is equivalent to external beam radiotherapy in primary efficacy, but the onset of response is slower than with radiotherapy. It delays the onset of new sites of pain. Its convenience as a simple outpatient injection treatment is attractive, although in most countries, it can only be administered by those licensed for its use by the appropriate authority. However, it must be emphasized that strontium-89 is applicable only in the palliation of pain from bony metastases and is not a substitute for external beam radiotherapy in the treatment or prevention of spinal cord compression and pathological fractures. Because of the risk of myelosuppression, it should be used with caution in patients in whom there could be bone marrow depression. The high costs of production inevitably make strontium-89 an expensive treatment. Although this cost is outweighed to an extent by a reduction in the costs of radiotherapy and especially in associated use of hospital beds, expense does limit its use.

Currently, strontium-89 provides a less toxic alternative to hemibody radiotherapy in patients with diffuse or multiple sites of pain. It should be considered for patients in whom further sites of pain occur following successful response to preliminary radiotherapy. In patients who live a long distance from a radiotherapy centre, the possibility of a single fraction of radiotherapy to the painful site to achieve the most rapid response combined with an injection of strontium-89 is worth considering.

FUTURE INVESTIGATION OF STRONTIUM-89

Because of the characteristic osteoblastic nature of prostatic bony metastases, most interest in the use of strontium has been in this disease. However, its use in breast cancer (and other primary sites) has been reported (Robinson *et al*, 1989) and is now under formal investigation. Identification of patients likely to respond to treatment would be useful, especially in view of the high cost of the isotope. In prostatic cancer, there is interest in its use earlier in the disease. Since long term exposure to radioisotopes may carry a risk of leukaemia (Archer, 1987), it would be unwise to use strontium-89 at a stage of the disease where a life expectation of more than a few years is possible. However, the isotope could be useful in symptom free patients in whom relapse following hormonal therapy is heralded by a rise in prostate specific antigen (PSA). In view of the definite delay in pain progression seen in patients with symptoms who are given strontium-89, a double blind trial using the isotope in those with rising PSA to assess whether this would delay the onset of pain would seem the next logical step in the sequence of investigation described in this paper.

SUMMARY

Strontium-89 is a beta emitting radioisotope, avidly taken up by osteoblastic metastatic prostatic cancer. In both open and controlled studies, it has been shown to palliate metastatic pain effectively. It is as effective as conventional radiotherapy in palliation of the primary site(s) of pain, but in addition, it seems to delay pain progression. Its role is confined to palliation of pain in the absence of actual or impending complications (cord compression or pathological fractures). Bone marrow suppression makes it unsuitable for myelosuppressed patients. Cost is the main limitation to its use. It is a useful alternative to hemibody radiotherapy and to local treatment in selected patients. Its use in other tumour types (especially breast cancer) is currently under investigation. Trials investigating its use to delay onset of pain in symptom free relapsing patients should be considered.

References

Ackery D and Yardley J (1993) Radionuclide-targeted therapy for the management of metastatic bone pain. *Seminars in Oncology* **20 (Supplement 2)** 27–31

Archer VE (1987) Association of nuclear fallout with leukemia in the United States. *Archives of Environmental Health* **42** 263–271

International Commission on Radiological Protection (1972) *Alkaline Earth Metabolism in Man,* Pergamon Press, Oxford

Laing AH, Ackery DM, Bayly RJ *et al* (1991) ^{89}Sr chloride for pain palliation in prostatic skeletal malignancy. *British Journal of Radiology* **64** 816–822

Lewington VJ, McEwan AJ, Ackery DM *et al* (1991) A prospective randomised crossover study to examine the efficacy of ^{89}Sr in pain palliation in patients with advanced prostate cancer metastatic to bone. *European Journal of Cancer* **27** 954–958

Porter AT, McEwan AJ, Powe FE *et al* (1993) Results of a randomised phase III trial to evaluate the efficacy of ^{89}Sr adjuvant to local field external beam irradiation in the management of endocrine resistant metastatic prostate cancer. *International Journal of Radiation Oncology Biology and Physics* **25** 805–813

Quilty PM, Kirk D, Bolger JJ *et al* (1994) A comparison of the palliative effects of strontium-89 and external beam radiotherapy in metastatic prostate cancer. *Radiotherapy and Oncology* **31** 33–40

Robinson RG (1986) Radionuclides for the alleviation of bone pain in advanced malignancy. *Clinical Oncology* **5** 39–49

Robinson RG, Blake GM, Preston DF *et al* (1989) Strontium-89: treatment results and kinetics in patients with painful metastatic prostatic and breast cancer in bone. *Radiographics* **9** 271–281

The author is responsible for the accuracy of the references.

UK Studies on Suramin Therapy in Hormone Resistant Prostate Cancer

ELIJAH O KEHINDE • TIM R TERRY • NATU MISTRY[1]
TERRY HORSBURGH[1] • DAVINDER P SANDHU • PETER R F BELL[1]
Departments of Urology and Surgery[1], University of Leicester, Leicester General Hospital, Leicester LE5 4PW

INTRODUCTION

Prostate cancer (CaP) that is no longer responsive to conventional hormonal manipulation is associated with a poor overall survival of 9–18 months irrespective of the subsequent therapeutic modality employed (Yagoda, 1989). Secondary hormonal manipulation may result in improvement of symptoms in about 38% of patients, but objective tumour response is less than 10% (Tannock *et al*, 1989). Similar objective tumour regression has been reported with cytotoxic chemotherapeutic agents (Tannock, 1985). Thus, an effective treatment for patients with hormone resistant prostate cancer is urgently needed.

To develop a novel therapy for hormone resistant CaP, a better understanding of the tumour biology of this cancer is required. It is now known that androgens are not the sole mitogens for CaP. Isaacs (1988) has shown that the growth of androgen independent CaP cells is under the influence of a number of polypeptide growth factors. Such non-androgenic growth factors have been

Cancer Surveys Volume 23: *Preventing Prostate Cancer: Screening versus Chemoprevention*

identified from conditioned media of human derived prostate cancer cell lines and from human malignant and benign prostate tissues. These growth factors include basic and acidic fibroblast growth factors (FGF), transforming growth factor (TGF), insulin like growth factor, epidermal growth factor (EGF), platelet derived growth factor (PDGF) and other unclassified mitogens (Connolly and Rose, 1990; Habib, 1990; Morton *et al,* 1990; Pienta *et al,* 1991). Although the actions and interactions of these growth factors are complex and the relative contribution of each factor alone or in combination is unknown, FGFs are likely to play a central part as they are present in the highest relative proportion and have been implicated in the angiogenesis, stromal growth, osteoblastic growth and malignant prostatic epithelial cell growth in vivo (Thompson, 1990). These non-androgenic growth factors behave in an autocrine, paracrine or endocrine manner to stimulate the growth of androgen independent prostate cancer cells. Anti-TGF and anti-EGF receptor monoclonal antibodies are capable of abrogating the proliferation of such tumour systems in vitro, suggesting a potential role for such moieties as components of systemic therapy (Hofer *et al,* 1991).

From a therapeutic point of view, interruption of the interaction between these growth factors and their receptors on prostate cancer cells may have some benefit. Drugs that have been shown to do this include suramin and somatostatin (Taneja *et al,* 1990; Kim *et al,* 1991; La Rocca *et al,* 1991; Kehinde *et al,* 1992).

SURAMIN: GROWTH FACTOR INHIBITOR

Suramin is a polysulphonated naphthylurea first synthesized in 1916 and used for treating African trypanosomiasis and onchocerciasis in the 1920s (Hawkins, 1978). Interest in the drug was rekindled when in 1979, it was found to reduce viraemia in patients with acquired immunodeficiency syndrome (AIDS) and to inhibit reverse transcriptase (De Clercq, 1979; Mitsuya *et al,* 1984). Suramin has since been shown to induce a cytostatic effect upon many tumour cells through various mechanisms, the most important of which appears to be its ability to inhibit the binding of various growth factors to their cell surface receptors (Stein *et al,* 1989). Recent studies have documented that suramin reduces the specific binding of TGF to prostate cancer cells in vitro. Suramin is also capable of increasing the percentage of such cells in the S-phase of the cell cycle, possibly via its ability to inhibit a variety of nuclear enzyme systems including DNA polymerase. Thus, suramin may be capable of inhibiting the proliferation of prostate cancer cells by the alteration of TGF mediated autocrine growth mechanisms and disruption of normal cell cycle kinetics. The latter observation suggests a potential role for the use of suramin and cell cycle specific chemotherapeutic agents. Furthermore, suramin is an adreno-corticolytic agent and thus may slow prostate cell proliferation by lowering circulating adrenal androgen levels. Other actions of suramin include inhibition of

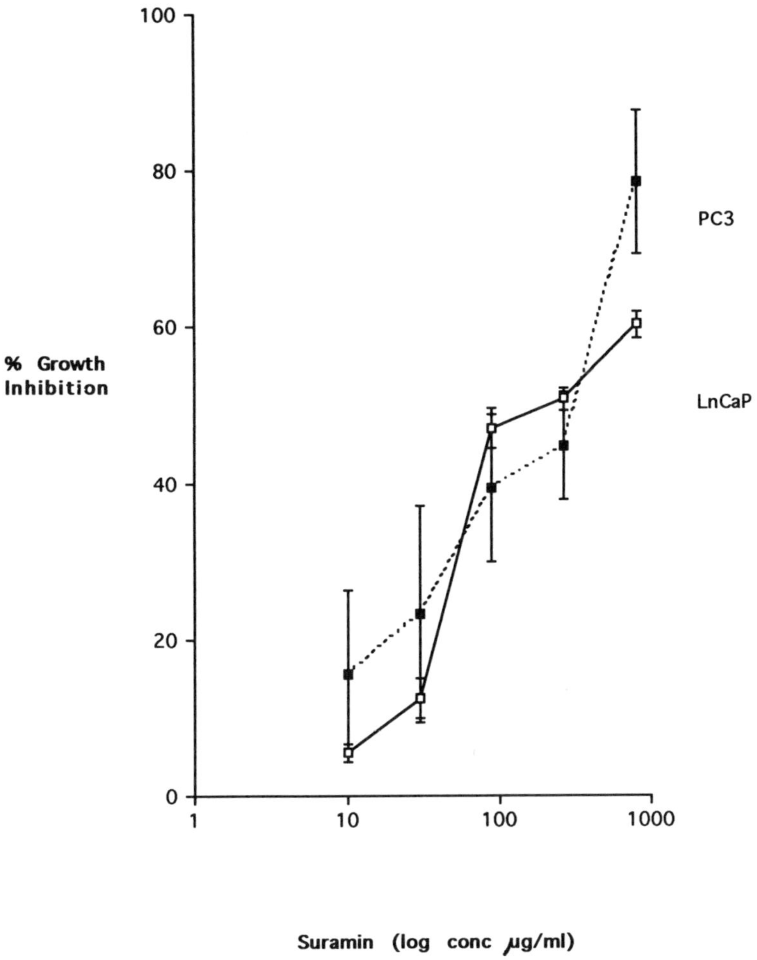

Fig. 1. Inhibition of PC-3 and LnCaP by suramin. Results represent mean of three experiments. Suramin inhibited the growth of LnCaP and PC-3 cell lines in a dose dependent manner

lysosomal enzymes, including hyaluronidase, glucuronidase and sphingoid hydrolases. The effect on lysosomal enzyme synthesis results in a systemic accumulation of glucosoaminoglycans, particularly in the serum, urine, kidney, liver and spleen, and explains some of the unique toxicities of this compound (Davies *et al,* 1971). Suramin is extensively protein bound and its action can be inhibited by albumin (Pollack and Richard, 1990).

EFFECTS OF SURAMIN ON ESTABLISHED HUMAN PROSTATE CANCER CELL LINES: IN VITRO STUDIES

In vitro experiments carried out in Leicester confirmed that suramin at a concentration of 0–270 µg/ml produced dose dependent growth inhibition on the following established prostate cancer cell lines: LNCaP (androgen dependent), PC3 and DU145 (androgen independent cell lines) (Fig. 1). At a concentration of 270 μg/ml, suramin produced 50%, 49% and 68% inhibition of growth of LNCaP, PC3 and DU145 cell lines, respectively, on day 6 (Kehinde *et al,* 1992). These results are similar to those reported previously (Stein *et al,* 1989; Kim *et al,* 1991; La Rocca *et al,* 1991). However, these effects are cytostatic as the withdrawal of suramin on day 6 after exposing the cells to 270 μg/ml leads to continuation of cell growth. The effects of suramin can also be reversed if the cells are grown in the presence of excess growth factors such as EGF and TGFA, indicating that a possible mechanism of action of suramin is by interference with growth factor induced cell proliferation of CaP cells.

In an attempt to improve the therapeutic profile of suramin, we carried out a series of in vitro experiments using combinations of growth factor inhibitors to see whether we could produce synergy with suramin, to render its action cytocidal. Firstly, we used a combination of suramin and somatostatin (SMS201–995). Somatostatin is a known growth factor antagonist that has been found to inhibit the proliferation of PC-3 cell lines in vitro (Taneja, 1990). Somatostatin is believed to antagonize centrosomal separation induced by EGF during cell division (Schally, 1988). Secondly, we tried a combination of suramin and estramustine phosphate (EMP). EMP is a drug that is claimed to be very effective in the treatment of hormone refractory CaP and has been shown to inhibit the proliferation of DU145 prostate cancer cells. EMP produces this effect because of its ability to combine with microtubule associated protein necessary for cell division (Hartley-Asp and Gunnarsson, 1982; Stearns *et al,* 1988). For in vitro combination therapies, the following combinations were used: (a) suramin and somatostatin (SMS201–995), (b) suramin and EMP and (c) EMP and SMS201–995.

The results are shown in Tables 1 and 2. As Fig. 2 shows, the only combination that produced a synergistic effect was EMP and suramin. Suramin at a concentration of 10 μg/ml produced a 14% growth inhibition on the PC-3 cell line. The addition of EMP 12.5 μg/ml to suramin 10 μg/ml increased the percentage growth inhibition to 64% (p=0.001), a difference that is statistically significant. Further in vitro analysis in our laboratory has confirmed that suramin and EMP combined produced synergistic activity. The addition of SMS201–995 to suramin does not improve the growth inhibitory effect over either agent used alone, even though independently the two drugs produce dose dependent growth inhibition. In vitro studies by Fruehauf *et al* (1990) have also reported synergy between suramin and doxorubicin and tumour necrosis factor at concentrations that are well below those associated with significant toxicities in vivo for suramin—that is, less than 250 μg/ml.

EFFECTS OF SURAMIN ON PROSTATE CANCER CELLS OBTAINED BY PRIMARY CULTURE

A major limitation of applying the findings reported above is that even though established CaP cell lines are useful for evaluating the response of CaP cells to

TABLE 1. Growth inhibitory effect of combining suramin (Sur, μg/ml) with somatostatin (SMS, μg/mL) on LNCaP and PC-3 prostate cancer cell lines

% Growth inhibition	Sur 10	Sur 10 +SMS 20	Sur 90	Sur 90 +SMS 20	Sur 270	Sur 270 +SMS 20
LNCaP	14	25	58	68	85*	81*
PC-3	29	25	47	39	54**	46**

*$p<0.2$, N/S; **$p<0.35$, N/S (analysis of variance)
Suramin's growth inhibitory effect was not significantly enhanced by the addition of somatostatin on either cell line
Results represent the mean of three experiments

chemotherapeutic agents, repeated passaging of cells can lead to loss of tumour characteristics (Otto *et al,* 1988). However, cells obtained by primary culture of CaP might provide a more relevant in vitro model. The previous experiments were therefore repeated using cells obtained by primary culture.

We found that in primary epithelial growth medium (WAJC 404 medium based), suramin inhibited the clonal growth of CaP cells in a dose dependent fashion. In addition, the effect of suramin on CaP cells obtained by primary culture was cytostatic and reversible more than 24 hours after the cells were exposed to suramin. These findings agree with those of Peehl *et al* (1991). A combination of suramin and EMP produced more growth inhibition on cells obtained by primary culture than suramin alone. The effect of suramin and EMP is also cytostatic and reversible—although to a lesser extent than to suramin alone—24 hours after exposure to the two drugs.

RESULTS OF CLINICAL TRIALS USING SURAMIN AS MONOTHERAPY IN PATIENTS WITH HORMONE RESISTANT PROSTATE CANCER

The results of our studies suggest that it is likely that suramin may have a role in the treatment of patients with hormone resistant CaP. Since 1990, reports

TABLE 2. Growth inhibitory effect of combining suramin (Sur, μg/ml) with estramustine phosphate (EMP, μg/mL) on prostate cancer cell lines LNCaP and PC-3

% Growth inhibition	Sur 10	Sur 10 + EMP 12.5	Sur 90	Sur 90+ EMP 12.5	Sur 270	Sur 270 + EMP 12.5 μg/0.5 ml	EMP 12.5
LNCaP	3.3*	75*	59	89	76*	93	86
PC-3	14**	64**	51	86	63	92	60

*$p<0.1$; **$p<0.002$ (analysis of variance)
Estramustine phosphate significantly enhanced the growth inhibitory effect of suramin on LNCaP and PC-3 prostate cancer cell lines
Results represent the mean of three experiments

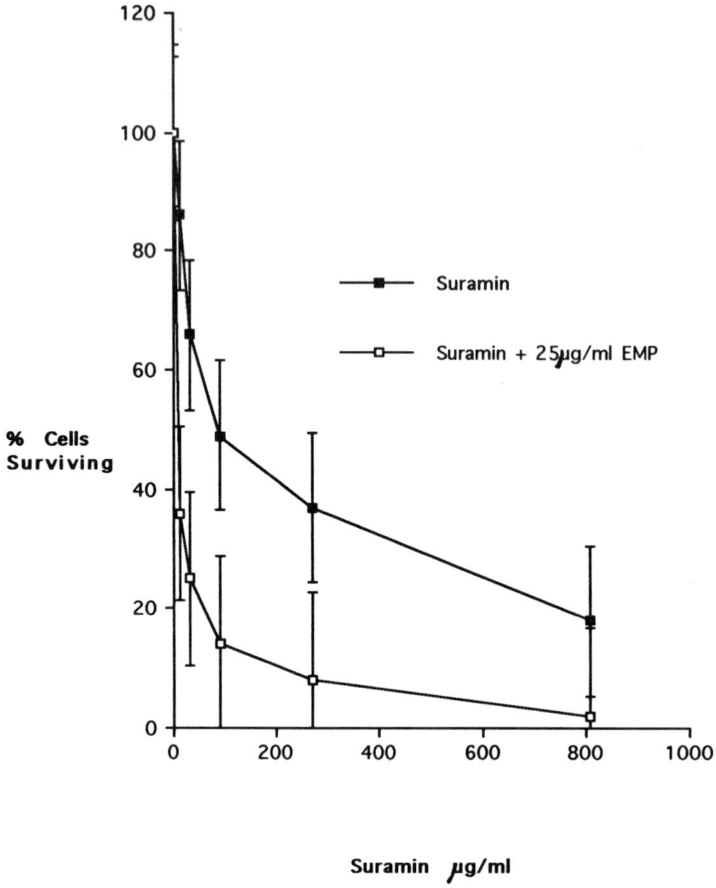

Fig. 2. Effect of suramin and estramustine phosphate on the proliferation of PC-3 cell line. Estramustine phosphate enhances the growth inhibitory effect of suramin

of clinical trials with suramin in patients with metastatic CaP have been published. In the first clinical trials, suramin was used as monotherapy and these will be discussed first (La Rocca *et al,* 1991; Eisenberger *et al,* 1992; Manyak *et al* 1992).

La Rocca *et al* (1991) first established that for suramin to be used as monotherapy for metastatic CaP, a serum suramin concentration of between 250 and 300 µg/ml was necessary. To achieve this, suramin was given as a continuous infusion, and serum suramin concentration was monitored daily. Using this regimen, Manyak *et al* (1992) and Eisenberger *et al* (1992) reported a response rate in patients with measurable lesions, more than a 75% decrease in prostate specific antigen (PSA), good improvement in symptoms and an overall response rate of 53%. However, at a serum concentration of 300 µg/ml, suramin caused many side effects, which included abnormal reversible coagulopathy (73%), rashes (42%), malaise (34%), reversible peripheral neuropathy (30%), reversible vortex keratopathy (8%) and suppression of adrenal activity necessitating replacement doses of hydrocortisone (10–30 mg/day) (La Rocca *et al,* 1991). The use of suramin in the USA was not associated with any mortality in the first 95 patients treated. However, Van Oosterom *et al* (1990), in Belgium, reported seven of nine patients dying of malignancy within 9 weeks of starting suramin infusion, but noted partial responses in four of nine patients and reported that the side effects of suramin were dose dependent. Hence, it could be argued that suramin as monotherapy in metastatic hormone resistant CaP produces modest short term responses, but at the cost of significant toxicity when a therapeutic serum level of 250–300 μg/ml is used.

RESULTS OF CLINICAL TRIALS USING SURAMIN IN COMBINATION WITH OTHER CHEMOTHERAPEUTIC AGENTS

Despite suramin's obvious activity in patients with hormone resistant metastatic CaP, its clinical use is limited by its toxicity and short duration of response. One therapeutic strategy to overcome this is to combine suramin with other drugs that are effective against CaP. This will allow use of lower doses of suramin without losing anti-tumour activity. Rapoport *et al* (1993) have combined suramin with mitomycin C.

Suramin and Mitomycin C

Suramin 350 mg/m^2 daily was given for 5 days, followed by 350 mg/m^2 weekly starting on day 4. Mitomycin C 12 μg/m^2 was given every 5 weeks starting on day 14. During induction of treatment, the median serum suramin level was 140 μg/ml (range 93–270 μg/ml). In 32 patients, one complete and six partial responses were observed, and in 15 patients, the disease had stabilized. The median time to treatment failure (rising PSA, reduced performance status) was 103 days and the median survival was 209 days. Significant side effects noted included haematological toxicities (59%), fatigue (34%), neurotoxicity (31%), proteinuria (28%) and skin rashes (25%). Rapoport *et al* concluded that the combination of suramin and mitomycin C has therapeutic activity but causes significant toxicity in patients with hormone resistant CaP. However, the level of toxicity they found using the combination of drugs and lower levels of suramin was less than that reported for high doses of suramin alone.

Suramin and EMP: The Leicester Regimen: Phase II Clinical Trial: Preliminary Report

In vitro studies on the established human CaP cell lines LNCaP, PC-3 and DU145 and on CaP cells obtained by primary culture in Leicester confirmed that suramin and EMP produce synergistic activity against cell growth. We decided to carry out a clinical trial on patients with metastatic hormone resistant CaP using this combination.

Patients and Methods

Patients with known metastatic prostate cancer, treated by maximal androgen blockade, goserelin or orchidectomy and flutamide, or cyproterone acetate, and who have subsequently had two successive rises in PSA, the last level being over 40 μg/l, were randomized into two treatment arms. Group A received EMP 280 mg twice a day orally for 3 months and group B received EMP 280 mg twice a day orally plus a weekly intravenous infusion of 1 g suramin for 6 weeks. Group C were suitable patients who refused consent and were therefore allowed to continue with their current treatment, mainly orchidectomy or goserelin + cyproterone acetate or flutamide.

The following baseline investigations were performed: full blood count, urea, electrolytes, liver function tests, glucose screen, chest X ray, PSA, bone scan, ultrasound of bladder for residual urine and para-aortic lymph nodes, urinalysis to exclude albuminuria and quality of life assessment using the Karnofsky Score.

Measurement of Serum Suramin Levels. Hawkins (1978) has shown that using suramin 1 g weekly for 6 weeks provides a peak serum suramin concentration of under 200 μg/ml and a trough level of about 10–15 μg/ml 3–6 months after discontinuation of suramin injections. In Leicester, high pressure liquid chromatography was used to determine suramin levels weekly for the first 7 weeks and at 2 month intervals subsequently. The next dose of suramin was to be omitted if the previous week's trough level was more than 300 μg/ml. The aim of this regimen was to keep a peak serum suramin concentration of under 200 μg/ml during induction of treatment and a trough concentration of over 15 μg/ml at 3 or 6 months. The first dose of suramin was given in hospital. Urinalysis was done during each visit before suramin injection. If albuminuria was detected, and serum suramin was more than 200 μg/ml, the next dose of suramin was not given.

Follow-up of Patients. Patients in group B receiving suramin were seen weekly for the first 8 weeks. All patients in groups A, B and C were seen once a month in outpatients, and blood samples were taken for full blood count, liver function tests and PSA. Repeat bone scan was obtained after 6 months of treatment.

Results

Details of the patients in this clinical trial as well as the treatment the patients had before developing hormone resistant CaP are shown in Table 3. Response to treatment is shown in Table 4. The mean baseline PSA for patients in groups A and B was 54 and 58 μg/l, respectively. The mean PSA 3 months after treatment was 15 and 4.1 μg/l for patients in groups A and B, respectively, compared to 159 μg/l for patients in group C. After 6 months of treatment, the mean PSA was 61 μg/l and 4.0 μg/l for patients in groups A and B, respectively, compared to 181 μg/l for patients in group C.

TABLE 3. Profile of patients with hormone resistant prostate cancer undergoing clinical trials with estramustine phosphate (EMP) or EMP and suramin

Patient characteristics	Treatment groups A	B	C
Number	6	6	6
Mean age (range)	68 (64–74)	71 (62–74)	70 (60–73)
Mean duration of previous therapy (months)	72	79	84
Previous hormonal manipulation			
Bilateral subcapsular orchidectomies ± cyproterone acetate ± flutamide	2	3	1
Luteinizing hormone releasing hormone ± cyproterone acetate ± flutamide	4	3	5
EMP	0	1	1
Previous radiotherapy	2	2	1
Stilboestrol ± aspirin	2	1	2

A steady rise in mean serum suramin was seen from 39 μg/ml (range 27–52) on day 7 of treatment to 120 μg/ml (range 105–150) on day 42 of treatment (Fig. 3). The mean value of serum suramin 3 months after the start of treatment was 65 μg/ml.

Side Effects. The side effects found in this study are listed in Table 5. None of the patients in group B (EMP and suramin) developed albuminuria. However, EMP produced significant side effects necessitating discontinuation of EMP therapy in four of six patients in group A and in one of six patients in group B before the third month of treatment. None of the patients in group B developed skin lesions.

One patient in each group had proven deep vein thrombosis. One death occurred in group B 3 months after treatment; the cause of death was not established.

TABLE 4. Response to treatment based on changes in PSA in patients with hormone resistant prostate cancer in groups A, B and C

Group	No of patients	Mean PSA (μg/l) before treatment	after 3 months' treatment	after 6 months' treatment
A	6	54	15*	61**
B	6	58	4.1*	4.0**
C	6	70	159	181

*$p<0.05$; **$p<0.001$

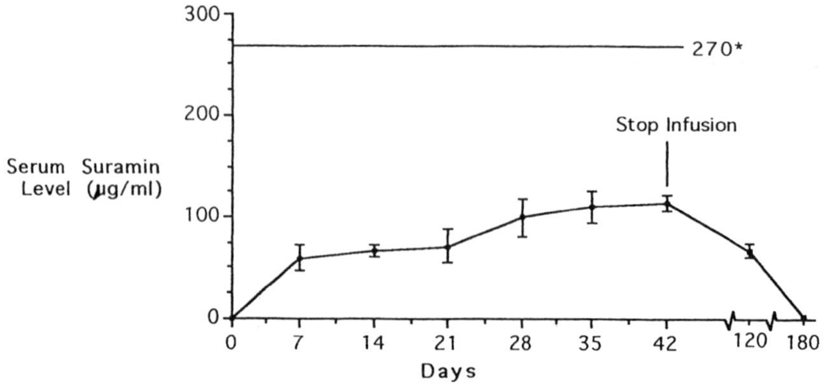

Fig. 3. Trough suramin levels in patients with hormone resistant prostate cancer receiving 1 g intravenous suramin weekly for 6 weeks. * At serum suramin concentration of >270 µg/ml, suramin produced significant toxicity

Response to Treatment. As Table 4 shows, there was a statistically significant fall in the mean value of PSA in group B patients (4.1 µg/l) compared to group A patients (15 µg/l) at the end of 3 months of treatment ($p<0.05$). At the end of 6 months of treatment, the differences in the mean PSA between group A (61 µg/l) and group B (4.0 µg/l) became more significant ($p=0.001$). The PSA started to rise again in group A patients before the end of 6 months of treatment. Two patients in group B and one patient in group A did not have bone pain before they started treatment. Four patients in group B who had bone pain reported a significant reduction in bone pain and in the requirement for analgesics, but none of the five patients in group A reported this. A bone scan 6 months after treatment revealed no change in bony metastases in three patients in group B, whereas in two patients in group A, there was progression of disease. Bone scan analysis has not yet been completed in the remaining seven patients in both groups at the time of this report. There were no bidimensionally measurable metastases in the 12 patients.

Discussion

The results of this pilot study show that the combination of EMP and suramin seems to be better tolerated than EMP alone. Furthermore, the response to treatment as judged by the fall in PSA, the reduction in bone pain and the reduced requirement for analgesics was much better with the combination of EMP and suramin than with EMP alone. The difference in the changes in PSA at the end of 6 months of treatment is statistically significant ($p<0.001$, Fisher's).

Furthermore, EMP and low dose suramin produced fewer side effects than suramin and mitomycin as reported by Rapoport *et al* (1993) and far fewer side effects than high dose suramin alone (La Rocca *et al,* 1991). The side effects produced by the combination of EMP and suramin were probably due to the EMP component. It is tempting to speculate that since suramin and

TABLE 5. Side effects of treatment in patients with hormone resistant prostate cancer receiving EMP alone (group A) or EMP and suramin (group B)

Side effects	Group A (n=6)	Group B (n=6)
Nausea/vomiting	4	0
Cardiovascular		
clinical DVT	1	1
fluid retention	5	4
Abnormal LFT	0	0
Albuminuria	0	0
Gynaecomastia	2	0
Mortality	0	1[a]
Discontinue EMP before 3 months	4	1

DVT = deep vein thrombosis
LFT = liver function test
[a]Died suddenly at home. Responding to treatment at the time of death

EMP show synergisitic activity in vitro, a further reduction in the EMP dose to say 280 or 140 mg daily plus low dose suramin might produce the same clinical response as 560 mg daily of EMP and suramin. We intend to pursue this line of investigation in a phase III clinical trial. One main advantage of our regimen is that EMP is given orally and can also be given to patients who have had previous irradiation for bony metastasis; this is in contradistinction to mitomycin C, which is given intravenously and is not advisable for patients with compromised bone marrow reserve. None of the patients in group B developed the albuminuria or dermatological lesions usually seen with high dose suramin (Rapoport *et al,* 1993). This regimen also obviates the need to use hydrocortisone for adrenal replacement therapy as is necessary with high dose suramin.

The conclusions from this study are that in reasonably matched groups of six patients, EMP and suramin significantly reduced PSA at 6 months compared to continued maximal androgen blockade ($p<0.001$) and secondline EMP alone ($p<0.001$). Side effects from low dose suramin (<200 μg/ml) seemed to be minor and most side effects in group B patients were due to EMP. There was also a significant reduction in bone pain and requirements for analgesics in group B patients compared to patients in groups A and C. Survival figures and bone scan analysis were not available at the time of this report.

Further studies to determine whether other drug regimens using suramin in combinations can produce clinically acceptable results with less toxicity than high dose suramin monotherapy for patients with hormone resistant CaP are warranted.

SUMMARY

New insights regarding the biology of hormone resistant CaP have shown that major growth factors other than testosterone are responsible for cellular proliferation of androgen resistant prostate cancer cells. In vitro studies have confirmed the efficacy of growth factor inhibitors such as suramin in reducing cellular proliferation of androgen dependent LNCaP and independent PC-3 CaP cell lines as well as CaP cells obtained by primary culture. Initial clinical trials using high dose suramin (peak serum concentration 250–300 μg/ml) as monotherapy in patients with hormone resistant CaP have shown some promise, but the duration of response to therapy has been short lived and suramin toxicity is a problem. To minimize toxicity without reducing anti-tumour activity, studies evaluating its use in combination with other cytotoxic drugs are attractive in CaP.

Suramin and doxorubicin, tumour necrosis factor and EMP have shown synergy in vitro. However, in a phase II clinical trial using combination therapy with low dose suramin (140 μg/ml) and mitomycin C in 32 patients, there was one complete response and six partial responses, and in 15 patients, the disease had stabilized. The median time to treatment failure was 103 days, and the median survival was 209 days. This regimen caused significant toxicities.

The present study has shown that the combination of EMP 280 mg twice a day and suramin 1 g weekly infusions for 6 weeks, compared to EMP 280 mg alone, showed a statistically significant difference in the rate of depression of PSA levels after 3 and 6 months of treatment ($p<0.01$) and a statistically significant reduction in bone pain and requirement for analgesics in patients on combination therapy—100% compared to 0% for patients on EMP alone.

References

Connolly JM and Rose DP (1990) Production of epidermal growth factor and transforming growth factor alpha by the androgen-responsive LNCaP human prostate cancer cell line. *The Prostate* **16** 209–218

Davies M, Lloyd JB and Beck F (1971) The effect of trypan blue, suramin and autothiomalate on the breakdown of 125 I-labelled albumin within rat liver lysosomes. *Biochemical Journal* **121** 21–76

De Clercq E (1979) Suramin: a potent inhibitor of the reverse transcriptase of RNA tumour viruses. *Cancer Letters* **8** 9–22

Eisenberger MA, Sinibaldi V, Jodrell D *et al* (1992) Activity of suramin in hormone refractory prostate cancer: University of Maryland experience. *Journal of Urology* **147** 418A

Fruehauf JP, Myers CE and Sinha BK (1990) Synergistic activity of suramin with tumor necrosis factor alpha and doxorubicin on human prostate cancer cell lines. *Journal of the National Cancer Institute* **82** 1206–1209

Habib FK (1990) Peptide growth factors: a new frontier in prostate cancer. *Progress in Clinical and Biological Research* **357** 107–110

Hartley-Asp and Gunnarsson PO (1982) Growth and cell survival following treatment with estramustine, non-nitrogen mustard, and estradiol, and testosterone of a human prostatic cancer cell line DU145. *Journal of Urology* **127** 818–822

Hawkins F (1978) Suramin: with special reference to onchocerciasis. *Advances in Pharmcology and Chemotherapy* **15** 281–322

Hofer DR, Sherwood ER, Bromberg WD *et al* (1991) The functional role of transforming growth factor alpha as an autocrine growth factor in androgen independent human prostatic carcinoma. *Cancer Research* **51** 2780–2785

Isaacs JT (1988) Therapeutic implications of the new tumor biology of cancer of prostate, In: Aumuller G and Krieg M (eds). *New Aspects in Regulation of Prostatic Function,* pp 45–48,

W Zuckschwerdt Verlag, Munich

Kehinde EO, Horsburgh T, Mistry N, Terry T and Donnelly PK (1992) Inhibitors of growth factors in the therapy of hormone resistant prostate carcinoma. *British Journal of Surgery* **79** 1240

Kim JH, Sherwood RE, Sutkowski DM, Lee C and Kozlowski JM (1991) Inhibition of prostate tumor cell proliferation by suramin: alterations in TGF alpha-mediated autocrine growth regulation and cell cycle distribution. *Journal of Urology* **146** 171–176

La Rocca RV, Cooper MR, Uhrich M *et al* (1991) Use of suramin in treatment of prostatic carcinoma refractory to conventional hormonal manipulation. *Urology Clinics of North America* **18** 123–129

Manyak MJ, Aligen JD, McNeills RJ *et al* (1992) Treatment of hormone resistant metastatic carcinoma of prostate with continuous infusion of suramin. *Journal of Urology* **147** 418A

Mitsuya H, Popovic M, Yardoan R *et al* (1984) Suramin protection of T cells in vitro against infectivity and cytopathic effect of HTLV-III. *Science* **226** 172–174

Morton RA, Isaacs JT and Isaacs WB (1990) Differential effects of growth factor antagonists on neoplastic and normal prostatic cells. *The Prostate* **17** 327–336

Otto U, Wagner B, Koppel G, Baisch H and Klosterhalfen H (1988) Animal models for prostate cancer, In: Klosterhalfen H (ed). *New Developments in Biosciences 4. Endocrine Management of Prostatic Cancer,* pp 29–37, Walter de Gruyter, Berlin

Peehl DM, Wong ST and Stamey TA (1991) Cytostatic effects of suramin on prostate cancer cells cultured from primary tumours. *Journal of Urology* **145** 624–630

Pienta KJ, Isaacs WB, Vindirich D and Coffey DS (1991) The effects of basic fibroblast growth factor and suramin on cell motility and growth of rat prostate cancer cells. *Journal of Urology* **145** 199–202

Pollak M and Richard M (1990) Suramin blockade of insulin-like growth factor-I stimulated proliferation of human osteosarcoma cells. *Journal of the National Cancer Institute* **82** 1349–1352

Rapoport BL, Falkson G, Ravats JI *et al* (1993) Suramin in combination with mitomycin C in hormone resistant prostate cancer: a phase II clinical study. *Annals of Oncology* **4** 567–573

Schally AV (1988) Oncological application of somatostatin analogues. *Cancer Research* **48** 6977–6985

Stearns ME, Ang M, Tew K and Prindler LF (1988) Estramustine binds MAP1-like protein to inhibit microtubule assembly in vitro and distrupt organization in DU145 cells. *Journal of Cell Biology* **107** 2647–2649

Stein CA, La Rocca RV, Thomas R *et al* (1989) Suramin: an anti-cancer drug with a unique mechanism of action. *Journal of Clinical Oncology* **7** 499–508

Taneja S, Kozlowski JM and Sherwood ER (1990) The in vitro growth inhibition of human prostate cancer cell lines DU145, PC3 by somatostatin analog RC 160. *Journal of Urology* **143** 225A

Tannock I (1985) Is it false evidence that chemotherapy is of benefit to patients with carcinoma of prostate? *Journal of Clinical Oncology* **3** 1013–1021

Tannock I, Gospodarowicz M, Meakin W *et al* (1989) Treatment of metastatic prostatic cancer with lower dose prednisolone: evaluation of pain and quality of life as prognostic indices of response. *Journal of Clinical Oncology* **7** 590–597

Thompson TC (1990) Growth factors and oncogenes in prostatic cancer. *Cancer Cells* **2** 345–354

Van Oeesterom AT, De Smedt EA, Denis LJ *et al* (1990) Suramin for prostatic cancer: a phase III study in advanced extensively pre-treated disease. *European Journal of Cancer* **26** 422

Yagoda A (1989) Prostate cancer, In: Wittess R (ed). *Manual of Oncologic Therapeutics,* pp 88–94, Lippincott, Philadelphia

The authors are responsible for the accuracy of the references.

American Studies on Suramin Therapy in Hormone Resistant Prostate Cancer

P ROSEN • A BELLDEGRUN
UCLA School of Medicine, Los Angeles, CA 90024-1738

Since the groundbreaking studies conducted over 50 years ago demonstrating the role of androgen deprivation in advanced prostate cancer, no equivalent advance has been generated for patients with disease refractory to primary hormonal management. Indeed, the median survival for patients with metastatic disease no longer responding to hormonal therapy approximates 8 months.

Suramin, a polysulphonated naphthylurea compound first developed early in the 20th century for the treatment of trypanosomiasis, has undergone recent extensive investigation in the USA and Europe as a novel approach to the treatment of hormone refractory prostate cancer. The initial results are encouraging. The development of suramin as an anti-tumour agent began fortuitously in the 1980s following an extensive search for compounds with anti-retroviral activity during the emerging AIDS epidemic. Clinical trials in AIDS patients failed to demonstrate significant anti-viral activity, but some patients with coincident low grade non-Hodgkin's lymphomas or Kaposi's sarcomas had remissions. Furthermore, unusual toxicities, including adrenal cortical necrosis, suggested a potential anti-tumour effect. These observations were supported by in vitro data suggesting protean effects of suramin, including binding to many established heparin binding growth factors, inhibition of glycosaminoglycan metabolism and inactivation of a variety of enzymes including some DNA polymerases and protein kinase C. The first clinical trial of suramin as a potential anti-tumour agent was conducted at the US National Cancer Institute (NCI) (Stein *et al*, 1989). In that study, only limited activity of the drug against adrenal cortical and renal carcinomas was suggested. However, activity of suramin against prostate cancer cell lines and inhibition of the fibroblast growth factor family's binding to their receptors (fibroblast growth factors arc thought to stimulate normal and malignant prostate cell growth) led to more extensive phase I and II testing of suramin in hormone refractory prostate cancer at the NCI, the University of Maryland and other institutions.

The specific pharmacological and toxicological properties of suramin, particularly its lack of metabolism, long terminal half life and significant neuro-

Cancer Surveys Volume 23: *Preventing Prostate Cancer: Screening versus Chemoprevention*

toxicity, had implications for dose schedule and the need for plasma drug level monitoring. Early observations suggested that sustained plasma levels exceeding 300 μg/ml correlated with a potentially life threatening peripheral neuropathy resembling the Guillain-Barré syndrome. The initial clinical trial in prostate cancer reported by Myers *et al* (1992) employed a continuous infusion of suramin with plasma level monitoring using a high performance liquid chromatography (HPLC) assay. Suramin was administered until the target level of 300 μg/ml was reached, usually in 2 weeks. At that point, treatment was withheld for approximately 8 weeks, and the patient was observed for response or toxicity before a second cycle of treatment was begun. In that study, impressive objective and subjective responses were noted, along with dramatic declines in prostate specific antigen (PSA) concentrations. Of 17 patients with bidimensionally measurable metastatic disease, 6 (35%) achieved a complete or partial response. Of the remaining 21 patients with metastases involving only bone, 15 (71%) had alleviation of pain. A decline of PSA by greater than 75% occurred in 34% of patients, and these patients survived significantly longer than the remaining group. Adverse reactions, including coagulopathies, were noted, but severe neurotoxicity was essentially averted, leading the way for further trials.

A second large trial involving suramin in hormone refractory prostate cancer was reported by Eisenberger *et al* (1993) at the University of Maryland. In that study, an alternative approach to dosing schedule based on the drug's long terminal half life was examined with plasma HPLC assays and Bayesian computerized modelling with an adaptive control strategy based on data obtained from a larger population plus the individual patient (Scher *et al,* 1992). Patients were treated with an intermittent bolus schedule. Objective responses paralleling those observed at the NCI were noted in the first cohort of 31 patients reported and confirmed in a larger series. The objective response rate for 12 patients with measurable disease was 50%; 83% of patients with bone pain experienced relief, and 55% of all patients had a decline in PSA of over 75%. Using the intermittent dosing schedule, coagulopathy was insignificant, and dose limiting toxicity consisted of a malaise-fatigue syndrome, which generally limited treatment to 10–12 weeks. Again, major neurotoxicity was avoided by careful plasma level monitoring.

At UCLA, our group has now treated 45 patients using an adaptive control strategy similar to the Eisenberger strategy. In an analysis of our first 36 patients, responses have been less frequent and probably less durable than those reported from the NCI and Maryland (Mendoza *et al,* 1994). In our experience, only 22% of patients achieved a greater than 75% reduction in PSA, and the measurable disease response rate was only 20%. Since we used an administration schedule very similar to that of the Maryland group, questions are raised regarding the reasons for the disparity in results.

Obviously, case selection, including the extent of previous treatment, might influence reported results, and it does appear that our patients might have had a less favourable prognosis on the basis of their higher median PSA levels and more extensive previous treatment. However, a potentially much more important variable that could explain much of the difference between studies is the so-called flutamide withdrawal syndrome, which had not been well recognized at the time of the NCI and University of Maryland studies. Scher and Kelly (1993) have reported that approximately 30% of patients with advanced prostate cancer experiencing disease progression on dual androgen blockade respond to withdrawal of flutamide with a decline in PSA, often accompanied by symptomatic relief and objective evidence of disease regression. This factor alone could account for much of the difference observed between our trial and the previously reported experiences. In our study, all patients had been withdrawn from flutamide at least 1 month before suramin was started and had disease progression despite cessation of flutamide.

A final caveat regarding the independent activity of suramin in prostate cancer has been the concomitant use of hydrocortisone, usually in the dose of 40 mg/day, in order to manage the potential associated adrenal insufficiency seen with suramin. Hydrocortisone or other corticosteroids even at doses approximately equivalent to 40 mg/day of hydrocortisone may have significant anti-tumour activity in hormone refractory prostate cancer. Reports by Tannock, corroborated by others, suggest a 35–40% response rate for corticosteroids as single agents (Tannock *et al,* 1989). Whereas it was previously felt that the replacement dose of hydrocortisone was about 37.5 mg/day, more recent data suggest that physiological replacement doses may be as low as 12 mg/day. Thus, our so-called replacement doses are in fact pharmacological. To assess the independent activity of suramin in hormone refractory prostate cancer, a randomized multicentre trial is now being conducted in the USA. In this trial, a double blind placebo controlled scheme is used, in which all patients will receive 40 mg/day of hydrocortisone and half will also receive suramin. If, after 6 weeks, patients are symptomatically progressing, the code may be broken, and those patients on placebo will be offered suramin. Until the results of this study are known, we should remain cautious in interpreting the earlier literature on suramin activity in hormone refractory prostate cancer.

References

Eisenberger MA, Reyno LM, Jodrell DI *et al* (1993) Suramin, an active drug for prostate cancer: interim observations in a phase I trial. *Journal of the National Cancer Institute* **85** 611–621

Mendoza E, Belldegrun A, Landaw E *et al* (1994) Suramin efficacy and toxicity in hormone refractory metastatic prostate cancer. *Proceedings of American Society of Clinical Oncology Annual Meeting* **13** [Abstract]

Myers C, Cooper M, Stein C *et al* (1992) Suramin: a novel growth factor antagonist with activity in hormone-refractory metastatic prostate cancer. *Journal of Clinical Oncology* **10** 881–889

Scher HI and Kelly WK (1993) Flutamide withdrawal syndrome: its impact on clinical trials in hormone refractory prostate cancer. *Journal of Clinical Oncology* **11** 1566–1572

Scher HI, Jodrell DI, Iversen JM *et al* (1992) Use of adaptive control with feedback to individualize suramin dosing. *Cancer Research* **52** 64–70

Stein CA, LaRocca RV, Thomas R *et al* (1989) Suramin: an anticancer drug with a unique mech-

anism of action. *Journal of Clinical Oncology* **7** 499–508
Tannock I, Gospodarowicz M, Meakin W *et al* (1989) Treatment of metastatic prostate cancer with low-dose prednisone: evaluation of pain and quality of life as pragmatic indices of response. *Journal of Clinical Oncology* **7** 590–597

The authors are responsible for the accuracy of the references.

Multiple Primary Cancers in Association with Prostate Cancer

H S PANDHA • J WAXMAN

Department of Clinical Oncology, Hammersmith Hospital, Du Cane Road, London W12 ONN

INTRODUCTION

The observation that the successful treatment of many primary tumours may be followed by the induction of second malignancies has prompted the investigation of this phenomenon in prostate cancer. The majority of published work is based on information from tumour registries, which is in turn based on death certification. This provides conflicting views as to whether there is or is not a real increase in the risk of second tumours in association with prostate cancer. It is not surprising that the data are contradictory, because they depend on second or third hand information, where the investigators have had no primary contact with the patients. The identification of patients at risk of the development of second tumour is important, particularly so in the context of prostate cancer, whose incidence has doubled during the past 20 years and is now the second most common cause of male cancer deaths. It may be that more intensive follow-up policies are warranted in order to facilitate the early detection of second malignancies. In this chapter, we review published information relating to second tumours occurring in patients with carcinoma of the prostate and present our own data.

Cancer Surveys Volume 23: *Preventing Prostate Cancer: Screening versus Chemoprevention*

HISTORICAL PERSPECTIVE

The phenomenon of multiple primary cancers occurring in the same patient was first described by the German surgeon Billroth in 1989. Forty years later, Warren and Gates collated and published details of 1259 patients with multiple primary malignant neoplasms (Warren and Gates, 1932) and attempted a classification of multiple tumour syndromes. Interest in this phenomenon has increased, and in the literature, there are now over 35 000 reported cases of patients with two separate malignancies.

MULTIPLE CANCERS

The study of multiple primary cancers has led to the identification of tumour groupings based on possible aetiological factors (Table 1). In many cases, the application of reductionist principles to this phenomenon may be simplistic, and a combination of genetic and environmental factors may be causal. For example in breast cancer diet, parity and family history are all important and may be linked to the development of uterine and colonic tumours in the same patient (Scottenfeld, 1982).

Although it is unlikely that hereditary cancers contribute substantially to the overall incidence of the majority of second tumours in cancer patients, some complexes of tumours clearly result to a large extent from genetic factors. Furthermore, specific abnormalities at a number of genetic levels are now being recognized. These new "syndromes" affect predominantly patients aged under 50 years and often include cancers of tissue from different embryological origins, but none include prostate cancer. Indeed, the occurrence of prostate cancer has been regarded as so inevitable by many authors that it has been excluded from many series reporting multiple tumour occurrence. Li and Fraumeni in 1969 described a syndrome affecting young patients, inherited in autosomal dominant fashion, in which there was the predisposition to the development of multiple tumours such as soft tissue sarcomas, leukaemias, adrenocortical, breast and brain tumours. It is now known that this syndrome is due to germline transmission of a mutant allele of the tumour suppressor gene *TP53* on chromosome 17 (Li and Fraumeni, 1988). Mutation of the *APC* gene on chromosome 5 is the cause of adenomatous polyposis coli, in which there is a predisposition to colorectal cancer, as well as malignant neoplasms of the stomach, duodenum, thyroid and brain (Table 2) (Jagelman *et al*, 1988).

Despite well defined chromosomal or germline genetic abnormalities, a number of well documented associations remain intriguing and as yet have no identifiable defect at the genetic level. These include the association between bilateral breast cancer and colorectal cancer and malignancies of the breast and ovary (Fraumeni, 1977).

During the past 20 years, the number of cancer patients successfully treated with radiation and chemotherapy has increased sharply, and the study

TABLE 1. Aetological factors involved in multiple primary cancers

Factor	Associated cancer sites
Treatment effects	
Radiotherapy	Carcinoma of rectum after radiotherapy for carcinoma of cervix; carcinoma of colon after pelvic radiotherapy
Chemotherapy	Acute non-lymphocytic leukaemia following Hodgkin's disease, non-Hodgkin's lymphoma, myeloma, ovary, breast, bladder, gastrointestinal, lung
Hormones	Endometrial and uterine corpus carcinoma after treatment for breast cancer
Immunological effects	Melanoma after chronic lymphatic leukaemia
Endocrine and/or dietary factors	Multicentric cancers of the colon, bilateral breast cancer, clusters of breast, ovary and colonic carcinoma
Environmental factors	
Tobacco and alcohol	Respiratory tract carcinomas and upper gastrointestinal cancers
Genetic predisposition	
Li-Fraumeni syndrome	Breast, soft tissue sarcomas, adrenocortical, brain, leukaemia
Family Cancer Syndrome	Colon, other gastrointestinal sites, ovary, uterus, renal tract, pancreas, breast
Familial Adenomatous Polyposis/ Gardner's syndrome	Colorectal, other gastrointestinal sites, thyroid, brain

of therapy related second cancers has become more important. The risk of second cancers developing after multimodal therapy has been best described in patients with Hodgkin's disease, for whom we can now closely observe large cohorts of "cured" patients over many years. Survivors of Hodgkin's disease have an increased risk of developing any second cancer, but this is by far most commonly leukaemia or non-Hodgkin's lymphoma. The overall relative risks of developing a second cancer due to radiotherapy or chemotherapy are 1.9 and 3.5, respectively, at 10 years, with a relative risk of 2.1 after 10 years if combined modality treatment is given (van Leeuwen *et al,* 1994b). Other important examples of treatment induced second cancers include the increased risk of colorectal cancer after pelvic radiotherapy for carcinoma of the cervix (Boice *et al,* 1985), stomach cancer after radiotherapy for testis cancer (van Leeuwen *et al* 1993), osteosarcoma after radiotherapy for Ewing's sarcoma (Greene *et al,* 1979) and endometrial cancer after either ovarian radiotherapy or more than 2 years of tamoxifen therapy for breast cancer (van Leeuwen *et al,* 1994a). Alkylating agents have been associated with extremely high risks of subsequent acute non-lymphocytic leukaemia following treatment for carcinoma of the ovary, breast, bladder, lung, multiple myeloma, Hodgkin's and non-Hodgkin's lymphomas and paediatric cancers (Lerner, 1978; Bergsagel *et al,* 1979; Greene *et al,* 1982). The risks of second cancers after treatment with epidophyllotoxins such as etoposide are being recognized, as well as second

TABLE 2. Hammersmith Hospital study: patient details

	Prostate cancer alone	Second tumours
Number of patients	196	30
Age at diagnosis	70.1 years	68.9 years
Follow up	28.9 months	30.4 months
Deaths from prostate cancer	97	13
Deaths from second malignancy	–	5

cancers in recipients of bone marrow transplants secondary to immunosuppression (Fuchs *et al,* 1981; Diámond *et al,* 1988; Kumar, 1993). However, in prostate cancer, none of these aetiological factors are significant.

REVIEW OF STUDIES

Five major studies have been published to date, plus several small studies. All are based on information from tumour registries. In general, these registries allow surveillance of the cancer incidence and mortality experience of particular geographical areas or entire countries and permit estimates of the risk of second cancers developing in relatively large and unselected populations of cancer patients. Although these provide information on large numbers of patients, interpretation of their findings has to be guarded because of a number of sources for potential error. Thus, registry information may be skewed by specific patterns of referral, local environmental factors, local treatment practices and demographical variation. The long periods during which data are gathered often encompass many eras of treatment, during which the response rate and survival from a particular malignancy may have improved dramatically.

The tumour registry information gathered is usually based on information from death certification, recordings of clinical details are often incomplete (as medical records themselves are not available) and the actual recordings may be made by clerical rather than health service personnel. Important information, such as tumour grading, review of histology to exclude recurrence of the same tumour and details of treatment and/or response to one or both of the primary tumours, is usually better documented in hospital based studies than registries. For example, in two of the four multicentre studies discussed below, more than 15% of the patient cohorts had incomplete information even regarding patient age. The conclusions from data analysed from long term follow-up of patients on long established registries such as in Denmark and Connecticut may be complicated further in that during the follow-up period, there may have been profound changes in the lifestyle of the population under scrutiny as a result of increased awareness of health issues such as diet, exercise, smoking, occupational hazards, environment, the concept of inherited or familial cancer and cancer screening. These factors may not be taken into account in the bare statistics compiled from registry information.

The incidence of second primary cancers associated with prostate cancer has been noted to be 27% in an autopsy based study by Hadju and Hadju (1968) and 20% in a clinical series by Lynch *et al* (1966). The average incidence of multiple primary malignant neoplasms, disregarding primary site, is 5%, again based on autopsy information (Hadju and Hadju, 1968).

Connecticut Tumor Registry

In 1985, Curtis *et al* reported second tumour incidence in cancer patients from data collected by the Connecticut Tumour Registry, one of the oldest and best established registries (Curtis *et al,* 1985). This centre evaluated 250 000 patients between 1935 and 1982, with follow-up of more than 40 years in some cases. Compared with the rest of the Connecticut population, cancer patients had a 31% increased risk of developing a second cancer overall and a 23% increased risk of cancer at a different site. Little variation was seen for the first 20 years of follow-up. However, there was a 51% risk of second cancers for females after 20 years and 45% for males. Patients with prostate cancer were the only ones found to be at significantly lower risk for second cancer development. In this registry, the risk of prostate cancer has been expressed in two ways: either by recording and following all patients registered with prostate cancer and observing the development of subsequent cancers or by the occurrence of prostate cancer after other primary tumours.

Schoenberg published an interim analysis of data also from this registry in 1977 and found a 29% excess risk of second cancers among 120 195 patients, and in particular a 34% increased risk of prostate cancer (Schoenberg, 1977). Kleinermann *et al,* in a reassessment of the same data in 1985, evaluated the risk of second cancers in 18 135 men with prostate cancer with an average follow-up of 4 years (Kleinerman *et al,* 1985). Curiously, any second cancers occurring within 1 month of the primary tumours were excluded, so the overall incidence of second cancers was probably underestimated. There was an excess of salivary tumours (relative risk 2.7, 95% confidence interval [CI] 1.3–4.8) and leukaemia (relative risk 1.3, 95% CI 1–1.6) in patients followed up for more than 10 years. A total of 1053 cancers were observed, a figure significantly less than the expected incidence of 1241 on the basis of general population rates. The reasons for the deficits of second cancers apart from leukaemia and salivary tumours were not clear. There was equal incidence of chronic lymphatic leukaemia and acute non-lymphocytic leukaemia, but these all occurred in prostate cancer patients who had not received radical radiotherapy. A number of authors have used data from this registry and defined the risk of prostate cancer as the second tumour:

Digestive system cancer: Hoar *et al* (1985) found an increased risk of most cancers in 64 000 patients evaluated and a twofold increased relative risk (95% CI 1.6–2.4) of prostate cancer. There was an increased relative risk of prostate cancer after oesophageal carcinoma (relative risk 3.5, 95% CI 2.35–3.65), small bowel tumours (relative risk 2.8, 95% CI 2.2–3.5) and colorectal cancer (relative risk 1.8, 95% CI 1.25–2.35).

Respiratory system carcinomas: Boice *et al* (1985) found a twofold increased relative risk (95% CI 1.5–2.5) of prostate cancer in 30 000 patients with lung cancer.

Lymphatic and haemopoietic malignancies: Greene *et al* (1985) found a 1.7 increased relative risk (95% CI 1.2–2.2) in 19 000 patients, which was present only for the first 4 years of follow-up in only those with leukaemia. There was no excess risk of prostate cancer in patients with lymphoma.

Testis cancer: Curtis *et al* (1985) found an increased relative risk of 2.1 (95% CI 1.7–2.3) in 1446 patients with testis cancer (Kleinerman *et al,* 1985).

Danish Tumour Registry

Of the cohort of 19 886 patients with prostate cancer evaluated by Osterlind *et al* between 1943 and 1980, 594 second cancers were detected (Osterlind *et al,* 1985). This was significantly less than the expected 1176 cases. Deficits were observed for tumours from all anatomical sites but reached statistical significance only for cancers of the lip, lung and gastrointestinal organs.

Japanese Study

Multiple primary cancers in patients with bladder cancer in Japan were evaluated by Kotake *et al* (1985). The source of data was clinical patient details from Japanese medical literature plus information for cases published in the *Annals of Pathological Autopsy* between 1941 and 1981; 372 cases of multiple primary tumours were found. Of these, there was a significantly increased incidence of prostate cancer (15.3% of total). Although the total number of second cancers of the stomach exceeded that of prostate cancer (27.4% of total), stomach cancer is common in Japan and this incidence did not represent a significant excess.

Georgia Center for Cancer Statistics Tumor Registry

Greenberg *et al* (1988) evaluated all men in metropolitan Atlanta who were initially diagnosed as having prostate cancer between 1975 and 1982. Of the cohort of 3675 men entered into the Georgia Center for Cancer Statistics Tumor Registry, 220 men developed second cancers, exceeding the expected number by 21.4%. Significant excesses of second cancers in the urethra, kidney and bladder were found, as well as cutaneous melanoma. The increased risk of second malignancy was generally greater in men aged under 70 years. Associated genitourinary malignancies tended to occur within 3 years of the prostate cancer.

Columbia-Presbyterian Medical Center Tumor Registry

Liskow *et al* (1987) evaluated 983 patients with prostate cancer through the tumour registry based at Columbia-Presbyterian Medical Center, New York, between 1970 and 1979. Of 919 patients who were evaluable, 106 (11.5%) patients had developed second cancers by January 1986. A total of 74 second tumours were found, including three in each of six patients with two in four. Prostate cancer was the first tumour diagnosed in 59.4% of cases. Comparing the observed incidence rates with expected rates on the basis of the Surveillance, Epidemiology and End Results data from the National Cancer Institute, urinary bladder cancer and malignant lymphoma appeared in excess numbers. The types of bladder cancer found were not recorded (ie superficial v. invasive), but according to the authors, the excess numbers were explained by the detection bias due to the routine use of cystoscopy. However, no explanation for excess numbers of lymphoma cases was apparent; 31.7% of patients with multiple malignancies had the second cancer diagnosed within 6 months of the prostate cancer.

Hammersmith Hospital Study

This is the only hospital based series from a single institution of which we are aware. All patients with prostate cancer assessed and treated from January 1986 to December 1993 inclusive were evaluated. In many cases, the second malignancy had been diagnosed elsewhere, and the pathology was reviewed in these. Patients who failed to continue attending the follow-up clinics were traced through the local hospice service, patients' families, family doctors or the local family practitioner committee. In all cases of second malignancy, the second primary tumour was accepted only when the lesions involved were non-contiguous and had differing morphologies. Multiple foci of tumour within the prostate were regarded as only one malignancy because it could not be established whether these lesions occurred independently. Average age at diagnosis referred to the diagnosis of prostate cancer; average duration of follow-up was defined as the interval in months between diagnosis of prostate cancer and death or last contact. The patients with third and fourth malignancies were counted only as one case of second cancer. Complete response of the prostate cancer to treatment was defined on National Prostate Cancer Project criteria (Schmidt *et al,* 1980), with normalization of tumour markers, reduction in prostatomegaly to normal size and no clinical or radiological evidence of metastatic disease.

TABLE 3. Hammersmith Hospital study: treatment modalities and response

Treatment	Prostate cancer alone (%)	Second malignancies (%)
Prostatectomy	0.5	0
Orchidectomy	13.2	6.6
Radical radiotherapy	7	11.5
Palliative radiotherapy	38	28
Hormonal therapy	84.2	70.1
Response to treatment of prostatic tumor:		
complete response	6.2	0
partial response	69.7	89.4
no response	24.1	0
Responses to treatment of second malignancy:		
complete response	–	69.2
partial response	–	7.8
no response	–	7.8
not evaluable	–	15.2

RESULTS

There were 226 patients in the study. The data were first standardized using person years, the standardized mortality ratio was then calculated, giving the ratio of deaths in the study cohort over the expected number given the national incidence. These differences were tested, taking into account that the data were not directly comparable, since they dealt with different time periods (Breslow and Day, 1987). Thirty patients had second malignancies; myelofibrosis and "benign monoclonal gammopathy" were included because their potential for malignant transformation is high. Of the patients with two or more malignancies, 17 developed prostate cancer first and 11 the second malignancy first, and in two cases, the two tumours occurred within 1 month of each other. There was no statistical difference between average age at diagnosis; the range of ages was also similar in the two groups—50 to 90 years in the prostate cancer only group and 52 to 88 years in the group with second malignancy. Follow-up averaged 1 week to 145 months and 1 month to 80 months, respectively (Table 2).

The two groups were similar in most clinical variables, including the proportion of each group who died of prostate cancer and partial response to hormone manipulation. However, there was a statistically significant difference between the proportion of patients showing no response to treatment of their prostate cancer: 47 patients in the single malignancy group did not respond, compared with only one patient in the second malignancy group ($p < 0.0191$, difference in proportions 0.2013 [95% CI 0.1062–0.2963]). Most patients with second tumours had a complete response to treatment (Tables 2 and 3).

TABLE 4. Hammersmith Hospital study: second malignancies observed

Tumour	Observed	Observed/ 100 000/yr	Expected/per 100 000/yr[a]
Basal cell	2	885	233.22
Lung	3	1327	427.57
Bladder	5	2212	123.09
Piriform fossa	1	442	3.77
Parotid	1	442	2.79
Squamous cell (skin)	1	442	115.11
Cholangiocarcinoma	1	442	7.57
Oesophageal	1	442	48.71
Caecal/colonic	5	2212	123.27
Carcinoid	1	442	0.66
Rectal	3	1327	90.86
Hairy cell leukaemia	1	442	0.33
Myelofibrosis	1	442	12.22
Myeloma[b]	3	1327	22.21
Chronic lymphatic leukaemia	2	885	15.01
Acute myeloid leukaemia	1	442	16.95
Haematological (all)	8	3539	54.52

[a]Calculated for male population above 45 years: 5693 100 (1981 census)
[b]Includes plasmacytoma and BMG

Table 4 compares the incidence of second tumours compared with the expected incidence according to Office of Population, Censuses and Surveys data in men above 50 years in England and Wales. All tumours except lung and squamous tumours of the skin occurred more frequently than expected, and this difference was statistically significant.

DISCUSSION

There are several explanations for the findings in this and previous studies. It is possible that certain second cancers may not have been discovered without intensive surveillance for the prostate cancer and bladder tumours. In our cohort, the three cases of bladder carcinoma preceded prostate cancer. Comparison against the cancer risk of men in the general population would then have suggested that the patients with prostate cancer had increased risk of second malignancies. This detection bias does not apply to the majority of our patients: 11 patients had malignancy before prostate cancer, and in all but one of the remainder, the second tumour presented to a different clinical team for treatment, in many instances at a different hospital. The possibility that the type of treatment of one tumour caused the second tumour must be carefully evaluated. In the group with other tumours before detection of prostate cancer, two patients had haematological malignancies that were treated successfully with alkylating agents 8 years and 2 years previously. There was no difference in the proportion of patients receiving radical radiotherapy to the prostate. In the remaining patients, there was no anatomical or temporal relationship between the two tumours, nor did any tumours arise within areas of radiotherapy.

The incidence of cancer rises with age, and this includes the occurrence of multiple tumours in the same patient. The finding of asymptomatic prostate cancer during surveillance for a specific primary cancer or health screening programmes may reflect more aggressive investigation in a predominantly older age group. This close scrutiny may indicate that the true incidence of asymptomatic prostate cancer may have been previously underestimated. Alternatively, with the increased survival from prostate cancer with hormonal manipulation and subsequent closer surveillance, the appearance of second tumours may be expected with increased age. The third possibility is that patients with prostate cancer have a specific response to environmental and/or genetic factors that may predispose them specifically to the development of second cancers.

There is no specific or unique genetic abnormality that is associated with prostate cancer, either in its "sporadic" form or as associated with second cancers. Molecular studies during the past decade suggest that activation of specific oncogenes separately or with the inactivation of certain tumour suppressor genes allows uncontrolled cellular proliferation and leads to tumorigenesis. Abnormalities in the *TP53* tumour suppressor gene has been seen in a variety of adult solid tumours, including prostate cancer, and is thought to be the most common genetic abnormality seen in human tumours (Malkin *et al,* 1990). Aberrant expression of another tumour suppressor gene, the retinoblastoma (*RB*) gene, has also been associated with prostate cancer and with the occurrence of multiple tumours (Bookstein *et al,* 1990). Although a number of abnormalities of oncogene expression have been described with prostate cancer, they are not seen consistently enough to have diagnostic, prognostic or therapeutic value for the management of prostate cancer. Furthermore, up to now, a fuller understanding of the molecular genetics of prostate cancer has been hampered by the difficulty in establishing suitable cell lines in the laboratory. At present, there are only four prostate carcinoma cell lines available to study.

SUMMARY

Patients with prostate cancer are at a significant risk of either having a preceding tumour or developing a second malignancy. The precise mechanism by which second cancers develop is not clear but may be the result of exposure to a shared mutagen, abnormalities in oncogene activation or the aberrant expression of tumour suppressor genes. In the recent past, case reports and tumour registry studies on the risk of second cancer development have been important and have alerted the clinician that careful surveillance in this group of patients is required. More prospective hospital based studies are required to delineate the true risk of second malignancies in association with prostate cancer.

References

Bergsagel DE, Bailey AJ, Langley GR *et al* (1979) The chemotherapy of plasma cell myeloma and the incidence of acute leukaemia. *New England Journal of Medicine* **301** 743–748

Billroth T (1889) *Die Allgemeine Churigische Pathologie und Therapie,* p 908, Reimer, Berlin

Boice JD and Fraumeni JF Jr (1985) Second cancer following cancer of the respiratory system in connecticut, 1935-1982. *National Cancer Institute Monograph* **68** 83–98

Boice JD, Day NE, Andersen A *et al* (1985) Second cancers following radiation treatment for cervical cancer. *Journal of the National Cancer Institute* **74** 955–975

Bookstein R, Rio P, Madreperta S *et al* (1990) Promotor deletion and loss of Rb gene expression in human prostate cancer. *Proceedings of the National Academy of Sciences of the USA* **87** 7762–6

Breslow NE and Day NE (1987) *Statistical Methods in Cancer Research,* Vol II, p 69, International Agency for Research on Cancer, Lyon

Curtis RE, Boice JD, Kleinerman R *et al* (1985) Multiple primary cancers in Connecticut 1935-82. *Nattional Cancer Institute Monograph* **68** 219–232

Diámond CA and Matthay KK (1988) Childhood acute lymphoblastic leukaemia. *Paediatric Annals* **17** 156–161

Fraumeni JF Jr (1977) Clinical patterns of familial cancer, In: Mulvihill JJ, Milber RW and Fraumeni JF Jr (eds). *Genetics of Human Cancer,* pp 223–233, Raven Press, New York

Fuchs EF, Key R, Poole R *et al* (1981) Uroepithelial carcinoma in association with cyclophosphamide ingestion. *Journal of Urology* **126** 544–545

Greenberg RS, Rustin E and Scott-Clark W (1988) Risk of genitourinary malignancies after cancer of the prostate. *Cancer* **61** 396–401

Greene MH and Wilson J (1985) Second cancer following lymphatic and haemopoietic cancers in Connecticut, 1935-1982. *National Cancer Institute Monograph* **68** 191–217

Greene MH, Olanbiger DL, Mead D *et al* (1979) Subsequent cancer in patients with Ewing's sarcoma. *Cancer Treatment Reports* **63** 2043–2046

Greene MH, Boice JD, Greer BE *et al* (1982) A cute non-lymphocytic leukaemia after treatment with alkylating agents for ovarian cancer. *New England Journal of Medicine* **307** 1416–1421

Hadju SI and Hadju EO (1968) Multiple primary malignant tumours. *Journal of the American Genetic Society* **16** 16–26

Hoar SK, Wilson J, Blot WJ *et al* (1985) Second cancer following cancer of the digestive system in Connecticut 1935-1982. *National Cancer Institute Monograph* **68** 49–82

Jagelman DG, De Cosse JJ and Bussey HJR (1988) Upper gastrointestinal cancer in familial polyposis coli. *Lancet* **i 0** 1149–1151

Kleinerman RA, Lieberban J and Li F (1985) Second cancer following cancer of the male genital system in Connecticut 1935-1982. *National Cancer Institute Monograph* **68** 139–147

Kotake J and Kiyohara H (1985) Multiple primary cancers associated with bladder cancer. *Japanese Journal of Clinical Oncology* **15 (Supplement)**

Kumar L (1993) Epipodophyllotoxins and secondary leukaemia. *Lancet* **342** 819–820

Lerner H J (1978) Acute myelogenous leukaemia in patients receiving chlorambucil as long-term adjuvant chemotherapy for stage II breast cancer. *Cancer Treatment Reports* **62** 1135–1138

Li FP, Fraumeni JF Jr *et al* (1988) A cancer family syndrome in 24 kindreds. *Cancer Research* **48** 5358–5362

Liskow A, Neugut A, Benson M *et al* (1987) Multiple primary neoplasms in association with prostate cancer in black and white patients. *Cancer* **59** 380–384

Lynch HT, Larsen AL, Mangnusin CU and Krusch AJ (1966) Prostatic carcinoma and multiple primary malignancies. *Cancer* **19** 1981–1987

Malkin D, Li FP, Strong LC and Fraumeni JF Jr (1990) Germline p53 mutations in a familial syndrome of breast cancer, sarcomas and other neoplasms. *Science* **250** 1233–1238

Osterlind A, Rorth M and Prener A (1985) Second cancer following cancer of the male genital system in Denmark, 1943-1980. *National Cancer Institute Monograph* **68** 341–347

Schmidt JD, Scott WW, Gibbon R *et al* (1980) Chemotherapy programs of the National Prostate Cancer Project (NPCP). *Cancer* **45** 1937–1946

Schoenberg BS (1977) Multiple primary neoplasms: The Connecticut Experience 1935-1964. *Recent Results in Cancer Research* **58** 1–173

Scottenfeld D (1982) Multiple primary cancers, In: Schottenfeld D and Fraumeni JF Jr (eds). *Cancer Epidemiology and Prevention,* pp 1025–1035, Philadelphia Saunders

van Leeuwen FE, Satiggelbout AM, Vandenbeltdusebout AW *et al* (1993) Second tumours after radiation treatment of testicular germ-cell tumours. *Journal of Clinical Oncology* **11** 2286–2287

van Leeuwen F, Benraadt J, Coebergh J *et al* (1994a) Risk of endometrial cancer after tamoxifen treatment of breast cancer. *Lancet* **343** 448–452

van Leeuwen FE, Klokman WJ, Hagenbeek A *et al* (1994b) Second cancer risk following Hodgkin's disease: a 20 year follow-up study. *Journal of Clinical Oncology* **12** 312–325

Warren S and Gates O (1993) Multiple primary malignant tumours: a survey of the literature and statistical study. *American Journal of Cancer* **16** 1358–1414

The authors are responsible for the accuracy of the references.

Gene Therapy: Principles and Potential

SAMIR S TANEJA • SHEN PANG • PEJMAN COHAN
ARIE BELLDEGRUN

Division of Urology, Department of Surgery, UCLA School of Medicine, Los Angeles, California 90024-1738

INTRODUCTION

The recent exponential growth of recombinant DNA technology along with our increasing knowledge of the molecular genetics of human disease has paved the way for a new approach to the therapy of human cancers. Gene therapy offers a renewed hope of utilizing the differential characteristics of normal and malignant tissue in constructing treatment strategies. Several gene therapy protocols have been used in the treatment of metabolic disorders such as cystic fibrosis and adenosine deaminase deficiency. From lessons learned in these early trials, we now venture into the application of gene therapy techniques to the treatment of malignant disease (Table 1).

Gene therapy involves the alteration of phenotypic expression of a targeted cell through the alteration of the cell's genotypic content. Through the addition of functional genes, or the functional deletion of a pre-existing gene, the behaviour of a target cell can be altered in order to achieve a desired therapeutic effect. In the case of neoplastic disease, the desired effect is the slowing or stopping of tumour growth or, ideally, destruction of the cell itself.

In effecting a successful gene therapy strategy, several fundamental issues must be addressed. An appropriate method of inserting genes into the desired

Cancer Surveys Volume 23: *Preventing Prostate Cancer: Screening versus Chemoprevention*

TABLE 1. Examples of clinical protocols for cancer gene therapy

Transferred gene	Target cell	Disease	Institution
Tumour necrosis factor (*TNF*)	tumour infiltrating lymphocytes	malignant melanoma	National Institutes of Health
TNF	tumour cells	advanced cancer	National Institutes of Health
Interleukin 2 (*IL2*)	tumour cells	advanced cancer	National Institutes of Health
Herpes simplex thymidine kinase	ovarian cancer cells	ovarian cancer	University of Rochester, New York
HLA-B7	in vivo	malignant melanoma	University of Michigan
Herpes simplex thymidine kinase	in vivo	brain tumour	National Institutes of Health
IL2	bone marrow cells	neuroblastoma	St Jude Children's Research Center, Tennessee
IL2	tumour cells	renal cell carcinoma	Memorial Sloan-Kettering Cancer Center, New York
IL4	tumour cells	malignant melanoma	University of Pittsburgh, Pennsylvania
Anti-sense *RAS* or *TP53*	in vivo	non-small cell lung cancer	University of Texas, MD Anderson Cancer Center

target cell must be identified. Traditional methods of plasmid transfection have largely been replaced by the use of replication deficient viral vectors, which provide consistently higher efficiency in the transfer of genes. Individual characteristics of each viral vector designate its utility in a given gene therapy strategy. Once an appropriate gene transfer vector is selected, a method of selectively delivering the potentially toxic gene to sites of cancer must be designed. Several potential methods have been devised for ex vivo, organ directed, or in vivo systemic delivery of genes. The chosen method must be tailored to the specific tumour and patient being treated. Finally, an appropriate gene for insertion must be selected. Such a gene must be capable of altering the biological behaviour of the cancer cell in order to slow growth, reduce local invasive potential or induce apoptosis. Individual molecular characteristics of the tumour will dictate the selection of an appropriate gene.

The application of gene therapy to prostate cancer has brought with it many challenges unique to this malignancy. The tumour is slow growing, making tumoricidal intervention difficult by standard methods. In addition, prostate cancer carries great heterogeneity in tumour morphology between both individual tumours and various cell populations within a single tumour. Such heterogeneity makes alteration of cell behaviour within an entire tumour difficult with a single genetic manipulation. Careful analysis of cells from prostate tumours within multiple sites from many patients may ultimately provide a common genetic intervention.

In this chapter, we discuss the various vectors suitable for prostate cancer gene therapy, suggested methods for delivery of genes to sites of cancer metastasis and genes potentially suitable for effective alteration of cell behaviour.

VECTOR SELECTION

Multiple methods of gene transfer exist ranging from the delivery of naked DNA to the use of replication deficient viral vectors genetically reconstructed to carry functional genes. The appropriate method must be chosen to meet the needs of the desired outcome of gene therapy. Traditional methods of plasmid transfection (Neumann *et al,* 1982; Chen and Okayama, 1988; Jaffee *et al,* 1993) carry significant limitations with regard to their application to in vivo gene therapy protocols. Such methods require targeted cells to be in culture prior to transfection and often result in extremely low and inconsistent rates of transfection. Although plasmid transfection does carry some potential for use in gene modified tumour vaccine protocols, several limitations specific to prostate cancer exist. The intrinsic difficulty in passaging prostate cancer cells in vitro makes the practical application of plasmid transfection virtually impossible in a reproducible fashion. Reported rates of transfection efficiency following plasmid transfection in human prostate cancer cell lines have been extremely low. In addition, we have found that viral gene transfer results in 1000 to 10 000 times greater expression of the inserted gene when compared to plasmid transfection by electroporation or calcium phosphate precipitation. Cytotoxicity is also highly prevalent, with cell death ranging from 50% to 90% with plasmid transfection of prostate cancer cell lines LNCaP, DU145 and PC-3, depending on the transfection method used.

Retroviral Vectors

Jaffee and co-workers have described the use of MFG retroviral vectors to achieve highly efficient gene transfer in several cell lines. High levels of mRNA are generated through use of Moloney murine leukaemia virus long terminal repeat sequences driving full length viral mRNA and subgenomic viral envelope mRNA containing the inserted gene. Recombinant MFG vectors are constructed by inserting the desired gene precisely at the point of initiation codon for the deleted gene encoding for envelope mRNA (Fig. 1). In the first studies reported of the use of MFG replication deficient retroviral vectors in prostate cancer, the MFG retroviral vector was used for the transfer of the β-galactosidase gene to various prostate cancer cell lines (Sanda *et al,* 1993). Single transduction experiments with the MFG vector resulted in transfer of the functional gene to 22–54% of cells in culture depending on the prostate cancer cell line tested. Gene transfer rates of 80% could be achieved through serial transduction. Little cytotoxicity was reported, with no significant effect on cell growth when compared to sham controls. Furthermore, transduction of two cell lines generated from radical prostatectomy resulted in gene transfer rates of approximately 50%.

Despite efficient gene transfer, the application of retroviral vectors to prostate cancer therapy is perhaps limited to use in tumour vaccine strategies. The high percentage of stable integration into the host cell genome seen with

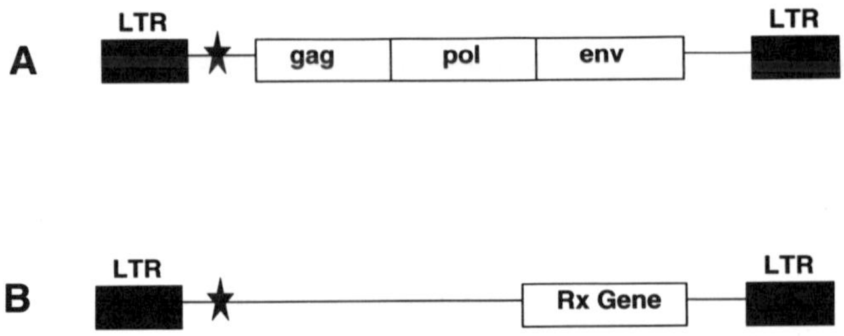

Fig. 1. Genetic structure of naturally occurring (A) and recombinant (B) retroviruses. (A) Genetic structure of the Moloney murine leukaemia virus with long terminal repeat (LTR) sequences directing viral transcription and mediating integration into the host cell genome. The star sequence is necessary for encapsidation. The *gag*, *pol* and *env* genes encode viral core proteins, reverse transcriptase and envelope glycoproteins, respectively. (B) The genetic structure of an MFG vector with inserted therapeutic gene (Rx gene) replacing the genes of viral replication. The vector is rendered replication defective requiring a packaging cell line for active replication

the retrovirus makes it ideal for the introduction of immunostimulatory cytokine genes into cultured cells in vitro. The ultimate goal of inducing an anti-tumour immune response upon reinfusion of transduced cells is likely to be achieved more easily with the prolonged expression of the inserted gene seen following stable transduction. This is especially obvious when compared to other vectors resulting in predominantly transient transfection with genomic integration rates of 1–5%. The requirement of rapid cell division for efficient retroviral gene transfer poses a potential limitation specific to prostate cancer. This is largely due to the morphological heterogeneity of these tumours with subpopulations of slower growing cells usually present in vivo. This would certainly limit the ability to achieve efficient gene transfer within sites of prostate cancer in situ with systemic delivery of the vector.

Adenoviral Vectors

The replication deficient adenoviral vector may offer a promising alternative to the retroviral vector for strategies involving systemic delivery of genes. The adenovirus has several characteristics that make it ideal for use in prostate cancer gene therapy. The virus is capable of entering cells through a receptor mediated mechanism, providing significant tropism to cells of epithelial origin. Unlike the retrovirus, efficient gene transfer can be achieved in non-replicating cells or even in tissue not in culture simply through virus to cell contact. Adenovirus has already been used in human gene therapy protocols for cystic fibrosis and adenosine deaminase deficiency, thus ensuring its safety for use in prostate cancer. Finally, due largely to its efficient entry into replicating and non-replicating cells of epithelial origin, adenovirus may be ideal for in vivo systemic therapy provided an effective avenue of delivery to sites of metastatic cancer can be devised.

In constructing a replication deficient adenoviral vector, the serotype 5 adenovirus has been used. By deleting the E1a and/or E1b regions of the early

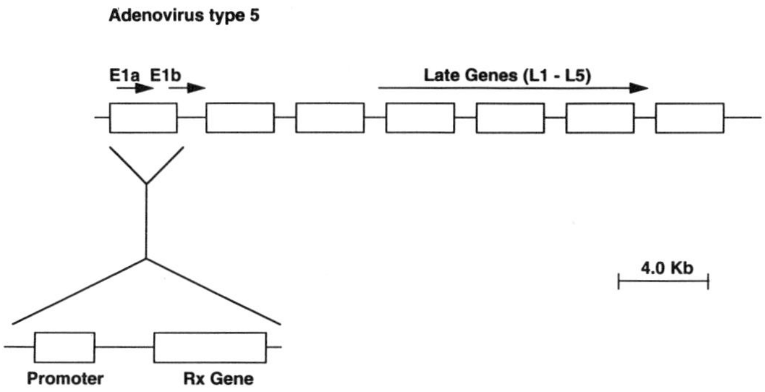

Fig. 2. Naturally occurring genome of the adenovirus carries both early and late domains. Early elements of the genome encode for proteins necessary for viral replication, whereas late elements encode structural components used in viral construction. In genetic reconstruction, the E1a and E1b early region is replaced with an expression cassette carrying the desired therapeutic gene driven by a promoter sequence. The virus is thereby rendered replication deficient, requiring a packaging cell line, carrying the early viral regions in trans, for active replication

viral domain, the virus is rendered incapable of replication without a packaging cell line carrying the E1a region in trans (Berkner, 1988; McGrory *et al,* 1988; Levrero *et al,* 1991). The deleted region is then the site of insertion of an ap-

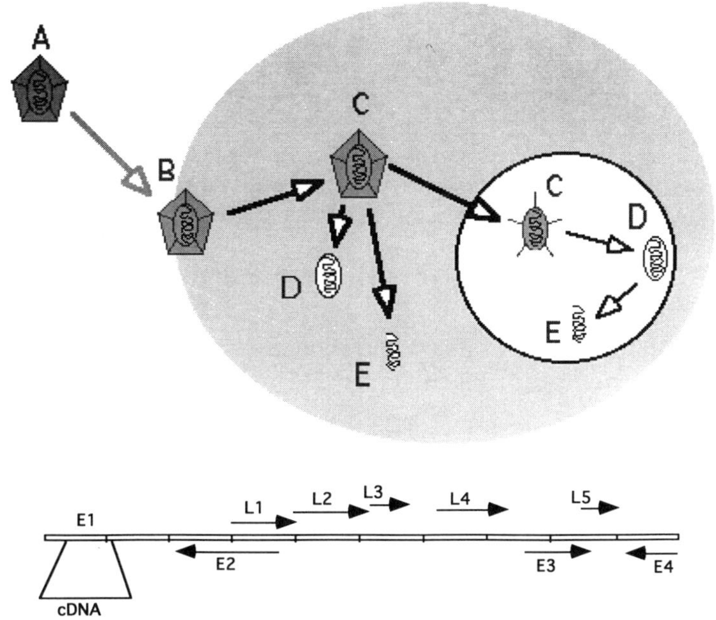

Fig. 3. Mechanism of adenoviral infection. (A) Reconstructed replication deficient virus carrying inserted gene. (B) Attachment of adenovirus to host cell membrane through ligand receptor mechanism. (C) Internalization of adenovirus within an endosome. (D) The adenovirus migrates into the host cell nucleus shedding capsid proteins leaving only DNA. This can occur within the cytoplasm through joining of endosome and lysosome. (E) The episomal adenovirus DNA uses the host cell transcriptional and translational enzymes to transcribe early viral domains and produce the inserted therapeutic protein

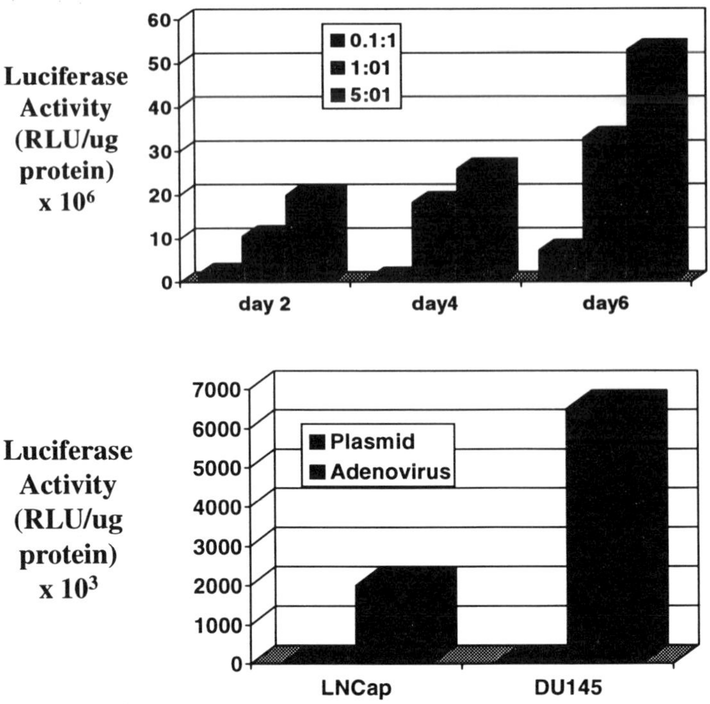

Fig. 4. (*Top*) Human prostate cancer cell line LNCaP is infected with adenoviral vector Ad-CMV-Luc, carrying expression cassette of cytomegalovirus promoter driven firefly luciferase gene, in increasing multiplicities of infection (MOI). Increasing levels of expression are noted throughout the first week following infection as well as with increasing MOI. (*Bottom*) Peak expression at day 2 following adenoviral infection of two human prostate cancer cell lines is compared to peak expression achieved at day 2 following plasmid transfection by electroporation using identical expression cassette. A 1000 to 10 000 times greater expression is achieved with adenoviral infection

propriate expression cassette consisting of promoter and therapeutic gene (Fig. 2). Although the virus is capable of high rates of transfection, the transfection is generally transient with low rates of genomic integration (usually less than 5%). Expression is carried out from the episomal virus using the host cell transcriptional machinery (Fig. 3).

We have performed preliminary studies of adenovirus mediated gene transfer in prostate cancer cell lines LNCaP, DU145 and PC-3 (Taneja *et al*, 1994a). Using an expression cassette of cytomegalovirus promoter driven firefly luciferase, we have noted high levels of expression (up to 10^8 relative luminescence units/μg protein) with relatively low multiplicity of infection. Even at a multiplicity of infection of 0.1 viral particles per cell, luciferase expression is consistently several times greater than in standard plasmid transfection methods. Expression appears to peak at days 2 to 6 depending on the cell line and rate of cell replication (Fig. 4). Rapidly proliferating cell lines appear to have a diluting effect on expression level due to inconsistent passage of inserted genes to progeny at time of cell division. Expression persists throughout 2 weeks following infection. Infection of cell lines derived from a radical

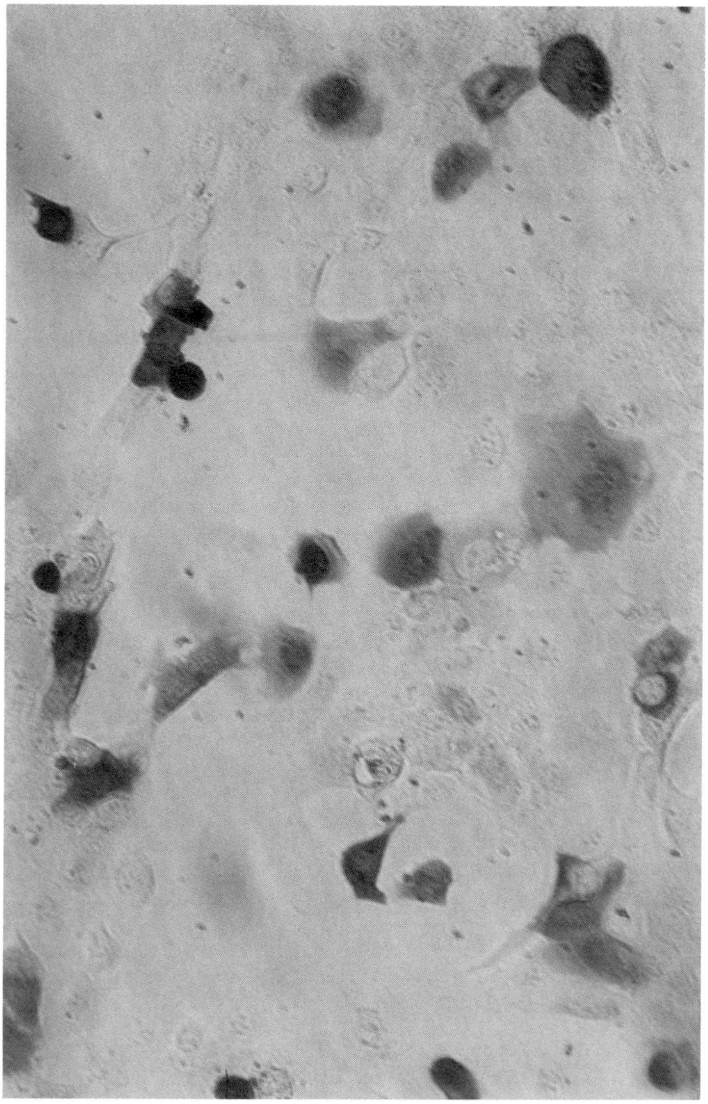

Fig. 5. Human prostate cancer cell line DU145 following infection with adenoviral vector Ad-CMV-B-gal carrying expression cassette of CMV promoter driven β-galactosidase gene. Cells were infected at MOI of 3:1 and incubated in culture for 2 days. Cells were then fixed and stained for β-galactosidase activity. Even at low MOI, significant cell staining is noted following a 1 hour infection. Some cytotoxicity is noted with focal disruption of the adherent cell monolayer

prostatectomy specimen resulted in similar transfection efficiencies. Cells were infected during the fourth or fifth passage, with peak expression occurring at days 4 to 6. With infection using an expression cassette carrying the β-galactosidase gene, cell staining revealed transfection rates of up to 65% at a multiplicity of infection of 10:1 (Fig. 5). Transfection rates increase with increasing multiplicities of infection as does cytopathic effect. Prolonging infection time also increases the transfection rate without significantly increasing cytotoxicity.

The shortcomings of the adenoviral vector are largely due to the relatively short duration of expression. This limitation makes the adenovirus a poor choice for tumour vaccine protocols requiring stable expression of the inserted cytokine. Use in protocols designed for in vivo directed gene delivery may require repetitive delivery of genes to generate an adequate therapeutic effect. In addition, the high incidence of previous exposure to most adenovirus serotypes seen in adults results in overwhelming humoural immunity to circulating adenovirus. This in combination with high levels of hepatic deposition of circulating virus would make unprotected systemic delivery of adenoviral particles an extremely inefficient avenue of delivering virus to sites of metastatic cancer in vivo.

Other viral vectors including herpesviruses and adeno-associated viruses (AAV) have been proposed for use in prostate cancer gene therapy. The use of AAV remains to be investigated as previous experience in other tumour models has been fraught with difficulty in viral expansion and handling. Vieweg *et al* (1994a) recently reported the use of liposome-DNA complexes containing an interleukin 2 (IL2) expressing AAV. Cells of the Mat-ly-lu Dunning rat model were transduced with the liposome-AAV construct, resulting in stable IL2 expression for 12–14 days, with IL2 levels comparable to those of retrovirally transduced cells. Transduction rates were reported to be 45%, indicating relatively efficient gene transfer.

STRATEGIES FOR GENE THERAPY

The majority of gene therapy strategies studied so far have fallen into one of three categories: (a) gene modified tumour vaccines, (b) direct local gene delivery and (c) systemic directed gene therapy. Selection of an appropriate method must rely on knowledge of the biology of the tumour to be treated, the response of the tumour to immune modulation, the desired therapeutic gene and its mechanism of action, as well as the stage and extent of disease to be treated.

Tumour Vaccines

The concept of the tumour vaccine is perhaps the most developed of these methods and has been used within clinical protocols in other tumour models. Cells are extracted from a patient with metastatic cancer and are transfected ex vivo with one of several functional cytokine genes. Following irradiation, the cells are reinfused into the patient in an effort to induce an enhanced target specific immune response to tumour sites throughout the body. Depending on the cytokine inserted, the immune response may be major histocompatibility complex class I or II restricted.

Initial reports of induction of immune response arose in murine models using colon and melanoma cell lines known to be poorly immunogenic (Fearon

TABLE 2. Effect of gene modified R11 cells on tumorigenicity of parental R11 cells in mice (Bellegrun *et al*, 1993)

Tumour cells injected into		No of mice with tumour/No of mice given injections
right flank	**left flank**	
Experiment 1		
Parental R11	–	11/14
R11 control vector	–	7/10
R11 *IL2* + *INFA*	–	1/10
Experiment 2		
–	parental R11	3/4
R11-*IL2* + *INFA* + parental R11	–	0/5
R11-*IL2* + *INFA*	parental R11	5/5
Parental R11+ exogenous human *IL2* and *INFA*	–	2/3

et al, 1990). Cells were transfected ex vivo with murine IL2 and reinjected subcutaneously into syngeneic mice. Tumour cells producing IL2 failed to grow, and mice initially exposed to these IL2 producing tumour cells were conferred protective immunity against subsequent tumour challenge. Failure of transfected tumour cells to grow in $CD4^+$ depleted mice confirmed the ability of gene modified tumour vaccines to bypass T helper cell function. Many other cytokines have ultimately been tested with variable results.

Use of gene modified tumour vaccines in human tumour cell lines reveals similar results. Belldegrun *et al* (1993) transfected the R11 renal cell cancer cell line with *IL2* and/or interferon alpha (*IFNA*). Cells were injected subcutaneously into T cell deficient mice revealing significant reduction in tumour growth within the cytokine transfected cell lines when compared to non-transfected parental R11. With co-injection of transfected cells with parental R11 at the same site, local cytokine production suppressed parental cell line growth. The same effect could not be achieved through co-injection at distant sites or systemic administration of cytokine (Table 2). Cell surface evaluation revealed enhanced HLA class I expression in *IFNA* transfected cell lines. Increased peripheral blood lymphocyte mediated cell killing was noted in vitro in all transfected lines. This apparent natural killer cell (NK)/lymphokine activated killer cell mediated tumour immunity further emphasizes the value of local cytokine production within tumour sites as well as in tumour vaccine formation.

Dranoff *et al* (1993) evaluated several immunomodulatory genes inserted into the MFG retroviral vector for their ability to stimulate anti-tumour immunity against the B16 malignant melanoma cell line. Cells transduced with the retroviral vector were injected subcutaneously into C57BL/6 mice (the B16 syngeneic host) and animals were subsequently evaluated for tumour formation. Although several cytokines induced mild reduction/delay in tumour formation, only IL2 transduced cells were completely rejected. Long term immunity to subsequent challenge with non-transduced cells was only achieved through co-transfection with IL2 and granulocyte macrophage colony stimulating factor (GM-CSF) but not with IL2 alone.

These observations led researchers to postulate that the role of IL2 was the rejection of the injected inoculum of transduced cells and not the initiation of long term cell specific immunity. This hypothesis was perhaps confirmed through irradiation of the transduced cells prior to inoculation. Irradiated cells transduced with GM-CSF alone conferred long term immunity to inoculated animals with subsequent exposure to non-transduced cells several months after initial inoculation. Depletion of $CD4^+$ and $CD8^+$ lymphocytes confirmed the induction of immunity to require both T helper and cytotoxic T lymphocytes and not NK cells. The target specificity of induced immunity was shown through the failure of animals inoculated with GM-CSF transduced B16 cells to reject subsequent injection with other non-transduced murine tumour cell lines. Inoculation with GM-CSF murine Lewis lung cancer cell line failed to induce immunity to non-transduced B16.

Sanda *et al* (1994) have recently described the use of a GM-CSF transduced MFG retroviral tumour vaccine in the Dunning rat model of prostate cancer. The gene modified tumour vaccine consists of GM-CSF transduced irradiated Mat-ly-lu cells. Injection into animals simultaneously inoculated with parental Mat-ly-lu cells in the contralateral limb resulted in delayed tumour formation and a reduction in the size of subsequently formed tumours when compared to controls injected with the parental cell line only. With injection of vaccine producing higher levels of GM-CSF, regression of established tumours was noted, with a 30% cure rate. Prolonged survival compared to non-treated controls was noted in all animals, including those with residual tumours. Serial transduction resulted in increased production of GM-CSF among transduced cells. Also noted was a lack of tumorigenesis inhibition with co-injection of parental cells and GM-CSF. Although this may illustrate the distinct advantage of GM-CSF production by the vaccinating cells over local injection of GM-CSF, modification of the injected GM-CSF dose may certainly produce very different results.

Vieweg *et al* (1994b) have evaluated the efficacy of an IL2 producing gene modified tumour vaccine in the same Dunning rat prostate cancer model. The IL2 vaccine was noted to produce regression of pre-established R3327 Mat-ly-lu tumours, resulting in both cure and prolonged immunity to subsequent challenge with Mat-ly-lu tumour cells. Tumour vaccine transduced with GM-CSF resulted in a diminished response when compared to the IL2 vaccine, and interferon gamma (IFNG) transduced vaccine produced little or no response against previously established tumours. The disparity in response noted by each group using GM-CSF transduced vaccines may have related to transduction efficiency and subsequent levels of GM-CSF production.

Regardless of the cytokine used, the results of in vivo immunization with gene modified tumour vaccine in animal models of prostate cancer have been impressive so far. The demonstrated regression of Mat-ly-lu tumours is underscored by the non-immunogenic nature of the tumour as well as the relatively anaplastic nature of the tumour's phenotypic expression. The applicability of animal model data to human prostate cancer, despite the similarities of the malignancies, remains to be confirmed by both in vitro and in vivo studies. The finding of effective cytokine gene transfer to human prostate cancer cells by serial transduction must be followed with in vitro studies of alteration in antigen expression and induction of HLA expression. Such findings would perhaps reaffirm the potential utility of cytokine based gene therapy in human prostate cancer prior to the initiation of in vivo protocols.

Direct Vector Injection

Due to the biological nature of metastatic prostate cancer, the role of direct injection of gene vectors into sites of tumour may have limited applications. Owing to the absence of defined arterial supply to the majority of in situ prostate cancer deposits, intra-arterial gene delivery is technically difficult. However, the ability of the adenovirus to infect cells in situ provides a new means towards immunization of tumour bearing patients by direct injection into solid tumour sites. Such an in situ tumour vaccine could potentially result in an efficient means of inducing anti-tumour immunity through repetitive injections of genes into accessible sites of metastasis. Transrectal injection of the prostate gland itself may provide an additional means towards the induction of anti-tumour immunity as well as the treatment of locally confined disease. Such therapeutic means may be especially valuable in patients with low volume metastatic disease or locally advanced disease without metastatic extension. Perhaps most provocative is the use of direct intraprostatic injections of cytokine genes as a means of immunizing patients prior to surgical resection in a neoadjuvant fashion. To date, direct transfection of in situ tumours has been used most in malignancies arising in easily accessible organs (ie lung and bladder). The application of such methods to solid tumours such as prostate cancer relies on the development of vectors capable of effecting high transfection rates with local intratumoural delivery. No studies have yet addressed these issues in models of prostate cancer in vivo.

Tissue Specific Promoters

Perhaps the most promising but least used method of gene therapy is the systemic delivery of genes with subsequent directed transfection of tumour sites. Such a method would require both protecting gene vectors in circulation from humoural immunity and a means of subsequently selectively delivering the potentially toxic genes to sites of tumour. Previous attempted methods of selective delivery have included packaging vectors within liposomes carrying anti-tumour monoclonal antibodies within the lipid membrane as well as binding vectors themselves, through polylysine tails, to monoclonal antibodies or ligand specific for tumour receptors (Fig. 6). These methods have resulted in

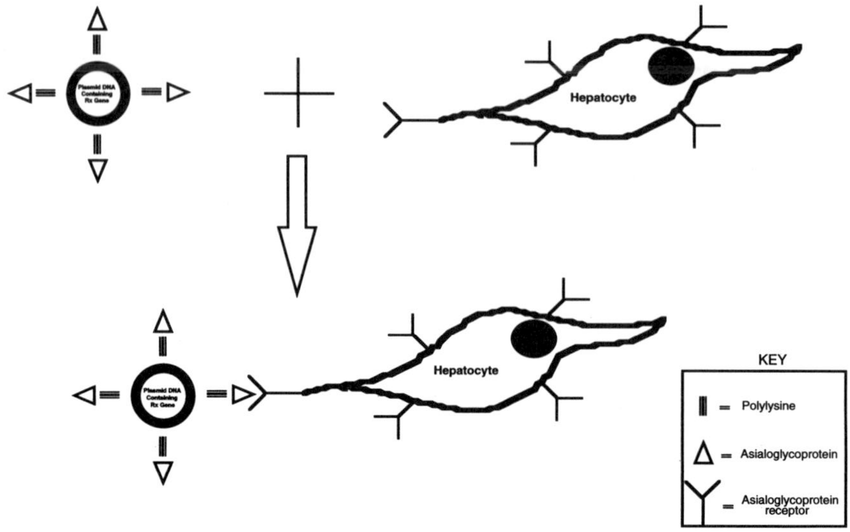

Fig. 6. Highly schematized diagram illustrating receptor-mediated gene transfer. Plasmid DNA containing the therapeutic gene (Rx) is conjugated to a protein ligand (asialogycoprotein) via polylysine. Upon in vivo delivery, the conjugate will target to tissues that express the appropriate receptor (in this case liver hepatocytes)

relatively dismal outcomes, with a large fraction of the vectors being delivered to non-cancer sites (Nicolau *et al,* 1983; Gao *et al,* 1993; Zhu *et al,* 1993).

The use of tissue specific promoters in providing selective cancer specific gene expression offers new promise for in vivo directed gene therapy protocols (Hatzoglou *et al,* 1990; Smith *et al,* 1994). The promoter sequence of genes selectively expressing within tumour tissues in vivo can theoretically be used selectively to express inserted genes within the same tumour tissue. The use of tumour specific promoters has been limited in practical application by the overlap of expression within related normal tissues (ie expression of surfactant gene in normal lung tissue and lung cancer tissue or the expression of carcinoembryonic antigen in normal gastrointestinal tissues and colonic or pancreatic malignancies). The prostate specific antigen (*PSA*) gene provides a unique promoter due to its specific expression in prostatic (and to a lesser extent seminal vesical and urethral) tissues. The human PSA promoter has previously been cloned and shown to carry a specific androgen responsive element within the 630 basepair 5′ flanking region of the *PSA* gene (Riegman *et al,* 1991).

We have evaluated the ability of the human PSA promoter to produce selective gene expression within PSA producing tissues (Taneja *et al,* 1994b). Prostate cancer cell lines LNCaP, DU145 and PC-3 were transfected with plasmid vector BM20-PSA-Luc carrying an expression cassette of firefly luciferase driven by a 630 bp cloned segment of the human PSA promoter. Preliminary results suggest expression of luciferase is limited to the PSA producing prostate cancer cell line LNCaP, with relatively low levels of expres-

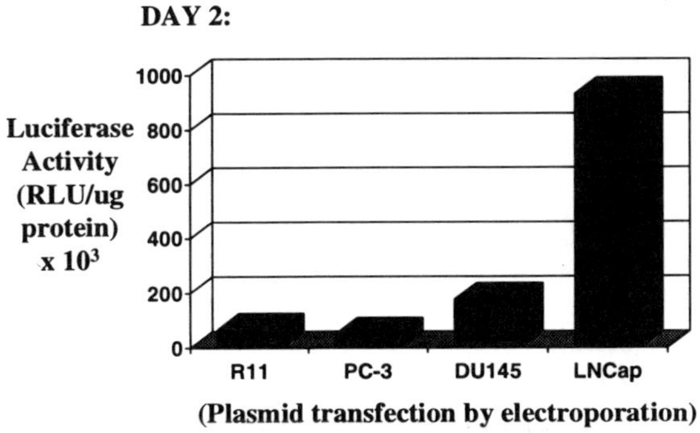

Fig. 7. Various cell lines transfected by electroporation with plasmid vector BM20-PSA-Luc carrying expression cassette of human PSA promoter driven firefly luciferase gene. Significant expression of luciferase at day 2 following transfection is noted only in PSA producing prostate cancer cell line LNCaP. Non-PSA producing prostate cancer cell lines DU145 and PC-3, as well as renal cancer cell line R11, show little or no expression

sion in non-PSA producing prostate cancer cell lines (Fig. 7). Further transfection of breast cancer cell MCF7 (with functional native androgen receptor) and renal cancer cell line R11 revealed virtual shutdown of PSA promoter directed expression. With the addition of increasing concentrations of androgen to transfected LNCaP cells, corresponding increases in luciferase expression are noted within the physiological range of androgen production, mimicking increases in PSA production. Although these studies remain to be validated by in vivo studies, the great potential for selective expression within sites of metastatic prostate cancer in vivo is evident. Further studies will be directed at defining the elements of the promoter sequence responsible for initiation, enhancer activity, androgen responsiveness and prostate specificity. Identification of such elements may allow construction of highly specific promoters capable of high levels of gene expression.

The limitations of PSA promoter directed gene expression may largely be secondary to an inability to deliver the promoter containing vector to all sites of metastatic cancer throughout the body. Vectors such as the adenovirus are often consumed within the circulation by humoural immune mechanisms with systemic delivery. In addition, a significant percentage of surviving virus will infect the liver upon initial contact due to known hepatotropism leaving a small amount of residual virus to infect the remainder of the body. To be truly effective, the vector should theoretically infect nearly all cells in the body expressing its toxic gene product only in cells of prostate origin. Additional problems may arise from the heterogeneous level of PSA production among cells within any given prostate malignancy. A subclonal population of cells producing little or no PSA secondary to transcriptional shutdown may certainly escape the intended effect of PSA promoter directed gene therapy. Conversely, simple delivery of the vector to a site of metastatic cancer where both PSA producing and non-producing cells co-exist may provide sufficient local toxicity through local bystander effect to influence the entire malignant cell population.

Other prostate selective tissue specific promoters including the probasin and prostate specific membrane protein promoters exist. Use of these promoters has been limited, but they do provide further potential for the execution of directed in vivo gene therapy.

SELECTION OF THE IDEAL GENE

The ideal gene for creating an alteration in the biological behaviour of prostate cancer remains to be identified and perhaps may depend on the desired outcome of a given gene therapy strategy. Strategies intended to enhance host immune recognition of cancer cells will rely on the use of cytokine genes capable of inducing alterations in cell surface antigen presentation. Strategies intended to treat localized disease may utilize genes capable of metastasis suppression or reduction in invasive potential. Directed in vivo strategies will focus on identification of genes capable of direct cytotoxicity to tumours resulting in cessation of growth or tumour destruction.

The molecular characterization of prostate cancer remains in its infancy with few consistently recognized unique features present in tumours capable of metastasis. Recent reports of potential putative metastasis suppressor genes and markers of metastasis are indeed exciting because they provide for the first time insight into the mechanism of prostate cancer progression. With the understanding of the role of the androgen receptor in growth stimulation, growth regulation and apoptosis, an alternative approach to stopping tumour cell growth may be identified. Studies involving the transfer of functional androgen receptor to androgen insensitive cells have shown promise in imparting morphological and biological differentiation to the treated cells. The effect of cytokines on prostate cancer tumorigenesis, growth and antigen expression remains poorly understood. Attempts at systemic treatment with cytokines for metastatic prostate cancer have resulted in little response (van Haelst-Pisani *et al,* 1992), but anecdotal reports of tumour regression following cytokine administration continue to arise.

Cytokine Genes

Walsh *et al* (1994) postulated that potential for "immune evasion" of prostate cancer exists secondary to MHC class I antigen processing defects. Therefore, cytokines dependent on MHC class I mediated mechanisms for immunostimulatory effects (IFNG, IL4, IL6) may not serve as ideal agents for use in prostate cancer therapy. Walsh *et al* quantitated by polymerase chain reaction the expression of three fundamental components of MHC-I antigen processing in human prostate cancer cells. β_2-microglobulin expression was uniform in all tested cells. MHC-I heavy chain and transporter of antigen processing (TAP-2) expression was decreased in cells with defective antigen processing. Attempts to restore normal expression with IFNG treatment were successful only for heavy chain expression, indicating an inability to restore functional MHC-I mediated antigen processing. The group concluded that cytokines not dependent on MHC class I mediated antigen processing (IL2 and GM-CSF) were appropriate for human prostate cancer gene therapy.

We have evaluated the effect of various cytokines on prostate cancer cell lines LNCaP, PC-3 and DU145 by assaying for cell growth, antigen presentation and proto-oncogene expression. In early experiments, cytokines tumour necrosis factor alpha (TNFA), IFNG, IFNA and IL2 were added to cell culture in fixed concentration for a 3-day incubation period. Cells were then harvested and stained for fluorescence assisted cell sorting analysis quantitating cell surface expression of HLA class I and intracellular adhesion molecule (ICAM) 1 antigens. It appeared that TNFA significantly upregulated expression of HLA class I and ICAM1 at the delivered dose. Likewise, upon assaying cell growth by thymidine incorporation, TNFA had the greatest inhibitory effect when compared to non-treated controls. The clinical use of TNFA has traditionally been hampered by tremendous systemic toxicity. Certainly, the ability to produce TNFA locally within sites of tumour may provide a new role for the cytokine in cancer therapy, avoiding systemic toxicity and providing intratumoural toxicity.

Assay of proto-oncogene and secretory protein production of cytokine treated cells was performed by quantitative polymerase chain reaction. Cells treated with TNFA showed a reduction in c-*myc,* epidermal growth factor receptor (*EGFR*), *PSA* and androgen receptor (*AR*) expression far greater than the interferons or IL2. This suggests a virtual cell shutdown through direct cytotoxicity from the TNFA, indicating the potential value for the cytokine within in vivo directed gene therapy protocols as well as tumour vaccine formation. Although TNFA may appear to produce the greatest alteration in antigen presentation, invasive potential and cell growth, as well as the greatest direct toxicity, these findings remain to be confirmed in vivo. Although IL2 showed little or no effect in these studies, it may still show the greatest antitumour effect in vivo as it has historically served as the best immunomodulator of those cytokines tested.

Cell Surface Molecules/Phenotypic Alteration

Schalken and co-workers have described the characterization of E-cadherin as a marker of locally confined disease less likely to metastasize. In evaluating 92 samples of prostate cancer from sites of locally confined or metastatic cancer, 46 had reduced or absent E-cadherin staining when compared with benign prostate tissue, which always produced strong staining (Umbas *et al,* 1994). The E-cadherin gene does in fact map to a locus often noted to be involved in allelic loss in advanced cancers (Giroldi and Schalken, 1993). In comparing locally confined tumours to either locally invasive or metastatic cancer, an increase in the percentage of aberrantly staining samples was noted among the latter two groups. Loss of E-cadherin expression correlated with loss of differentiation. Interestingly, aberrant E-cadherin staining usually took the form of a mixed population of cells with various gradations of staining illustrating the heterogeneous morphology of the tumour. Subsequent studies have revealed aberrant staining in human prostate cancer cell lines (Morton *et al,* 1993). Although an understanding of the mechanism of loss of E-cadherin remains to be elucidated, one can extrapolate a potential role of E-cadherin transfection in non-expressing cells at early stages of disease.

The recent description of prostate specific membrane antigen as a putative metastasis suppressor gene mapping to chromosome 11, a frequent site of loss of heterozygosity, offers a potential new means for local control of aggressive tumours through gene transfer. Like *PSA, PSM* is expressed by LNCaP, but not by PC-3 or DU145 (Israeli *et al,* 1994b). Similarly, both benign and malignant tissues consistently express *PSM,* but subsequent studies have suggested a reduction in metastatic potential in tumours expressing *PSM*. Dunning rat prostate adenocarcinoma cell lines transfected with human chromosome 11p11.2-13, capable of suppressing metastatic ability of the Dunning tumour, are noted to express *PSM*, unlike the non-transfected cell lines (Israeli *et al,* 1994a). This suggests a mapping of the *PSM* gene to the PSM locus. Upon transfection of the *PSM* gene into PC-3, a non-expressing cell line, a reduction in growth rate in vitro is noted. Subsequent orthotopic implantation of transfected cells into nude mice resulted in a significant reduction in both tumour growth and frequency of metastasis. Those sites of metastasis occurring in animals inoculated with PSM transfected cells showed no expression of *PSM,* suggesting a loss or absence of expression in a subpopulation of cells.

A similar experiment involved the transfer of functional androgen receptor to PC-3, a prostate cancer cell line lacking any functional androgen receptor expression (Yuan *et al,* 1993). With androgen stimulation of transfected cells, a more histologically differentiated appearance was noted. Cell proliferation assay showed decreased growth rates among transfected cells. Cells also lost invasive capability within in vitro invasion assays. The more differentiated phenotype produced when compared to non-transfected controls suggests an aetiological role for the androgen receptor in the regulation of cell growth and metastatic capability.

Although the identification of genes such as those described above is provocative, it is still difficult to determine whether such genes are truly responsible for the production of the metastatic phenotype or are simply phenotypic changes resulting from another genetic alteration. Androgen receptor (AR), *PSM* and *E-cadherin* may all represent separate points within a single cascade of events resulting in the metastatic phenotype. Regardless of the difficulties in determining the true aetiological gene in metastatic progression, each of these studies provides promise and insight into the potential gene therapy of locally confined prostate cancer and prevention of metastasis.

Other Potential Genetic Interventions

Treatment of metastatic prostate cancer offers a separate challenge in identifying a gene responsible for the growth of the cancer. An appropriate genetic in-

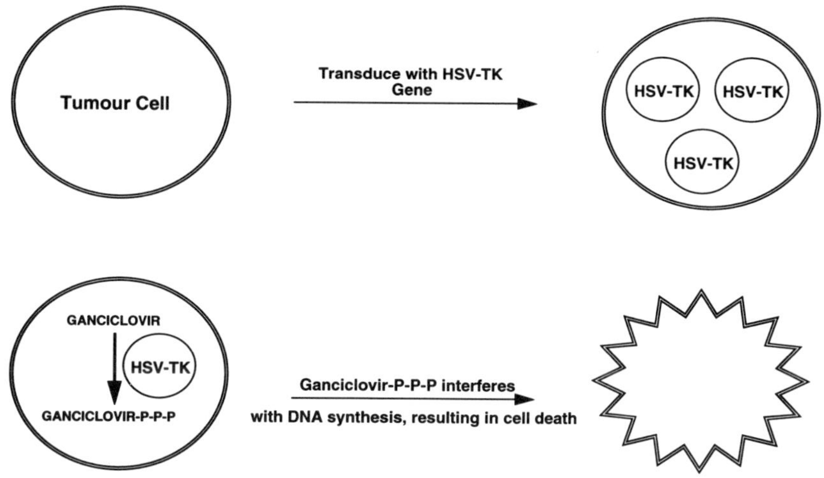

Fig. 8. Concept of tumour suicide genes. The herpes simplex virus thymidine kinase (HSV-TK) gene is transduced into tumour cells. The subsequent expression of HSV-TK results in the "lethal synthesis" of ganciclovir triphosphate from ganciclovir. This toxic metabolite interferes with DNA synthesis, thus killing the tumour cell. Obviously, the selective delivery of the HSV-TK into tumour cells is an essential prerequisite of this strategy

tervention must be capable of a cytocidal effect through depletion of gene products necessary for growth, or insertion of gene products toxic to cell growth. Investigation into the proto-oncogene expression of metastatic cancers continues, but oncogenes that consistently express remain to be found. Although many genes have been identified as part of a proposed tumorigenesis cascade, it is difficult to determine the true functional mechanism of these genes.

Various researchers have investigated the role of *TP53* as a mediator of prostate cancer tumorigenesis (Isaacs *et al,* 1991; Mellon *et al,* 1992). *TP53* maps to the p arm of chromosome 17 with loss of heterozygosity resulting in expression of a mutant allele (Miller *et al,* 1986). Loss of heterozygosity at the chromosome 17p locus of *TP53* has been noted to result in tumorigenicity in a number of tumour models. Mutant *TP53* expression has been found with some variability in a number of prostate cancer specimens. Transfection of wild type *TP53* into prostate cancer cell lines expressing mutant alleles results in loss of tumorigenic capability (Isaacs *et al,* 1991). Only cells expressing mutant *TP53* were capable of colony formation. This suggestion of a functional role of *TP53* in prostate tumorigenesis is an example of a potential mechanism for the suppression of widespread disease. Further identification of similar genes acting in a larger number of cancers may provide the ideal gene for therapeutic manipulation.

The use of tumour "suicide" genes offers an additional approach to the treatment of metastatic disease. Although not yet tested in prostate cancer models, such genes render cancer cells vulnerable to systemic agents not normally used for cancer therapy. The classically described "suicide" gene, herpes simplex virus thymidine kinase, renders actively replicating cells vulnerable to therapy with systemically delivered ganciclovir (Fig. 8) (Oldfield *et al,* 1993). The accumulation of toxic metabolites interferes with DNA synthesis, resulting in cell death. Such a strategy requires an efficient method of delivering genes to sites of cancer throughout the body. With the application of the methods mentioned above, the "suicide" gene may provide the most definitive answer to the treatment of malignancy through genetic intervention.

SUMMARY

Gene therapy is a new and provocative means of treating human malignancy. Insight into the mechanisms of growth and growth regulation within cancer cells has offered multiple potential methods for genetic intervention. The application of gene therapy to prostate cancer is in its infancy. The development of both adenoviral and retroviral replication deficient vectors has provided the ability consistently to transfer genes into cancer cells. Although the ideal gene for transfer has not yet been clearly identified, many genes capable of altering the biological behaviour of prostate cancer exist. Selection of the appropriate gene is highly dependent on the desired therapeutic outcome. A gene therapy strategy, whether dependent on ex vivo or in vivo transfection, must ultimately be tailored to meet the specific needs of the disease to be treated. The potential to treat locally confined disease, preventing subsequent metastasis, or widespread metastatic disease exists. The ultimate success of a prostate cancer gene therapy strategy will rely on comprehensive investigation of the biology of the tumour and careful planning of an effective intervention.

References

Belldegrun A, Tso CL, Sakata T *et al* (1993) Human renal carcinoma line transfected with interleukin-2 and/or interferon-α genes: implications for live cancer vaccines. *Journal of the National Cancer Institute* **85** 207–216

Berkner KL (1988) Development of adenovirus vectors for the expression of heterologous genes. *Biotechniques* **6** 616–629

Chen C and Okayama H (1988) Calcium phosphate mediated gene transfer: a highly efficient transfection system for stably transformed cells with plasmid DNA. *Biotechniques* **6** 632–638

Dranoff G, Jaffee E, Lazenby A *et al* (1993) Vaccination with irradiated tumor cells engineered to secrete granulocyte-macrophage colony-stimulating factor stimulates potent, specific and long-lasting anti-tumor immunity. *Proceedings of the National Academy of Sciences of the USA* **90** 3539–3543

Fearon ER, Pardoll DM, Itaya T *et al* (1990) Interleukin 2 production by tumor cells bypasses T-helper function in the generation of an anti-tumor response. *Cell* **60** 397

Gao L, Wagner E, Cotten M *et al* (1993) Direct in vivo gene transfer to airway epithelium employing adenovirus-polylysine-DNA complexes. *Human Gene Therapy* **4** 17–24

Giroldi LA and Schalken JA (1993) Decreased expression of the intercellular adhesion molecule E-cadherin in prostate cancer: biological significance and clinical implications. *Cancer Metastasis Reviews* **12** 29–37

Hatzoglou M, Lamers W, Bosch F, Wynshaw-Boris A, Clapp DW and Hanson RW (1990) Hepatic gene transfer in animals using retroviruses containing the promoter from the gene for phosphoenolpyruvate carboxykinase. *Journal of Biological Chemistry* **265** 17285–17293

Isaacs WB, Carter BS and Ewing CM (1991) Wild type p53 suppresses growth of human prostate cancer cells containing mutant p53 alleles. *Cancer Research* **51** 4716–4720

Israeli RS, Powell T, Corr JG, Fair WR and Heston WD (1994a) Expression of the prostate-specific membrane antigen. *Cancer Research* **54** 1807–1811

Israeli RS, Rinker-Schaeffer C, Powell T, Isaacs JT, Fair WR and Heston WDW (1994b) Localization of the prostate specific membrane antigen (PSM) to the putative metastasis-suppressor region on human chromosome 11. *Journal of Urology* **151** 252A [Abstract]

Jaffee EM, Dranoff G, Cohen L *et al* (1993) High efficiency gene transfer into primary human tumor explants without cell selection. *Cancer Research* **53** 2221–2226

Levrero M, Barban V, Manteca S *et al* (1991) Defective and non-defective adenovirus vector for expressing foreign genes in vitro and in vivo. *Gene* **101** 195–202

McGrory WJ, Bautista DS and Graham FL (1988) A simple technique for the rescue of early region I mutations into infectious human adenovirus type 5. *Virology* **163** 614–617

Mellon K, Thompson S, Charlton RB *et al* (1992) p53, c-erb B-2, and the epidermal growth factor receptor in the benign and malignant prostate. *Journal of Urology* **147** 496–499

Mill C, Mohandas T, Wolf D, Prokocimer M, Rotter V and Koeffler HP (1986) Human p53 gene localized to short arm of chromosome 17. *Nature* **319** 783–784

Morton RA, Ewing CM, Nagafuchi A, Tsukita S and Isaacs WB (1993) Reduction of E-cadherin levels and deletion of the alpha-catenin gene in human prostate cancer cells. *Cancer Research* **53** 3585–3590

Neumann E, Schoeffer-Rider M and Wang Y (1982) Gene transfer into mouse lymphoma cells by electroporation in high electric fields. *EMBO Journal* **1** 841

Nicolau C, Le Pape A, Soriano P, Fargette F and Juhel MF (1983) In vivo expression of rat insulin after intravenous administration of the liposome-entrapped gene for rat insulin I. *Proceedings of the National Academy of Sciences of the USA* **80** 1068–1072

Oldfield EH, Ram Z, Culver KW, Blaese RM, DeVroom HL and Anderson WF (1993) Gene therapy for the treatment of brain tumors using intratumoral transduction with the thymidine kinase gene and intravenous gancicyclovir. *Human Gene Therapy* **4** 39–69

Riegman PHJ, Vlietstra RJ, van der Korput JA, Brinkmann AO and Trapman J (1991) The promoter of the prostate-specific antigen gene contains a functional androgen responsive element. *Molecular Endocrinology* **5** 1921–1930

Sanda MG, Jaffee L, Ayyagar S, Perdoll D, Mulligan R and Simons J (1993) MFG: A new vector for human prostate gene therapy. *Journal of Urology* **149** 222A

Sanda MG, Ayyagari SR, Jaffee EM *et al* (1994) Demonstration of a rational strategy for human prostate cancer gene therapy. *Journal of Urology* **151** 622–628

Smith MJ, Rousculp MD, Goldsmith KT, Curiel DT and Garver RI Jr (1994) Surfactant protein A-directed toxin gene kills lung cancer cells in vitro. *Human Gene Therapy* **5** 29–35

Taneja SS, Belldegrun A, deKernion JB and Pang S (1994a) Adenoviral vector mediated high efficiency gene transfer in prostate cancer cell lines. *Journal of Urology* **151** 253A [Abstract]

Taneja SS, Belldegrun A , Dardashti K, Cohan P, deKernion JB and Pang S (1994b) Construction of a prostate specific antigen promoter-driven gene transfer vector: a novel strategy for target specific gene therapy in prostate cancer. *Journal of Urology* **151** 491A [Abstract]

Umbas R, Isaacs WB, Bringuier PP *et al* (1994) Decreased E-cadherin expression is associated with poor prognosis in patients with prostate cancer. *Cancer Research* **54** 3929–3933

van Haelst-Pisani CM, Richardson RL, Su J *et al* (1992) A phase II study of recombinant human alpha-interferon in advanced hormone-refractory prostate cancer. *Cancer* **70** 2310–2312

Vieweg J, Rudoll T, Philip R *et al* (1994a) Gene transfer with DNA-liposome complexes for human prostate cancer gene therapy. *Journal of Urology* **151** 254A [Abstract]

Vieweg J, Rosenthal F, Bannerji R *et al* (1994b) Immunotherapy of prostate cancer in the Dunning rat model: use of cytokine modified tumor vaccines. *Cancer Research* **54** 1760–1765

Walsh J, Nelson W, Simons J and Sanda M (1994) Molecular characterization of heterogeneity in immune evasion by human prostate cancer cells: implications for prostate cancer gene therapy. *Journal of Urology* **151** 254A [Abstract]

Yuan S, Trachtenberg J, Mills GB, Brown TJ, Xu F and Keating A (1993) Androgen-induced inhibition of cell proliferation in an androgen-insensitive prostate cancer cell line (PC-3) transfected with a human androgen receptor complementary DNA. *Cancer Research* **53** 1304–1311

Zhu N, Liggit D, Liu Y and Debs R (1993) Systemic gene expression after intravenous DNA delivery into adult mice. *Science* **261** 209–211

The authors are responsible for the accuracy of the references.

The Geography of Prostate Cancer and Its Treatment in Japan

KENJI OISHI[1]* • OSAMU YOSHIDA[1] • FRITZ H SCHROEDER[2]

[1]Department of Urology, Faculty of Medicine, Kyoto University, 53 Kawahara-cho, Shogoin, Sakyo-ku, Kyoto; [2]Department of Urology, Erasmus University Rotterdam, Dr Molewaterplein 50, Rotterdam

INTRODUCTION

The incidence of prostate cancer increases rapidly with age, and the disease is detected in about 40% of men aged 80 years or more at autopsy. The incidence rate of clinically manifest prostate cancer in the USA and in Europe is high and is second only to skin cancer in this region. In fact, the American Cancer Society predicted that 35 000 men would die from prostate cancer in the USA in 1993. In Japan, the incidence rate of clinically manifest prostate cancer, although increasing exponentially, is still quite low by comparison with western countries. About 4700 men are expected to die from prostate cancer in 1995 (Tominaga *et al*, 1993). The results of epidemiological studies in immigrants suggest that unknown environmental factors might play some part in the development and/or progression of prostate cancer. In this connection, it would be interesting to know the rates of latent prostate cancer, prostate cancer found by mass screening, incidental prostate cancer, clinically manifest prostate cancer and mortality from the disease.

Many risk factors for prostate cancer have been suggested, but some of the data are inconsistent. There is a suspicion that we have been interpreting data from various sources with different backgrounds. In this context, an international co-operative epidemiological study using a single study design would be helpful. We have carried out such a study in Japan and the Netherlands. Some

*Present address: Department of Urology, Nishi-Kobe Medical Center, 5-7-1 Koji-Dai, Nishi-Ku, Kobe.

Cancer Surveys Volume 23: *Preventing Prostate Cancer: Screening versus Chemoprevention*
 0-87969-466-1/95. $5.00 + .00

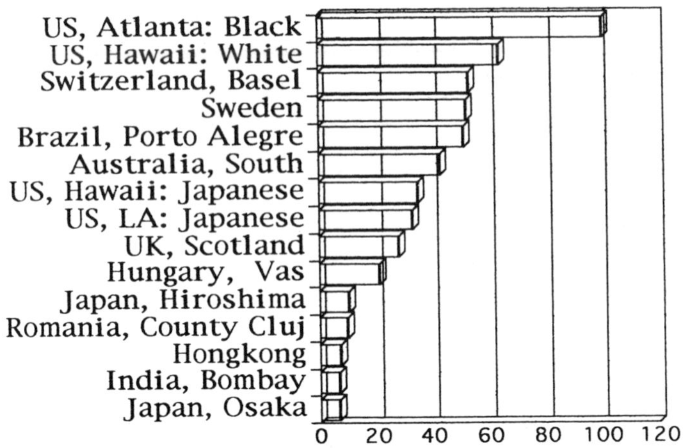

Fig. 1. Age adjusted incidence rates of prostate cancer (per 100 000 male population in selected areas in 1985, adjusted to world population (Tominaga *et al*, 1993)

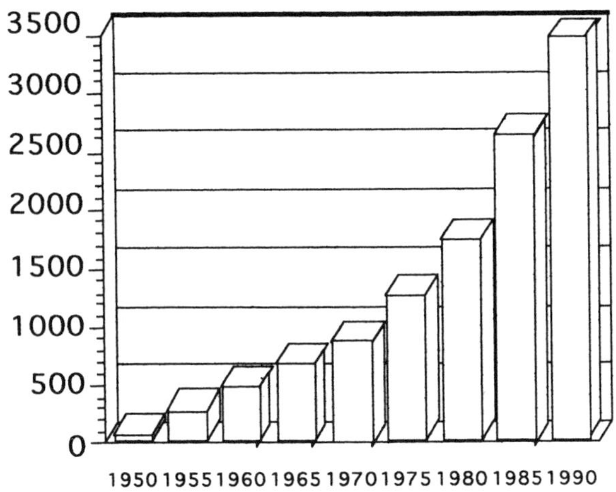

Fig. 2. Deaths from prostate cancer, Japan, 1950–1990 (Tominaga *et al*, 1993)

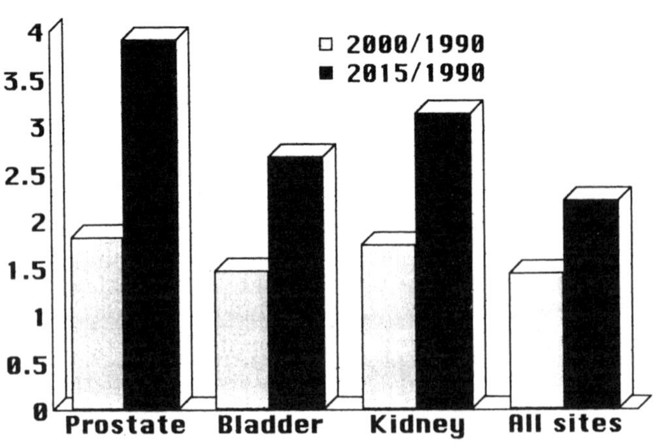

Fig. 3. Ratios projected (years 2000 and 2015) to 1990 cancer death rates (Tominaga *et al*, 1993)

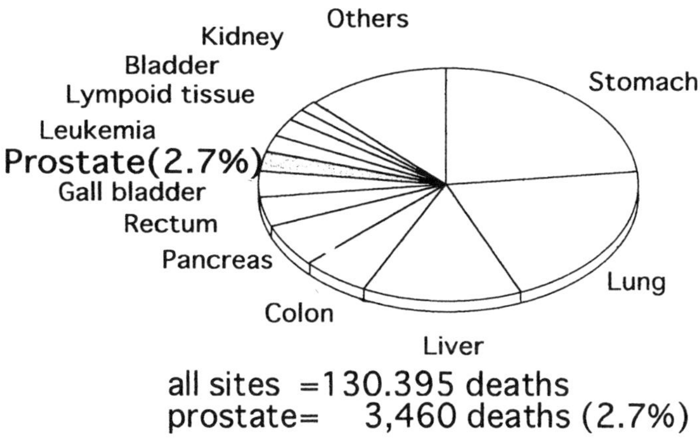

Fig. 4. Deaths from prostate cancer as a proportion of all cancer deaths, Japan, 1990 (Tominaga *et al*, 1993)

of the results of our case-control study have been reported elsewhere (Yamabe *et al*, 1986; Hayes *et al*, 1988; Ohno *et al*, 1988; Oishi *et al*, 1988a,b,c, 1989, 1990, 1992; Yoshida *et al*, 1988; de Jong *et al*, 1991).

EPIDEMIOLOGY

Prostate Cancer in Japan

Age adjusted incidence rates of prostate cancer for various parts of the world are shown in Fig. 1. The death rate from prostate cancer among Japanese in Japan was 3.3 in 1983–1987, which is about one eighth of that among US blacks. US whites have the second highest rate, followed by Japanese immigrants in the USA, then west Europeans and east Europeans.

Although the death rate from prostate cancer among Japanese in Japan is one of the lowest in the world, it has increased rapidly and exponentially during the past 40 years (Fig. 2). In Japan, 3485 men died from the disease in 1990 (Tominaga *et al*, 1993), and the numbers are expected to rise to 6289 in 2000 and 13 494 in 2015 (Tominaga *et al*, 1993). This expected increase of deaths of prostate cancer in Japan is most striking compared to other urological and all sites of malignancies (Fig. 3). The 3485 deaths from prostate cancer in Japan in 1990 accounted for 2.7% of 130 395 deaths from all malignancies (Fig. 4).

Latent and Manifest Prostate Cancer in Japan and USA

Data for rates of latent prostate cancer (autopsy cancers) (Guileyardo *et al*, 1980; Yatani *et al*, 1988; Furusato, 1990; Whittemore *et al*, 1991) (Table 1), prostate cancer found incidentally in specimens from patients with a diagnosis of benign prostatic hyperplasia (Sheldon *et al*, 1980; Yamabe *et al*, 1986;

TABLE 1. Influence of age on incidence of latent prostate cancer at autopsy

	45–59	60–69	70+		Total
Japanese 1980 (Yatani *et al,* 1988)	32	41	43		13
US White 1980 (Guileyardo *et al,* 1980)	23	32	41		7
US Black 1980 (Guileyardo *et al,* 1980)	20	34	44		16
	40–59	**60–69**	**70+**	**80+**	**Total**
Japanese 1990 (Furusato *et al,* 1990)	13	20	35	52	5
US White 1991 (Whittemore *et al,* 1991)	23	33	37	54	9
US Black 1991 (Whittemore *et al,* 1991)	19	38	49	57	9

Detection rates are age adjusted to the world population using techniques described by Tominaga *et al* (1993)

Uchida *et al,* 1987; Fujita *et al,* 1991) (Table 2), prostate cancer found at mass screening (screening cancer) (Mettlin *et al,* 1991; Moon and Clejan, 1991; Tsukamoto *et al,* 1991; Brawar *et al,* 1992; Imai and Yamanaka, 1993; Tsukamoto T, unpublished data) (Table 3), clinically manifest prostate cancer (clinical cancer) (Dhom, 1983; Mebane *et al,* 1990; Tominaga *et al,* 1993) (Table 4) and lethal prostate cancer (lethal cancer) (Tominaga *et al,* 1993) (Table 5) were reviewed. The detection rates of prostate cancer of each category were adjusted to the world population (Tominaga *et al,* 1993). The detection rates of autopsy cancer, BPH cancer, screening cancer, clinical cancer and lethal cancer per 100 000 male population are 9250, 228, 50, 6.5 and 3.3, respectively, in Japanese in Japan, 8050, 117, 153, 41.7 and 14.2, respectively, in whites in the USA and 1250, 378, 153, 68.3 and 26.5, respectively, in blacks in the USA (Table 6). Compared with the detection rate of lethal prostate cancer in Japanese men in Japan, the relative rates of autopsy cancer, BPH cancer, screening cancer, and clinical cancer in Japanese in Japan are 2803, 69, 15.2 and 2.0, respectively, those in white men in the USA are 2439, 35.5, 46.4 (whites and blacks), 12.6 and 4.3, respectively, and those in black men in the USA are 3797, 115, 46.4 (whites and blacks), 20.7 and 8, respectively.

Risk Factors for Prostate Cancer in Japan and the Netherlands

We have studied risk factors for prostate cancer in a case-control study carried out in Japan and the Netherlands, using the same study design in the two countries. The methods are described elsewhere (Yamabe *et al,* 1986; Hayes *et al,* 1988; Ohno *et al,* 1988; Oishi *et al,* 1988a,b,c, 1989, 1990, 1992; de Jong *et al,* 1991).

TABLE 2. Detection rate of BPH cancer of prostate (incidental cancer)

Age range	a	b	c	Detection rates of prostate cancer in BPH specimen (%)			
≥80	1000	34	35	19	22.2	15.7	37.1
70–79	3000	102	105	17	10.7	15	28.7
60–69	7000	237	245	7	8.3	10.1	18.5
50–59	9000	307	315	4	0	2.3	10.4
40–49	12 000	409	420				6.3
30–39	12 000	409	420				1.9
Total				0.055	0.04	0.055	0.153
Reference				Yamabe *et al* (1986)	Uchida *et al* (1987)	Fujita *et al* (1991)	Sheldon *et al* (1980)
Ethnic group				Japanese	Japanese	Japanese	USA
Year				1986	1987	1991	1980

[a]World population (Tominaga *et al*, 1993)
[b]Number of prostatectomies in USA by age in 1988; since operation rate was 1.5% of population, then 7.5% of population aged over 30 years
[c]Number of prostatectomies in Japan by age in 1988; since operation rate was 0.7% of population, then 3.5% of population aged over 50 years

TABLE 3. Detection rate of prostate cancer at mass screening

	Detection rate (%) of screening prostate cancer by age						
	2.94 (70+) 0.77 (60–69) 0.17 (50–59)	1.95 (80+) 1.19 (70–79) 0.49 (60–69) 0.2 (50–59)	2.1 (80+) 2.83 (70–79) 0.88 (60–69) 0.19 (50–59)	3.3 (66–70) 2.2 (61–55) 1.3 (55–60)	1.3 (50–59)	4.2 (50–59)	1.6 (80+) 3.01 (70–79) 3 (60–69) 0.9 (50–59)
Total[a]	0.216	0.283	0.185	0.239	0.117	0.378	0.397
Reference	Tsukamoto *et al* (1991)	Imai and Yamanaka (1993)	Tsukamoto T (unpubl.)	Mattlin *et al* (1991)	Moon and Clejan (1991)	Moon and Clejan (1991)	Brawer *et al* (1992)
Ethnic group	Japanese	Japanese	Japanese	USA	US white	US black	USA
Year	1991	1993	1993	1991	1991	1991	1992

[a]Age adjusted to world population (Tominaga *et al*, 1993)

TABLE 4. Incidence of clinical prostate cancer

Age	Incidence rate/100 000						
85+	283	927.6	726.3		961.5	877.2	
80–84	195.4	909.9	787.2		1486.2	1142.2	
75–79	156.6	708.9	552.2		1002.5	843.7	
70–74	84	470.8	406.6		992.6	767.4	
65–69	37.1	261.4	255.7		328.8	509.5	
60–64	18.7	138.4	105.8		241.6	276.3	
55–59	6.3	59.6	49.1		145.2	99.9	
50–54	1.7	13.7	14.5		37.3	45.5	
45–49	0.4	4.3	3.9		14.3	6.2	
40–44	0.1	1.7	0.3			1.6	
35–39	0.1		0.4			1.8	
Total[a]	6.5	36	31	58	61	59	95
Reference	Tominaga *et al* (1993)	Dhom (1983)	Dhom (1983)	Mebane *et al* (1990)	Dhom (1983)	Dhom (1983)	Mebane *et al* (1990)
Ethnic group	Japanese	US white[b]	US white[c]	US white	US black[d]	US black[e]	US black
Year	1988	1969–1971	1969–1971	1970	1969–1971	1969–1971	1970

[a]Age adjusted to world population (Tominaga *et al*, 1993)
[b]White in San Francisco
[c]White in Detroit
[d]Black in San Francisco
[e]Black in Detroit

TABLE 5. Death rate for prostate cancer[a]

	Death rate/100 000		
Total[b]	**3.3**	**14.2**	**26.5**
Ethnic group	Japanese	US white	US non-white
Year	1983–1987	1983–1987	1983–1987

[a]Tominaga *et al* (1993)
[b]Age adjusted to world population (Tominaga *et al,* 1993)

TABLE 6. Detection rate of autopsy, screening, BPH, clinical and lethal prostate cancer of Japanese men in Japan and white and black men in USA[a]

	Death rate/100 000 all men		
	Japanese in Japan	**US white**	**US black**
Autopsy cancer	9250 (2803)	8050 (2439)	1253 (3797)
references	Yatani *et al* (1990); Furusato (1990)	Guileyardo *et al* (1980); Ebstein *et al* (1988)	Guileyardo *et al* (1980); Ebstein *et al* (1988)
Screening cancer	228 (69.0)	117 (35.5)[b]	378 (115)[b]
references	Mettlin *et al* (1991) Tsukamoto *et al* (1991) Imai and Yamanaka (1993)	Moon and Clejan (1991)	Moon and Clejan (1991)
BPH cancer	50 (15.2)	153 (white and black)	46.4
references	Uchida *et al* (1987); Fujita *et al* (1991); Whittemore *et al* (1991)	Sheldon *et al* (1990)	Sheldon *et al* (1990)
Clinical cancer	6.5 (2.0)	41.7 (12.6)	68.3 (20.7)
references	Tominaga *et al* (1993)	Dhom (1983); Mebane *et al* (1990)	Dhom (1983); Mebane *et al* (1990)
Lethal cancer	3.3 (1)	14.2 (4.3)	26.5 (8.0)
references	Tominaga *et al* (1993)	Tominaga *et al* (1993)	Tominaga *et al* (1993)

[a]Figures in parentheses indicate the rate relative to the lethal cancer of Japanese. If more than one reference is given, averages of data are indicated
[b]Age range 50–59 only

TABLE 7. Odds ratios (95% confidential intervals) for risk factors for prostate cancer with same trend and with statistical significance in both Japan and the Netherlands (Tominaga *et al,* 1993)

	Odds ratio (compared with control groups)			
	Japan		Netherlands	
Risk factor	**BPH[a]**	**Hospital[b]**	**BPH[a]**	**Hospital[b]**
No morning erections now[c]	1.39	2.38[d]	2.5[d]	2.86[d]
(95% CI)	(0.75–2.70)	(1.18–4.76)	(1.45–4.35)	(1.64–5.00)

[a]Benign prostate hyperplasia patients as controls for prostate cancer patients
[b]Patients in same hospitals as prostate cancer patients
[c]Control category is "yes"
[d]Odds ratio with statistical significance

The risk factors investigated in our case-control study of prostate cancer can be divided into four groups according to the odds rations and their statistical significance. Group A includes the only factor (no morning erection) for which the odds ratio is greater than unity in both Japan and the Netherlands and is statistically significant compared with at least one control (Table 7); it also includes risk factors for which the odds ratios are greater than unity and statistically significant in Japan and which show the same trend without statistical significance in the Netherlands (Table 8) and risk factors for which the odds ratios are greater than unity and statistically significant in the Netherlands and which show the same trend without statistical significance in Japan (Table 9). Group B consists of risk factors with a statistically significant odds ratio in one country but not in the other. Group C consists of risk factors without a statistically significant odds ratio in either country. Group D consists of risk factors with odds ratios that are greater than unity in one country and less than unity in the other country, with or without statistical significance.

Group A includes "no morning erection now", "incidence of rectal cancer in brothers or colon polyp in patients", "level of education", "residence in rural area", "brothers", "marriages", "intake of water or β-carotene", "blood sex hormone binding globulin level", "orgasms during sexual intercourse", "frequent coitus during 4th decade", "foreplay", "episodes of sexually transmitted diseases", "level of blood testosterone or dihydrotestosterone" (Tables 7–9).

Group B includes two subgroups. Group B1 consists of risk factors with an odds ratio that is statistically significant in Japan but not in the Netherlands. Group B2 consists of risk factors with an odds ratio that is statistically significant in the Netherlands but not in Japan.

Group B1 includes "obesity index", "blood pressure", "appearance of pubic hair", "level of excitement during sexual intercourse in 6th decade", "occurrence of first nocturnal emission" and "body hair".

Group B2 includes "body weight at interview", "maximum body weight", "activity of work and leisure", "inhalation of smoking", "sisters", "intake of riboflavin" and "unsatisfactory sexual relations."

Group C consists of 75 items, including "occupation", "intake of protein, fat or carbohydrate", "total number of sexual partners" and "mental characteristics".

Group D consists of "age at cessation of body growth", "intake of fibre or ascorbic acid", "blood level of β-carotene" and "retinol and vitamin E".

DISCUSSION

Prostate cancer in Japan seems quite different in many respects from the disease in other parts of the world except Asia. Although both incidence and death rates of prostate cancer in Japan are among the lowest in the world (Fig. 1), they are rapidly increasing and are expected to continue increasing in the near future (Figs. 2 and 3).

TABLE 8. Odds ratios (95% confidential intervals) for risk factors for prostate cancer, statistically significant in Japan, with same trend but not statistically significant in the Netherlands (Yanabe *et al*, 1986)

	Odds ratios (compared with controls)					
	Japan			Netherlands		
Risk factor	Cut off point	BPH[a]	Hospital[b]	Cut off point	BPH[a]	Hospital[b]
Wife's education (95% CI)	Preliminary school or low	1.04 (0.56–1.94)	1.96[c] (1.02–3.77)	Preliminary school or low	0.97 (0.55–1.77)	1.32 (0.75–2.33)
Cancer in relatives (95% CI)	Colon	2.82 (0.38–)	23.7[c] (1.24–)	Colon	4.78 (0.53–43.5)	1.18 (0.29–4.28)
Orgasm (95% CI)	Rare	2.46[c] (1.05–5.82)	2.00 (0.83–4.91)	Rare	1.24 (0.40–2.64)	1.16 (0.41–3.81)
Coitus in 30s (95% CI)	>3 times/week	1.66 (0.80–3.45)	2.26[c] (1.03–4.95)	>3 times/week	1.03 (0.56–2.36)	1.24 (0.38–3.45)
Sexually transmitted diseases (95% CI)	No	2.27[c] (1.11–7.10)	0.55 (0.23–1.29)	No	3.37 (0.51–)	1.55 (0.13–)
Water intake (95% CI)	>1250 ml/day	1.69[c] (1.01–3.03)	1.33 (0.86–2.32)	<1460 ml/day	1.26 (0.56–3.24)	1.04 (0.34–2.45)
β-Carotene intake (95% CI)	<1720 μg/day	2.13[c] (1.20–3.77)	2.13[c] (1.20–3.77)	<1580 μg/day	1.17 (0.62–2.20)	1.89 (.099–3.57)
SHBG in serum (95% CI)	>53 μg/dl	2.04[c] (1.10–3.78)	1.27 (0.62–2.63)	>57 μg/dl	1.00 (0.52–1.91)	1.03 (0.54–1.95)

SHBG = sex hormone binding globulin
[a]Benign prostate hyperplasia patients as controls for prostate cancer patients
[b]Patients in same hospitals as prostate cancer patients
[c]Odds ratio with statistical significance

TABLE 9. Odds ratios (95% confidential intervals) for risk factors for prostate cancer with statistical significant in the Netherlands but not statistically significant in Japan (Oishi *et al*, 1988c)

	Odds ratios (compared with controls)					
	Japan			Netherlands		
Risk factor	Cut off point	BPH[a]	Hospital[b]	Cut off point	BPH[a]	Hospital[b]
Longest residence (95% CI)	Rural	1.38 (0.69–2.76)	1.01 (0.52–1.98)	Rural	2.10[c] (1.05–4.22)	2.16[c] (1.05–4.28)
No of brothers (95% CI)	4 or more	1.71 (0.61–4.83)	2.1 (0.70–6.27)	4 or more	2.05[c] (1.06–3.98)	1.84 (0.95–3.60)
No or previous marriages (95% CI)	0 or 1	1.31 (0.53–3.21)	1.09 (0.41–2.84)	0 or 1	2.47[c] (1.06–5.86)	2.42[c] (1.05–5.74)
Duration of foreplay (95% CI)	<2 min	1.52 (0.67–3.46)	2.42 (0.94–6.38)	<5 min	1.99[c] (1.09–3.66)	2.29[c] (1.25–4.24)
Plasma testosterone (95% CI)	<14.8 nmol/l	1.12 (0.57–2.22)	1.11 (0.57–2.179)	<16.8 nmol/l	1.98[c] (1.09–3.62)	1.94[c] (1.07–3.53)
Plasma dihydrotestosterone (95% CI)	<1.43 nmol/l	1.17 (0.57–2.23)	1.29 (0.66–2.56)	<1.42 nmol/l	1.59 (0.90–2.84)	2.04[c] (1.12–3.72)

[a]Benign prostate hyperplasia patients as controls for prostate cancer patients
[b]Patients in same hospitals as prostate cancer patients
[c]Odds ratio with statistical significance

Pathological evidence suggests that autopsy cancer, screening cancer, BPH cancer, clinical cancer and lethal cancer of the prostate gland cannot be separated. Pathological examination of total prostatectomy specimens of stage A cancer revealed that more than 90% of specimens contained cancer tissue after transurethral resection or enucleation of BPH tissue (Ebstein *et al*, 1988a; Greene *et al*, 1991). In addition, the rate of progression of stage A cancer to clinical cancer increases by grade and tumour volume (Ebstein *et al*, 1988b; Lowe and Listrom, 1988). It is thus plausible that small volume and well differentiated autopsy cancers have the potential to progress to poorly differentiated and large lethal cancers if the host lives long enough for this to happen. When cancer is detected at autopsy or in a BPH specimen, we call it "latent cancer" or "incidental cancer", but this does not mean that "latent" cancer is dormant forever.

Our analysis of data concerning descriptive epidemiology suggests that the detection rate of lethal cancer as a percentage of that of autopsy cancer is 0.21% for black men in the USA, 0.18% for white men in the USA and 0.036% for Japanese men in Japan. The detection rate of autopsy cancer in black men in the USA is 1.35 times higher than in Japanese men in Japan. This suggests that (a) prostate cancer takes longer to progress to clinically manifest or lethal cancer, (b) prostate cancer occurs at an earlier age in black mean and (c) cancer progresses more rapidly in black men in the USA and more slowly in Japanese men in Japan. Thus, it is likely that both initiation and progression factors are most prevalent in black men and less so in Japanese men in Japan.

The ratio of detection rate of screening cancer for the three ethnic groups is about the same as that for autopsy cancer and BPH cancer, but the ratios of clinical cancer and lethal cancer are somewhat higher between Japan and the USA. This suggests that some larger prostate cancers are overlooked in Japan, probably because of lack of education about prostate diseases and a low operation rate for BPH in Japan (Holtgrewe *et al*, 1993).

Although the incidence rate of prostate cancer is about five times higher in the Netherlands than in Japan, true risk factors for prostate cancer are likely to appear statistically significant in both countries (group A) or at least one country (group B). On the other hand, we must be very cautious in interpreting the results when factors appear to be risk enhancing in one country but risk reducing in the other (group D). Some group D factors would have been designated risk factors if the study had been carried out in only one region.

The factors included in groups A and B could be regarded as truly important and common risk factors. One factor in group A is "an absence of spontaneous penile erection during morning awakening when study subjects were interviewed." This result might be interpreted as a psychological consequence of having become a prostate cancer patient or as meaning that prostate cancer patients have lower blood concentrations of testosterone in both countries (de Jong *et al*, 1991) (Table 9). Group B includes environmental factors that are associated with dietary habits and sexual behaviour, factors related to colon polyp or colon cancer and biochemical factors such as blood concentrations of sex steroids.

The sexual behaviour of prostate cancer patients is characterized by poor quality of sexual life ("shorter foreplay" and "infrequent orgasm") and "more frequent coitus in the 30s and 40s." In this regard, the characteristics of patients' sexual behaviour and some other factors such as "rural residence" and "lower level of education" might be interrelated (Tables 8 and 9). Sexually sensational stimuli or erotic fantasies lead to spikes of blood testosterone (Fox *et al,* 1972). From the beginning of fourth decade or even in third decade of male life, autopsy cancers can be detected in black people in the USA (Haas, 1993). Thus, the fourth and fifth decades are important periods for the progression of tiny prostate cancers to large clinical cancers. Vigorous sex life during the fourth and fifth decades might lead to spikes of blood testosterone which in turn accelerate the promotion and progression of prostate cancers.

Plasma concentrations of testosterone and its derivative, dihydrotestosterone, were lower in prostate cancer patients (de Jong *et al,* 1991) (Tables 8 and 9) than in controls. But these can be considered as base levels after hospitalization. It might be that the larger difference between maximum and base level might promote the development of prostate cancer. High concentrations of plasma sex hormone binding globulin might result in lower concentrations of free testosterone, which can be absorbed and utilized by prostate cells, leading to lowering of basal testosterone concentrations. The increase in the incidence of clinical prostate cancer in the Netherlands has to be attributed to some factors other than testosterone and dihydrotestosterone.

Many risk factors associated with dietary habits have been reported in prostate cancer patients, such as high consumption of animal protein, fat or cereals. However, our case-control study revealed only one such risk factor, namely consumption of β-carotene. Lower consumption of green-yellow vegetables and lower blood concentrations of β-carotene (Hayes *et al,* 1988; Ohno *et al,* 1988; Oishi *et al,* 1988c) (Table 8) could be claimed to be risk enhancing factors for prostate cancer. β-carotene, a precursor of active vitamin A is contained predominantly in green-yellow vegetables and is converted to retinol in the body. Many A group vitamins have been tested for their effects on chemoprevention of several types of malignant tumours (Lippman *et al,* 1991).

All-*trans* retinoic acid is used for the treatment of acute promyelocytic leukaemia and produces a high complete remission rate (Lippman *et al,* 1991). Thus, combining our results with those from other investigators, some of the A vitamins are likely to play an important part in the prevention of prostate cancer development and promotion.

SUMMARY

The age adjusted death rate from prostate cancer in Japan is one of the lowest in the world but is rising steadily. The vast majority of cases of prostate cancer remain undetected during life, the prevalence of prostate cancer detected at autopsy being 2800 times that of lethal cancer in Japanese in Japan, 570 times in whites in the USA and 470 times in blacks in the USA.

A case-control study of prostate cancer carried out in Japan and the Netherlands revealed a number of statistically significant risk factors, including rural residence, more brothers, colon neoplasms in relatives, no morning erections, frequent sexual intercourse in 30s, episodes of sexually transmitted disease, lower plasma testosterone and dihydrotestosterone concentrations and lower β-carotene intake.

References

Brawer MK, Chetner MP, Bratie J, Buchner DM, Vessella RL and Lange PH (1992) Screening for prostatic carcinoma with prostate specific antigen. *Journal of Urology* **147** 841–845

de Jong FH, Oishi K, Hayes RB *et al* (1991) Peripheral hormone levels in controls and patients with prostatic cancer or benign prostatic hyperplasia: results from the Dutch-Japanese case-control study. *Cancer Research* **51** 3445–3450

Dhom G (1983) Epidemiologic aspects of latent and clinically manifest carcinoma of the prostate. *Cancer Research and Clinical Oncology* **106** 210–218

Ebstein JI, Oesterling JE and Walsh PC (1988a) The volume and anatomical location of residual tumor in radical prostatectomy specimens removed for stage A1 prostate cancer. *Journal of Urology* **139** 975–979

Ebstein JI, Oesterling JE and Walsh PC (1988b) Tumor volume versus percentage of specimen involved by tumor correlated with progression in stage A prostatic cancer. *Journal of Urology* **139** 980–984

Fox CA, Ismail AAA, Love DN, Kirkham KE and Loraine JA (1972) Studies on the relationship between plasma testosterone levels and human sexual activity. *Journal of Endocrinology* **52** 51–58

Fujita T, Kanimoto Y, Akino H and Okada K (1991) Study of incidental carcinoma of the prostate, Part 1, pathological analysis related to the clinical features. *Acta Urologica Japonica* **37** 695–703

Furusato M (1990) Natural history of latent prostatic carcinoma. *Tokyo Jikeikai Medical Journal* **105** 615–629

Greene DR, Egawa S, Neerhut G, Flanagan W, Wheeler TM and Scardino PT (1991) The distribution of residual cancer in radical prostatectomy specimens in stage A prostate cancer. *Journal of Urology* **145** 324–329

Guileyardo JM, Johnson WD, Welsh RA, Akazaki K and Correa P (1980) Prevalence of latent prostate carcinoma in two US populations. *Journal of the National Cancer Institute* **65** 311–316

Haas GP (1993) US-Japan Summer Seminar Urology—Update, Yokohama

Hayes RB, Bogdanovicz JFAT, Schroeder FH *et al* (1988) Serum retinol and prostatic cancer. *Cancer* **62** 2021–2026

Holtgrewe HL, Ackermann R, Bay-Nielsen H *et al* (1993) The economics of BPH. Cockett ATK, Khoury S, Aso Y *et al* (eds). *Proceedings of the 2nd International Consultation on Benign Prostatic Hyperplasia,* Digital Print, Paris

Imai K and Yamanaka H (1993) Screening examination for prostate cancer: early detection and mass screening. *Japanese Journal of Urology* **84** 1175–1187

Lippman SM, Hittelman WN, Lotan R, Pastorino U and Hong WK (1991) Recent advances in cancer prevention. *Cancer Cells* **3** 59–65

Lowe BA and Listrom MB (1988) Incidental carcinoma of the prostate: an analysis of the predictors of progression. *Journal of Urology* **140** 1340–1344

Mebane C, Gibbs T and Horm J (1990) Current status of prostate cancer in North American black males. *Journal of the National Medical Association* **82** 782–788

Mettlin C, Lee F, Drago J, Murphy GP and the Investigators of the American Cancer Society National Cancer Detection Project (1991) The American Cancer Society National Cancer Detection Project. *Cancer* **67** 2949–2958

Moon TD and Clejan S (1991) Prostate cancer screening in younger men: prostatic-specific antigen and public awareness. *Urology* **38** 216–219

Ohno Y, Yoshida O, Oishi K, Okada K, Yamabe H and Schroeder FH (1988) Dietary β-carotene and cancer of the prostate: a case-control study in Kyoto, Japan. *Cancer Research* **48** 1331–1336

Oishi K, Okabe T, Kawakita M and Yoshida O (1988) A mass screening and a case-control study on prostatic cancer. Proceedings of papers sponsored by Kyoei Seimei, Tokyo, 1–12

Oishi K, Okada K, Ohno Y and Yoshida O (1988) A case-control study on prostatic cancer in Kyoto: dietary risk factors. *Gann no Rinsho* **Supplement 15** 191–205

Oishi K, Okada K, Yoshida O, Yamabe H, Ohno Y and Schroeder FH (1988) A case-control study of prostatic cancer with reference to dietary habits. *Prostate* **12** 179–190

Oishi K, Okada K, Yoshida O *et al* (1989) A case-control study of prostatic cancer in Kyoto, Japan: demographic and some lifestyle risk factors. *Prostate* **14** 117–122

Oishi K, Okada K, Yoshida O *et al* (1990) A case-control study of prostatic cancer in Kyoto, Japan: sexual risk factors. *Prostate* **17** 269–279

Oishi K, Yoshida O, Ohno O and Schroeder FH (1992) Epidemiological study of prostatic cancer in Japan and the Netherlands. Proceedings of the Third Workshop on Prostate Cancer, 1992, pp 43–45

Sheldon CA, Williams R and Fraley E (1980) Incidental carcinoma of the prostate: a review of the literature and critical reappraisal of classification. *Journal of Urology* **124** 626–631

Tominaga S, Aoki K, Hanai A and Kurihara N (eds) (1993) *White Paper on Cancer and Statistics: Morbidity/Death/Prognosis,* Shinohara Shuppan, Tokyo

Tsukamoto T, Kumamoto Y, Umehara T and Takagi Y (1991) Study on frequency of prostate carcinoma and benign prostatic hypertrophy by mass screening in Hokkaido. *Japanese Journal of Urology* **82** 420–426

Uchida K, Ishikawa S, Nemoto R, Koiso K and Harada M (1987) Incidental prostatic carcinoma diagnosed by step-section technique of surgical specimen: histopathological analysis. *Japanese Journal of Urology* **78** 24–28

Whittemore AS, Keller JB and Betensky R (1991) Low-grade, latent prostate cancer volume: predictor of clinical cancer incidence? *Journal of the National Cancer Institute* **83** 1231–1235

Yamabe H, ten Kate FJW, Gallee MPW *et al* (1986) Stage A prostatic cancer: a comparative study in Japan and the Netherlands. *World Journal of Urology* **4** 136–140

Yatani R, Shiraishi T, Nakakuki K *et al* (1988) *Journal of the National Cancer Institute* **80** 68–82

The authors are responsible for the accuracy of the references.

The Geography of Prostate Cancer and Its Treatment in Africa

ELIJAH O KEHINDE

Department of Urology, University of Leicester, Leicester General Hospital, Leicester, LE5 4PW

INTRODUCTION AND HISTORICAL PERSPECTIVE

Epidemiological research has a proven value in understanding a number of urological cancers, for example bladder and scrotal cancer (Doll, 1972; Burkitt, 1973). The pattern of cancers in a community is related to environmental factors such as diet, climate, occupation and national customs as well as the genetic makeup of the population. Western doctors practising in Africa before 1900 thought that cancer was very rare in the indigenous population (des Ligneris, 1927). However, they soon realized that cancer was not a disease of "modern civilization" but that certain types of cancers had a very high incidence in Africans (Davies *et al*, 1964).

The study of cancer of the prostate in indigenous Africans has been rudimentary. Between 1925 and 1965, about 90 articles appeared in the world literature on various cancers in Africans. Of these, only one (Dodge, 1963) discussed cancer of the prostate. The initial series of articles on various cancers in Africans published between 1925 and 1950 never even mentioned prostate cancer. Between 1966 and 1993, only 41 articles were published on cancer of the prostate in indigenous Africans.

INCIDENCE OF PROSTATE CANCER IN AFRICA

Cancer of the prostate is the commonest urological cancer in Ibadan, Nigeria, (Lawani *et al*, 1982) and the second commonest urological cancer in Uganda

Cancer Surveys Volume 23: *Preventing Prostate Cancer: Screening versus Chemoprevention*

TABLE 1. Frequency distribution of urological cancers in different African countries

Type of cancer	Nigeria (%) Lawani *et al* (1979)	Uganda[a] Dodge (1963) Olweny (1982)	Zambia (%) Elem and Patil (1991)
Prostate	46.1	+++	26.2
Bladder	24.4	++	50.9
Penis	0.1	++++[b]	17.9
Kidney	20.9	+	4.3
Testis	6.6	+	0.7
Urethra	1.1	rare	rare
Ureters	0.3	very rare	rare

[a]Percentages not specified. ++++ commonest; +++ very common; ++ common; + not common
[b]Carcinoma of the penis is commonest in Uganda because circumcision is not practiced routinely, unlike in Nigeria where circumcision of infants is routinely performed

and Lusaka, Zambia (Table 1) (Elem and Patil, 1991). Interestingly, it appears that prostate cancer is rare in the Arabs of North Africa: in a current review of cancers in Libya, Akhtar (1993) found only nine cases in 664 cancers in the 5 year period analysed.

The age standardized incidence rate for prostate cancer was 32/100 000 in Zimbabweans, 9.7/100 000 in Nigerians, 4.4/100 000 in Senegalese and 4.3/100 000 in Ugandans compared to 59.8/100 000 in blacks living in Washington DC (Table 2) (Jackson *et al,* 1977; Lytton, 1993). In a comparative study of prostate cancer in a high risk black population (Washington DC) and a low risk population (Ibadan, Nigeria), Jackson *et al* (1977) found no difference between the two groups in the incidence of unsuspected, latent or occult carcinomas of the prostate as determined in autopsy studies. However, the incidence of clinically apparent or aggressive carcinomas was sixfold higher in American blacks compared to their Nigerian counterparts. This means that differences in genetic constitution among racial groups may function as a permissive factor for the development of prostate cancer but that environmental influences may cause such occult tumours to become clinically demonstrable neoplasms (Kozlowski and Grayhack, 1991).

The differences in incidence of prostate cancer in different parts of Africa can be explained partly by the differences in the socioeconomic status of the countries (Dayal *et al,* 1985). For example, the incidence in urban South African blacks and in Zimbabwe is 17/100 000 and 32/100 000 population, respectively, compared to 9.7 in Nigeria and 4.4 in Senegal. The gross national product per capital for South Africa and Zimbabwe was $2560 and $650, respectively, whereas for Nigeria and Uganda, it was $340 and $170, respectively, in 1991 (United Nations, 1993).

Similarly, because white South Africans are richer and have a longer life expectancy (73 years) than their black counterparts (63 years) (Slabber, 1992), the incidence of prostate cancer is 32.6/100 000, which is similar to the rates

TABLE 2. Economic status, life expectancy and incidence of prostate cancer in three African countries compared to the USA and UK (1991)

Countries	% Budgetary allocation to health care	Life expectancy: males	Incidence of carcinoma of prostrate/100 000 population
USA			
White	13	76	58
Black		73.6	71
UK			
White	11	75	32
South Africa			
White	11.2	73	32.6
Black		63	23.2
Zimbabwe	8	60	32
Nigeria	1	52	9.7
Senegal	1	48	4.4
Uganda	2	46	4.3

for whites in the UK (Lytton, 1993). Furthermore, male Zimbabweans have a life expectancy of 60 years and an incidence of 32/100 000. Hence, it could be argued that the life expectancy for blacks in Africa is much lower than for blacks in the USA (73.6 years), and therefore an insufficient number of men live long enough to develop the disease (Table 2). Life expectancy and socioeconomic status as well as survival from prostate cancer are strongly linked (Dayal *et al,* 1985). It is also the differences in life expectancy between Africans and their counterparts in the Western world that can explain why the peak age for development of cancer of the prostate in the Nigerian is 55–64 years, while for blacks in Washington DC, it is a decade later (Jackson *et al,* 1977).

The idea that prostate cancer is uncommon in Africans can be dismissed, as the high incidence in Zimbabwe shows. Of all "truly" black African countries, Zimbabwe spends the highest percentage (8%) of its total budget on health care (Table 2). It probably has the best health care delivery system for blacks in Africa. Until recently, the health care delivery system in South Africa has been geared towards whites only (Slabber, 1992). Moreover, Zimbabwe is politically stable, which means that accurate data can be collected. Hence, the incidence of cancer of the prostate in Zimbabwe of 32/100 000 probably represents the true incidence of this cancer for indigenous Africans in general when corrected for factors militating against accurate data collection in other African countries that have reported a lower incidence.

MODE OF PRESENTATION OF PROSTATE CANCER IN AFRICANS

Patients in Africa tend to present with advanced disease, and this is also true for prostate cancer. In a comparative review of prostate cancer in Ibadan

TABLE 3. Clinical features of prostate cancer at presentation in Ile-Ife, Nigeria (152 consecutive new cases 1982–1986)

Presenting symptoms	Percentage
Acute urinary retention	43.7
Chronic urinary retention	16.9
"Prostatism"	13.0
Haematuria	9.9
Paraplegia	8.6[a]
Bone pains	7.9

Patients in Ile-Ife, Nigeria, presented late compared with patients in Leicester, UK, as shown in Table 4
[a]All patients presenting with paraplegia made a full recovery on stilboestrol therapy

(Nigeria) and in blacks in Washington DC, Jackson *et al* (1977) found that 52% of Nigerians and 10% of American blacks at the initial presentation had early or stages I and II disease, whereas 48% of American blacks and 90% of Nigerians had stages III and IV (high stage) disease. A common mode of presentation of prostate cancer in Africans is spinal cord compression in about 10% of patients. The reasons for these are multifactorial; however, poverty and ignorance of the importance of symptoms are partly responsible. As Tables 3 and 4 show, 8.6% of patients in Ile Ife, Nigeria, presented with paraplegia but no patients in Leicester, UK, presented with paraplegia.

The pattern of skeletal metastasis in Africans is similar to that in whites; however, about 2% of patients in Africa may present with proptosis due to involvement of the orbital bone—a very rare occurrence in whites. The reason for this is unknown. Similarly, all metastases to the skull in Africans have been noted to be osteolytic in nature and the reasons are unknown (Nkposong *et al,* 1987).

TREATMENT OF PROSTATE CANCER IN AFRICA

The mainstay of treatment for disseminated cancer of the prostate is stilboestrol 1 mg three times a day. Not only is this a cheap and effective means of treating patients with cancer of the prostate, but, fortunately for most Africans, the cardiovascular complications produced by stilboestrol, which has made it unpopular with urologists in the Western world, are relatively rare in the African (Walker *et al,* 1994). The incidence of myocardial infarction, fluid retention and hypertension is much lower than in whites. However, 90% of patients given stilboestrol will develop painful gynaecomastia. Surgical orchidectomy is widely accepted as a treatment, especially in Nigerians (Okeke LI, personal communication). For obvious economic reasons, luteinizing hormone releasing hormone agonists are not widely used in Africa nor the other very expensive drugs used for hormonal manipulations in prostate cancer patients.

TABLE 4. Prostate cancer: presenting features in 126 consecutive new patients in Leicester, UK, 1993

Presenting features	Percentage
"Prostatism"	64
Chronic urinary retention	16.0
Acute urinary retention	12.8
Boney metastasis on plain X ray	3.2
Haematuria	1.6
Back pain	1.6
Anaemia	0.8

No patient in Leicester, UK, presented with paraplegia compared to 8.6% of patients in Ile-Ife, Nigeria, who presented with paraplegia (see Table 3)

PROGNOSIS OF PROSTATE CANCER IN AFRICANS

Cancer survival mirrors the quality of health care of any given community (Dayal *et al,* 1985). A combination of low socioeconomic status, late presentation and poor health care delivery systems in most African countries have contributed to the poor prognosis of cancer of the prostate in Africans.

It has often been said that health care is not the priority of most governments in Africa, as illustrated by the proportion of each country's resources that is devoted to health care (Table 2). At present, only South Africa rivals Western countries in budgetary allocation to the health sector. Currently, South Africa allocates 11.2% of its total state budget to health care, whereas in Nigeria, it is 1%, in Uganda 2% and in Zimbabwe 8%. The proportion for other developed countries is 13.8% in the USA and 18% in Germany (Slabber, 1992). It is hoped that when more of the African countries start to spend more money on medicine than on arms the situation will improve.

SUMMARY

Cancer of the prostate is perhaps the commonest urological malignancy affecting Africans. The incidence between different countries varies and mirrors very closely the socioeconomic status of the countries and the life expectancy. The disease has an early peak incidence at ages 55–64 years, compared to 65–74 years for whites. This is primarily due to the low life expectancy in Africans. Late presentation is a common feature in Africans. Stilboestrol is widely used in treating disseminated cancer of the prostate not only because it is cheap and effective, but also because the cardiovascular side effects of stilboestrol seem not to be serious in Africans compared to whites. Further study of cancer of the prostate gland in indigenous Africans should provide vital data on the epidemiology and aetiology of this important cancer and may shed light on why the clinical aggressiveness of the disease varies from one part of the world to another.

Acknowledgements

In preparing this chapter I made numerous inquiries of colleagues working in various parts of Africa. I wish to thank them for their cooperation and to mention in particular the help I received from the following colleagues: Professor EO Nkposong of Gizan, Saudi Arabia; Mr B Elem, FRCS, of Lusaka, Zambia; Mr IB Shittu, FRCS, Ibadan, Nigeria; Mr T Nkono, FRCS of Harare, Zimbabwe; Dr LI Okeke of Ibadan, Nigeria; and Dr Freddie Sitas of Johannesburg, South Africa.

References

Akhtar SS(1993) Cancer in Libya: a retrospective analysis. *African Journal of Medicine and Medical Sciences* **22** 17–24

Burkitt DP (1973) Distribution of cancer in Africa. *Proceedings of the Royal Society of Medicine* **66** 312–314

Davies JNP, Elmes S, Hutt MSR, Mtimavalye LAR, Owor R and Sharper L (1964) Cancer in an African community: 1897–1956. *British Medical Journal* **1** 259–341

Dayal HH, Polissar L and Dahlberg S (1985) Race, socio-economic status and other prostatic prognostic factors for survival from prostate cancer. *Journal of the National Cancer Institute* **74** 1001–1006

Des Ligneris MJA (1927) Cancer in South Africans. *Journal of the Medical Association of South Africa* **25** 102–104

Dodge OG (1963) Carcinoma of the prostate in Ugandan Africans. *Cancer* **16** 1264–1268

Doll R (1972) Cancer in five continents. *Proceedings of Royal Society of Medicine* **65** 49–55

Elem B and Patil PS (1991) Pattern of urological malignancy in Zambia. *British Journal of Urology* **67** 37–39

Jackson MA, Ahlawalia BS, Herson J *et al* (1977) Characterization of prostatic carcinoma among blacks: a continuation report. *Cancer Treatment Reports* **61** 167–172

Kozlowski JM and Grayhack TT (1991) Carcinoma of prostate, In: Gillenwater JY (ed). *Adult and Paediatric Urology,* pp 1277–1393, Mosby Year Book, St Louis, Missouri

Lawani J, Nkposong EO, Aghadiuno PU and Akute O (1982) Twenty years review of genito-urinary tract tumours in Ibadan, In: Solanke TF (ed). *Cancer in Nigeria,* pp 67–67, Ibadan University Press, Ibadan

Lytton B (1993) Epidemiology of prostate cancer. *Urology Topics* **10** 114–116

Nkposong EO, Lawani J, Kyalwazi SK *et al* (1987) Genito-urinary system, In: Adeloye A (ed). *Davey's Companion to Surgery in Africa,* pp 446–479, Churchill Livingstone, Edinburgh

Olweny CLM (1982) Cancer patterns in Nigeria and Uganda, In: Solanke TF (ed). *Cancer in Nigeria,* pp 239–249, Ibadan University Press, Ibadan

Slabber CF (1992) A new South Africa—a new health care strategy. *South African Journal of Medicine* **82** 388–391

Walker ARP, Walker BF and Glatthaan II (1994) Impoverished Africa: any hope for the future? *Journal of the Royal Society of Medicine* **87** 157–160

United Nations World Development Reports (1993), July, pp 238–295, United Nations, New York

The author is responsible for the accuracy of the references.

The Geography of Prostate Cancer and Its Treatment in Israel

H J BRENNER • P RATH • T TICHLER • B NUSSBAUM
Department of Oncology, Sheba Medical Center, Tel Hashomer 52621, Israel

With a total population of 5.5 million, Israel has a rate of 17.5 cases of prostate cancer per 100 000 per year, as measured by the Israel Cancer Registry for the period 1982–1986. In 1989, there were 532 newly reported cases. Of these, there were 143 cases in the Sephardi North African population, with a crude rate of 33.4. For the 389 cases of Ashkenazi European origin, the crude rate was 76.2. Seventy cases were seen in 1993 at the Sheba Medical Center affiliated to the Tel Aviv University (Israel Cancer Registry, 1982–1986).

There is as yet no policy for an organized early detection campaign. However, urologists and departments of urology use the triad of rectal examination, ultrasound (transrectal) and estimation of the prostatic specific antigen (PSA) to diagnose asymptomatic patients. Transrectal biopsies are carried out in our hospital, using random directions under ultrasound guidance.

When a diagnosis has been established, Gleason's prognostic criteria are determined. (At the University of Tel Aviv, attempts to evaluate the degree of malignancy as measured by S-phase estimations are in progress.)

Surgery, and specifically the nerve-sparing Walsh technique, vies with radiation as the definitive treatment for early stage cancers. The response rates are no different from those noted in the USA and Europe. The radiation techniques used in our department are, however, somewhat modified in that we do not use large pelvic portals, as suggested by the Stanford group, but three and four field techniques to a dosage of 45 Gy and a rotation cone down boost to raise the total dose to as near to 70 Gy as possible, being limited by the patient's symptoms. Iodine-125 implants are rarely used, but the technique is available. Orchidectomy and lately anti-androgens, such as cryproterone acetate and the luteinizing hormone releasing hormone (LHRH) agonists, form the backbone of hormone therapy for palliation in patients with metastatic disease.

Recently, some surgeons and radiation therapists have been experimenting with initial administration of LHRH agonists for stage C carcinoma of the prostate, in the hope that the reduction in tumour size will lead to a higher frequency of ablative surgery or smaller radiation portals will translate to better cure rates.

Hyperthermia has been used for the management of benign prostate hypertrophy, and there have been some clinical trials (limited in scope) in the

Cancer Surveys Volume 23: *Preventing Prostate Cancer: Screening versus Chemoprevention*

management of localized advanced prostatic cancers. The preliminary results seem promising (2nd International Workshop on Hyperthermia for the Prostate, 1993).

The use of chemotherapy in the adjuvant setting was pioneered in Israel by the Beilinson Hospital group, led by Professor C Servadio (Servadio *et al,* 1983, 1992). He has published 15 year follow-up reports on patients who received cyclophosphamide and 5-fluorouracil on a long term basis, with a 15-year survival rate of 40%.

The Sheba Medical Center chemotherapy trials for advanced metastatic prostate cancer were presented at the European Conference on Clinical Oncology 7 meeting. We have used continuous infusion of 5-fluorouracil (1000 $mg/m^2/24$ hr for 5 days) as the basic drug and supplemented this either with an infusion of mitomycin C 12 mg/m^2 every 6 weeks or with cisplatin 70 mg/m^2 by intravenous infusion every 3 weeks.

The results in 16 patients showed no complete responses, but excellent partial responses were seen in 6 of the 16 patients, with PSA and acid phosphatase levels reaching normal values. In 4 of the 16 patients, progressive disease was halted and stabilized, with marked symptomatic improvement. The duration of response was a median of 5.5 months (range 2–14 months). Only three patients were granulopenic, and only two patients had a grade II-III mucositis.

This regimen has proved useful, and it is hoped that when it is used earlier in the evolution of metastatic disease, better palliation and longer survival will be achieved seen (extrapolating from the Servadio results).

References

Israel Cancer Registry (1982–1986) *Cancer in Israel. Facts and Figures.*Israel Cancer Registry, Jerusalem

2nd International Workshop on Hyperthermia for the Prostate (1993) *Israel Journal of Medical Sciences* **29** 501, 506–550

Servadio C, Mukamel E, Lurie H and Nissenkorn I (1983) Early combined hormonal and chemotherapy for metastatic prostatic carcinoma. *Urology* **21** 493–495

Servadio C, Mukamel E and Nussbaum B (1992) 15 years' experience of combined hormone/chemotherapy in metastatic prostate cancer. *Urology* **39** 274–276

The authors are responsible for the accuracy of the references.

The Geography of Prostate Cancer and Its Treatment in Europe

D W W NEWLING
Free University Hospital (AZVU), Department of Urology, Amsterdam, The Netherlands

INTRODUCTION

In many European countries, the treatment of prostate cancer has been governed by a combination of scientific and economic factors. Probably one of the most important scientific papers on the subject was written in 1954 by Franks, who from a large postmortem series showed that only about 1 in 300 men with histological evidence of prostate cancer actually died of the disease. Other postmortem studies tended to confirm this and showed that if the disease was confined to the prostate gland, and particularly to one area of the gland, then no patients appeared to develop metastases and die of the condition.

In many European countries, there has been a lack of medical manpower and particularly a lack of specialist surgeons. Urology came relatively late as a specialty to countries such as the UK, and specialized urological operations, such as radical prostatectomy, were carried out only sporadically until a few years ago. In 1973, the results of the Veterans Administration Cooperative Urological Research Group's placebo controlled studies in stage C and D_1 prostate cancer indicated that there was no need to treat patients with prostate cancer until symptoms developed and that even after this wait a significant proportion of patients died of other conditions (Byar, 1973). The scientific evidence thus helped hard pressed health services with limited resources in the management of prostate cancer and supported the concept that for patients with very localized disease, radical treatment was unnecessary and for patients

 0-87969-466-1/95. $5.00 + .00

with more widespread disease, treatment was necessary only when symptoms developed.

During the past 20 years, there has been an expansion of good clinical research in the management of prostate cancer. In Europe, this has been mainly in the management of metastatic prostate cancer, and with the publication of the results of many consensus meetings, there appears to be some confluence of ideas on the way forward in the treatment of advanced disease at least. In addition, through the medium of the consensus meetings organized by the European Organization for Research on Treatment of Cancer (EORTC), there has been more coordination of studies, avoiding much overlap and useless repetition (Newling and Jones, 1990).

MANAGEMENT OF LOCALIZED AND INCIDENTAL DISEASE

In Europe until now, few prospective studies have been completed comparing immediate with deferred treatment in patients presenting with localized disease. Newling *et al* (1985), Chodak *et al* (1993) and others have done retrospective studies of a personal series of patients who for one reason or another were not treated, and all have shown that for the incidental T_1 (A_1 unifocal disease), there is really little justification for a radical approach. The Medical Research Council (MRC) attempted to carry out a study of patients with incidentally discovered unifocal and multifocal disease, but too few cases were collected and the study was prematurely terminated. Probably the most important study in this area is that of Johansson (1994) in Sweden, who has now followed up 223 patients over 17 years and has shown that there is an identifiable group who do not benefit from treatment and who remain free of symptoms and without evidence of metastases 10 years after diagnosis. At the present time, there are a number of important ongoing studies, at least two of which may include patients with incidentally discovered prostate cancer as well as patients with clinical prostate cancer. The MRC has just completed recruitment to a large study in which patients with all stages of localized prostate cancer and even metastatic cancer are randomized to receive immediate or delayed hormonal therapy. This study has just been closed to entry with 938 patients, of whom 397 have died, 72% from prostatic cancer. The first analysis has not yet been carried out (Kirk D and Shearer R, personal communication).

The EORTC has two studies of immediate versus deferred therapy at the present time. Study 30846 looks at patients for whom radical prostatectomy is planned but who are found to have positive lymph nodes at laparotomy. These patients are randomized to immediate or deferred hormonal therapy with orchidectomy or a luteinizing hormone releasing hormone (LHRH) agonist. The study has enrolled over 213 patients and requires 320. The second EORTC study, 30891, takes patients with only localized disease who are deemed unsuitable for radical prostatectomy and who are also randomized to immediate or deferred therapy with either orchidectomy or LHRH agonists. This study has recruited 360 patients but requires 750 patients for completion.

MANAGEMENT OF LOCALLY ADVANCED DISEASE

In the mid 1970s, when prostate cancer clinical trials in Europe began with the introduction of the first two EORTC studies on locally advanced and metastatic prostate cancer, it was felt that locally advanced disease always required systemic therapy and could only be treated palliatively with hormones. In studies 30761 and 30762, patients with localized disease, who were treated with one of four different hormonal therapies, diethylstilboestrol (DES) 3 mg/day, medroxyprogesterone acetate (MPA) 250 mg/day, cyproterone acetate (CPA) 250 mg/day or estramustine 280 mg/day, achieved reasonable responses, with some long term survivors at 5 years (Pavone Macaluso *et al,* 1986; Smith *et al,* 1986). The oestrogen containing compounds cause considerable cardiovascular side effects, and MPA was clearly used in too low a dose to be as effective as in subsequent studies (Bouffioux, (1979) and therefore was unfairly compared.

In an extensive MRC study of patients with localized prostate cancer (T_{2-3} and T_4) who were randomized to receive immediate orchidectomy, radiotherapy or a combination of the two, those who received the hormonal therapy, either alone or with radiotherapy, had a longer interval before the appearance of distant metastases than those treated with radiotherapy alone (Fellows *et al,* 1992). Survival statistics also supported the use of hormonal therapy in patients with advanced localized disease. With the more widespread use of radical prostatectomy, particularly with the introduction of laparoscopic pelvic lymph node dissection, we now know that about 50% of patients with T_3 tumours and 75% of those with T_4 tumours have positive lymph nodes (Austenfeld and Davis, 1990) and thus almost certainly will be considered for early hormonal therapy.

Apart from the ongoing EORTC and MRC studies, there is another important study being carried out in Europe at the present time. For some time, and probably originally based on work at the Mayo Clinic on the treatment of D_1 tumours, that is, patients with positive lymph nodes (Zincke, 1989), there has been a suggestion that combination therapy with hormones and radical surgery or radiotherapy may offer a significant survival advantage in patients with localized prostate cancer. At present, there is an ongoing European study in which patients with T_{2-4} prostate cancer are randomized to undergo radical prostatectomy with or without 3 months' prior treatment with total androgen blockade using LHRH agonists and a non-steroidal anti-androgen. Some 10% of the patients presenting with T_2 tumours who received total androgen blockade have shown no evidence of prostate cancer either in the lymph nodes or in the prostate gland itself after 3 months hormonal therapy (Debruyne FMJ, personal communication). It will, however, be at least 5 years before the impact of total androgen blockade on survival of these patients can be seen.

MANAGEMENT OF METASTATIC DISEASE

Many years ago it was realized that patients with metastatic disease who were treated with simple orchidectomy, stilboestrol or an anti-androgen responded for approximately 18 months before relapsing, and the median survival from diagnosis was a little under 3 years. The reason for the hormone relapse appeared to be a change in the sensitivity of the cells, some of which became completely refractory to hormonal therapy, others of which appeared to respond to a second line hormonal treatment. Labrie (1984) and others identified the adrenals as the apparent source of further androgen stimulation after orchidectomy, medical or surgical, and the concept of total androgen blockade as primary treatment began with Bracchi in Rome in 1978. In 1980, the EORTC launched its first study of total androgen blockade against standard therapy, protocol number 30805. Total androgen blockade with orchidectomy plus CPA, a steroidal anti-androgen, was compared with orchidectomy alone and DES 1 mg/day. The result of this study, as with protocol 30843, which compared CPA plus buserelin with orchidectomy or buserelin alone, showed no difference between any of the arms, and there was no improvement in survival compared with that of patients in previous studies, who had metastases at diagnosis (Robinson, 1988; Klijn *et al,* 1993). At the same time as these studies were carried out in North America, National Cancer Institute Intergroup study 134 showed a substantial improvement in time to progression and survival in a group of patients treated with the combination therapy of leuproline (leuprorelin), an LHRH agonist, and the non-steroidal anti-androgen flutamide (Crawford *et al,* 1989). This led to a positive explosion of protocols in Europe and elsewhere, attempting to prove or disprove the concept of total androgen blockade. Two identical studies, the Daproca study (Iverson *et al,* 1990) and EORTC 3085318 (Dennis *et al,* 1993), compared orchidectomy with goserelin and flutamide. The patients in the two studies appeared to be similar demographically, yet the 30853 study showed a considerable advantage in time to progression and survival, whereas the Daproca study showed no advantage.

These discrepancies led the EORTC to carry out a meta-analysis of 23 studies of combined androgen blockade against standard therapy, and although there is now undoubtedly a trend for improved survival and time to progression in those patients managed with combination therapy, the difference is so small that it is clearly only a small group of patients with metastatic disease who respond better. All the evidence points to the fact that these are patients with small volume metastatic disease, that is, fewer than five bony metastases, and their mean survival may well be 18 months longer than that of patients treated by orchidectomy alone (Dennis, 1992).

With the advent of total androgen blockade, many urologists and endocrinologists believed that the zenith of treatment of metastatic prostate cancer had been reached and that there were no further studies to be done. There are, however, a number of developments in endocrine therapy that may change our views in this respect and certainly need to be explored.

In Scandinavia, oestrogens have always remained a popular treatment despite their observed severe cardiovascular side effects when given orally (De Voogt *et al,* 1986). In Scandinavia, parenteral oestrogens have been shown to be relatively free of cardiovascular side effects, well tolerated and just as effective as any other form of simple androgen ablation—that is, orchidectomy (Tomic R, 1983).

It had been known from the early days of the VACURG study that oestrogens were more effective in preventing death from prostate cancer than orchidectomy. If the cardiovascular side effects can be eliminated, then clearly they may be a cheaper and superior therapy to orchidectomy alone or even to total androgen blockade. Whether or not they will prove to be superior to total androgen blockade in all patients with metastatic disease must await the results of an ongoing Scandinavian trial studying polystradiol against an LHRH agonist plus an anti-androgen.

The EORTC wishes to explore the possibility that a non-steroidal anti-androgen given in a high enough dose could be as effective as total androgen blockade, and there is a planned study of a non-steroidal anti-androgen against the same anti-androgen plus an LHRH agonist. The presently available non-steroidal anti-androgens have dose limiting side effect profiles, but "Casodex", presently undergoing phase III evaluation, probably does not (Shellhammer, 1992). Not only would this possibly provide a treatment as effective as the more expensive combination therapy, but patients would have the advantage of retaining their potency as well. This study would be open to all patients with metastatic disease and should be large enough to detect a 10% difference between the two treatment arms. Approximately 2500 patients would be needed to carry out this study.

Meanwhile in Canada, Buchowsky has suggested that intermittent hormonal therapy might provide the answer to the complications and expense of continuous hormone therapy that we are using now and prevent the development of hormone resistant cells (Buchowsky *et al,* 1990). Although this is being extensively looked at in the USA and Canada, there is no ongoing study in Europe at the present time.

Recent observations by Scher have led to a new concept of management of patients who relapse while receiving combination therapy (Scher and Kelly, 1993). Of 29 patients who had clear evidence of progression following combination therapy with an LHRH agonist and anti-androgen, 10 went back into remission if the anti-androgen alone was stopped, some for as long as 2 years. Not only was this subjective remission, with a falling prostate specific antigen (PSA) concentration, but there was also evidence of objective remission and objective response in those patients with measurable lesions. It is no coincidence that this secondary response is seen in a third of patients—almost exactly the same proportion of patients who on hormone relapse respond to single agent chemotherapy. Scher and Kelly have suggested that all patients who relapse on combination therapy should for a period of time, particularly if their PSA remains stable, stop treatment with the anti-androgen and be treated with LHRH only. If long term responses in these patients occur, then it is clear evidence that a clone of cells has been induced that has become dependent on that therapy. Thus, have we further indirect evidence that intermittent hormone therapy might provide a more satisfactory treatment for patients with metastatic disease?

MANAGEMENT OF HORMONE ESCAPED DISEASE

Despite the very large numbers of phase II studies and a few phase III studies investigating chemotherapeutic agents and combination chemotherapeutic hormonal agents, there is no effective chemotherapeutic agent that can be used in high enough concentrations in patients who have relapsed on hormonal therapy to induce a meaningful second response. With single agents such as cisplatin, methotrexate, mitomycin, epirubicin and vinblastine, and even the second line drug estramustine in high doses, the response rate is a maximum 30% and rarely lasts more than 6 months (Eisenberger and Abrams, 1988). In a phase III study of high dose estramustine against mitomycin in patients with objective progression following multiple previous hormonal therapies, no useful response was identified in either arm, and the systemic toxicity for both agents was considerable (Newling *et al,* 1993).

EORTC study 30853, which analyses progression in patients treated with combination hormonal therapy or orchidectomy, has shown that almost all patients who relapse with objective signs of progression after hormonal therapy have a rising PSA before relapse (Newling, 1993). If this finding is confirmed, then before patients become ill with a deteriorating performance status, increasing pain and objective evidence of new bony metastases, they could be treated with chemotherapeutic agents in doses that would give these agents a reasonable chance of success. The most promising combination of chemohormonal therapy emerging from some phase I and phase II studies appears to be a combination of estramustine and vinblastine (Akaza *et al,* 1988). The EORTC is planning to start a phase III study looking at this combination against estramustine alone in patients who have relapsed with a rising PSA following primary hormonal therapy.

CONCLUSION

The search for the most effective therapy for all stages of prostate cancer continues. The improvement of surgical techniques will undoubtedly lead to an improvement in survival and cure rates for localized prostate cancer. The possible combination of hormone therapy and surgery for patients with more advanced localized disease looks promising. The search for the most effective hormonal therapy is not over, and further basic scientific research is necessary on the development of hormone dependence and independence before the timing of this palliative treatment is perfected. There is little doubt that once a prostate cancer has become locally extensive, and certainly once it is metastasized, there are groups of cells within that cancer that can be killed only by chemotherapeutic agents, and therefore the search for effective chemotherapeutic agents, either to be used in combination as first line treatment or on relapse after primary hormonal therapy, must continue.

SUMMARY

The search for more efficient treatments for prostate cancer continues. In localized prostate cancer, the combination of neo-adjuvant or adjuvant hormone therapy with surgery may improve curability rates. In the palliation of advanced prostate cancer, novel concepts of varying forms of maximal androgen blockade, including the re-introduction of safer forms of oestrogen therapy, should be capable of lengthening the time to progression and improving the quality of life of patients with advanced disease. The chemotherapy of prostate cancer remains experimental, but its earlier introduction may enable better dosing schedules to further limit advanced disease.

References

Akaza H and Tokyo Estracyt Study Group (1988) A prospective randomized controlled study on the treatment of stage D and C prostatic cancer with Estracyt in combination with other therapeutic agents. *Japanese Journal of Clinical Oncology* **18** 343–355

Austenfeld MS and Davis BE (1990) New concepts in the treatment of stage D1 adenocarcinoma of the prostate. *Urologic Clinics of North America* **17** 867–884

Bouffioux C (1979) Le cancer du prostate. *Acta Urologica Belgica* **47** 189–195

Bruchowsky N, Goldenberg SL and Gleave M (1990) Intermittent androgen suppression in patients with metastatic prostate cancer. *Cancer Research* **50** 2275–2282

Byar DP (1973) The Veterans Administration Cooperative Urological Research Group studies of cancer of the prostate. *Cancer* **32** 1126–1130

Chodak GW, Visted R, Gerber G *et al* (1993) Multivariate analysis of outcome following observation—delayed therapy of clinically localized prostatic cancer. *Journal of Urology* **149** 396a–400

Crawford ED, Eisenberger MA, McCleod DJ *et al* (1989) A controlled trial of Luprolyte with and without Flutamide in prostatic carcinoma. *New England Journal of Medicine* **321** 419–426

Denis L (1992) Maximal androgen blockade: an overview, In: Murphy G, Khoury S, Chatelain C and Denis L (eds). *Proceedings of the 3rd International Symposium on Advances in Urological Cancer: Diagnosis and Treatment,* pp 137–145, Scientific Publications, Paris

Denis L, Carneiro de Moura JL, Bono A *et al* (1993) Goserelin acetate and Flutamide vs bilateral orchiectomy: a phase III EORTC trial (30853). *Urology* **42** 119–130

De Voogt HJ, Smiths PH, Pavone Macalus M, De Pauw M, Suciu S and members of the EORTC GU-Group (1986) Cardiovascular side effects of diethylstibestrol, CPA, MPA and estramustine phosphate used for the treatment of advanced prostatatic cancer results for EORTC trials 30761 and 30762. *Journal of Urology* **135** 303–307

Eisenberger MA and Abrams JS (1988) Chemotherapy for prostatic carcinoma. *Seminars in Urology* **6** 303–310

Fellows GJ, Clark PB, Beynon LL *et al* (1992) Treatment of advanced localised prostate cancer by orchiectomy, radiotherapy, or combined treatment. *British Journal of Urology* **70** 304–309

Franks LM (1954) Latent carcinoma of the prostate. *Journal of Pathology* **68** 617–621

Iverson P, Suciu S, Sylvester R, Christensen and Denis L (1990) Zoladex and Flutamide vs orchiectomy in the treatment of patients with advanced carcinoma of the prostate, a phase III trial. *Cancer* **66** 1067–1073

Johansson JE (1994) Watchful waiting for early stage prostate cancer. *Urology* **2** 138–142

Klijn JGM, De Voogt, HJ, Studer UE *et al* (1993) Short term vs long term addition of CPA to Buserelin therapy in comparison with orchiectomy for metastatic prostatic cancer (EORTC trial 30843). *Cancer* **72 (Supplement 12)** 3850–3862

Labrie F (1984) A new approach in the hormonal treatment of prostate cancer complete instead of partial blockade of androgens. *International Journal of Andrology* **7** 1–4

Newling DWW and Jones WG (eds) (1990) *Prostate Cancer and Testicular Cancer* EORTC GU-Group Monograph No 7, pp 151–235, Wiley Liss, New York

Newling DWW, Hall RR, Richards B, Robinson MRG and Hetherington JW (1985) The natural history of prostatic cancer, the argument for a no treatment policy, In: Pavone Macaluso M, Smith PH and Bagshaw MA (eds). *Testical Cancer and Other Tumors of the Genitourinary Tract,* pp 443–449, Plenum Publications, New York

Newling DWW, Fossa S, Tunn U, Kish KH, DePano M and Sylvester R (1993) Mitomycin C vs estramustine in the treatment of hormone resistant metastatic prostatic cancer. *Journal of Urology* **150** 1840–1844

Pavone Macaluso M, De Voogt HJ, Vaggiano G *et al* (1986) Comparison of DES, CPA and MPA in the treatment of advanced prostatic cancer: final analysis of a randomized phase III trial of EORTC urological group. *Journal of Urology* **136** 624

Robinson MRG (1988) EORTC protocol 30805: a phase III trial comparing orchiectomy versus orchiectomy and CPA and low dose stilboestrol in the management of metastatic carcinoma of the prostate, In: Pavone Macaluso M and Smith PH (eds). *Management of Advanced Cancer of Prostate and Bladder,* EORTC GU-Group Monograph No 4, pp 101–110. Allen R Liss, New York

Scher HF and Kelly W (1993) Flutamide withdrawal syndrome its impact on clinical trials in hormone refractory prostate cancer. *Journal of Clinical Oncology* **11** 1566–1572

Shellhammer PF (1992) Casodex: the phase II results, In: Murphy G, Khoury S, Chatelain C and Denis L (eds). *Proceedings on the 3rd International Symposium on Advances in Urological Cancer: Diagnosis and Treatment,* pp 116–120, Scientific Publications, Paris

Smith PH, Suciu S, Robinson MRG *et al* (1986) Comparison of the effects of DES with low dose Estramustine phosphate in the treatment of advanced prostate cancer: final analysis of a phase III trial of the EORTC Urological Group. *Journal of Urology* **136** 619

Tomic R (1983) Some effects of orchiectomy, oestrogen treatment and radiation therapy in patients with prostatic carcinoma. *Scand. J. Urol. Nephrol.* Suppl. **77** 1–37

Zincke H (1989) Extended experience with surgical treatment of stage D1 adenocarcinoma of the prostate. *Urology* **33** 27

The author is responsible for the accuracy of the references.

Overviews

A Basic Science Perspective

WALTER F BODMER
Imperial Cancer Research Fund, 44 Lincoln's Inn Fields, London WC2A 3PX

This meeting emphasized for me four major points:

- How little is known about the biology and genetics of prostate cancer. Molecular approaches have been applied only quite recently.
- How very limited are the epidemiological clues about prostate cancer, apart from the striking evidence for ethnic differences.
- What a major problem there is in deciding which tumours, if any, picked up early by the prostate specific antigen (PSA) test are truly likely to have malignant potential, raising the enormously difficult question of how individuals with elevated PSA should be treated.
- The lack of consensus on how to treat prostate cancer, and when or even whether to treat.

I have no doubt that further exploration of the fundamental biology and genetics of prostate cancer will be the key to answering these questions.

The one striking result of the epidemiology is the extraordinary indications of large ethnic variation. This clearly needs further analysis, including what has been done, for example, for breast cancer—namely the analysis of migrant populations. There also needs to be careful standardization of diagnosis and the interpretation of death rates.

Many approaches that have been used in the study of other tumours can contribute to elucidating the genetics of prostate cancer. Loss of heterozygosity studies suggest the possibility of interesting genes at 8p22, 16q22 and 17p13.3. The study of prostate cancer cells in culture can reveal dominant oncogene and tumour suppresser gene mutations and has shown the potential importance of alterations in attachment molecules such as E cadherin. In addition, attachment to extracellular matrix via integrins and the role of proteolytic enzymes involved in degrading extracellular matrix components are important, as well as the signalling mechanisms that follow attachment.

There are some clues, as in other cancers, to the existence of clear-cut Mendelian dominant families. There is a question as to whether prostate cancer is associated with the breast and ovarian cancer families connected with the *BRCA1* gene, and it surely would be worth doing the PSA test on such families. It is also worth looking for a possible role for mutator genes. Obviously, once clear-cut families and linkage involving them are established, posi-

Cancer Surveys Volume 23: *Preventing Prostate Cancer: Screening versus Chemoprevention*

tional cloning should provide important clues to any new genes. Perhaps further emphasis could be put on the search for families, using early age of onset as a major clue.

There is the clear possibility of the existence of relatively high frequency, low penetrance alleles that could be detected by sib pair analysis in families that do not give clear-cut Mendelian inheritance. The role of candidate genes can then be tested by looking at the population associations between prostate cancer incidence and polymorphisms for such genes. As in other cancers, plausible candidates include the dominant and recessive oncogenes, genes for metabolism such as the P450 enzymes and genes controlling DNA repair processes. For such studies, it is essential to have good normal population controls, especially taking into account the evidence for ethnic variation in the incidence of prostate cancer.

The aim must be eventually to use the genetics to distinguish which early tumours detected, for example, by the PSA test are benign and which have significant malignant potential and should be treated. It is important here to emphasize the collection of material for such studies, especially biopsies. However, it may also be possible to pick up the signatures of genetic changes from cancer cells circulating in the blood, and perhaps especially in the bone marrow. There is also the possibility of screening urine and semen for cancer cells, given the sensitivity of polymerase chain reaction based assays.

What are the differences between the 90% of cancers picked up by PSA screening that are not lethal if untreated and the minority that are. A second level of evaluation is needed to reduce the frequency of false positives after detection of a PSA in the range 4–10 ng/ml. One possibility is to use monoclonal antibodies against surface antigens specific to prostate cancer for immunoscintigraphy, and eventually perhaps targeted antibody based therapy.

To pursue effectively the cell biology and genetics, there is an urgent need for new sources of cell lines from prostate cancers. Transformation of prostate cells should be tried, using the various approaches that are now available. This would at least preserve their major genotype and probably many other features, such as production of growth factors and expression of growth factor receptors. The few cell lines now available clearly do not seem to be representative of the general population of prostate cancers.

What growth factors are really critical for prostate cancer? Can hormone dependence and resistance be effectively sorted out? There is also a need for good animal models, which no doubt can come from transgenic mice once more is known about the genetics. What, if any, is the functional significance of PSA?

A variety of approaches are being discussed for gene therapy for cancer. On the one hand, these involve either non-specific immune stimulation using, for example, cytokines and accessory attachment molecules and, on the other hand, drug based approaches that depend on significant bystander killing. Targeting to a cancer can be achieved by using tissue specific promoters, and for this, the novel prostate specific surface antigen, for which there is now a monoclonal antibody, is a potentially interesting target as well, of course, as PSA. To pursue the immune therapies, it would be valuable to have information on the distribution of HLA class I and class II molecules, which can provide evidence for the existence of immune attack. There are now many potential novel approaches to T cell based therapy, including against *TP53* mutations.

Tumour proliferation is a balance between the rate of division and the rate of cell death (apoptosis). The particular role of *TP53* mutations selected for during carcinogenesis seems to be to counteract apoptosis, whose incidence may otherwise be increased by some of the earlier changes selected for during tumour initiation and progression. It seems possible that other genetic changes are also involved in decreasing cell death rate and so increasing tumour proliferation rate. This may, for example, be the role of the mutator mismatch repair gene mutations found in colorectal and many other cancers. New approaches to treatment based on influencing apoptosis should offer considerable promise.

In conclusion, I believe there are many clear-cut directions for novel research in the laboratory on the cell biology and genetics of prostate cancer and that these will provide a way forward to improving diagnosis, early detection and treatment of this disease.

An Historical Perspective of the Pathology and Treatment

L M FRANKS
13 Allingham Street, London N1 8NX

INTRODUCTION

Although history may have much to teach us, we do not in fact learn much from history, but the fault is ours. When I first became interested in prostatic cancer when I was appointed to a new ICRF unit to investigate human cancer in 1951, a few weeks in the library showed me the depths of my ignorance. In spite of a medical training and some years in practice, I was unaware of—and did not believe—much that I found. My own subsequent work, set up to demonstrate the errors of my predecessors, confirmed almost everything that had been known and published many years before. Forty years on it is interesting to compare two excellent reviews from 1994 (Dearnaley, 1994) and 1985 (Kirk, 1985) with earlier reviews of my own (Franks, 1954a,b) and to find that the questions that were asked in the past are still being asked today. In this chapter, I give a brief survey of these earlier findings and identify some questions that remain to be answered.

Many of the features of prostatic cancer are a consequence of the anatomical site of origin, whilst others are a consequence of the biological behaviour of the tumour.

SITE OF ORIGIN AND ITS CONSEQUENCES

There are two main groups of prostatic glands—inner and outer. Benign enlargement arises from the inner glands, but cancers begin in the outer glands. The site of origin of prostatic cancer has two main consequences. The first is that the disease is difficult if not impossible to diagnose in its early stages. It may be present for a considerable time before it involves any structure that

Cancer Surveys Volume 23: *Preventing Prostate Cancer: Screening versus Chemoprevention*
 0-87969-466-1/95. $5.00 + .00

might produce symptoms. The second consequence is that invasion of the capsule is early, and tumour cells soon involve lymphatics and blood vessels. The extent of spread is almost invariably greater than the clinical assessment has suggested. Jewett (1949) found that only about 4% of his patients were thought to have tumours confined to the gland, but even in this group, over half were found to have extraprostatic spread on histological examination. Distant spread is equally common and almost invariable in patients dying of the disease. (Franks, 1956a). Clifton *et al* (1952) found that at least a third of patients had tumour cells in the bone marrow.

BIOLOGICAL ACTIVITY OF PROSTATIC CANCER

Under the microscope and to the naked eye, all prostatic cancers are similar, but biologically, that is in the patient, two types can be distinguished, the active or clinical cancer and the latent or unsuspected cancer. The incidence of clinical cases is about 16 per 100 000 in Caucasians, but there is considerable racial variation. In the West, it causes about 7–8% of tumour deaths in men over 50 years old. At least 30% of prostates removed at autopsy from men over this age who have died of some other disease are found to have carcinomas that are indistinguishable histologically from active clinical cancers, yet they have not grown or killed the patient. A distinction must be made between the disease prostatic cancer and these latent, apparently inactive tumours. The microscope in this instance gives us no guide to the biological malignancy of the tumour. Both clinical and latent tumours are rare before age 50 but become increasingly frequent with age. There is some evidence that biological malignancy of the tumours and their metastases may be reduced in older patients (Franks, 1956a), but this has not been confirmed.

ASSESSING THE RESULTS OF TREATMENT

The results of treatment must be assessed against this biological and pathological background. There may be a very small group of patients with tumours confined entirely to the gland. It is logical to consider radical surgery for this group, although in view of the high incidence of local and distant spread, the numbers are likely to be small. Most patients must be given some form of general treatment, whether it be endocrine, radiation or other. But there are problems.

The first is that we do not know at what stage any given tumour is at the time of diagnosis. For example, let us assume that a disease has a natural history of 6 years. Patient A, by chance or otherwise, notices a lump and has it removed within the first year. Patient B does not seek treatment until the tumour has been present for 3 years. Both die with recurrences after the tumour has been present for 6 years, but the survival period after treatment for the first patient is 5 years, whereas the second survives for only 3 years, although both had the same type of tumour and the same treatment. The onset of symptoms and early diagnosis may depend more on the precise site of origin of the tumour than on its biological malignancy.

A second problem is that we have no method of assessing the biological malignancy of tumours. Some cases of prostatic cancer diagnosed clinically may be biologically latent. As might be expected, these are often cases in which the tumour is discovered accidentally, for example patients with benign enlargement in whom cancer is found incidentally on microscopy or in patients in whom a small nodule is found on routine rectal examination. Cancers of this type have a long survival period whatever form of treatment is given. In an earlier study (Franks *et al,* 1958), we were unable to find any reliable prognostic feature except for the not altogether surprising fact that the presence of metastases indicated a poor outcome, yet even this was not absolute since some of our long term survivors lived for many years even though metastases were present when first seen. Histological grading is now regarded as a guide to prognosis. I think that this is true in general terms—that is, a group of patients with well differentiated tumours will have a better prognosis than a group with anaplastic tumours, but it may not give a reliable guide in individual cases.

RESULTS OF TREATMENT

Since hormones were first shown to have an effect on the prostate, they have been considered to have a primary role in prostatic carcinogenesis, although the evidence for this is slight. I think that it is reasonable to assume that the main part played by hormones is to stimulate the development and maintenance of prostatic epithelium so that enough cells are present in which malignant change can occur. Hormones may play no part in the actual process of carcinogenesis. Once a tumour has developed, the neoplastic cells may remain responsive to the factors that control normal growth provided the cells still retain these particular normal differentiated characters.

The response of many prostatic cancers to anti-androgenic treatment is dramatic. Clinically, primary and secondary tumours may become progressively smaller and some almost disappear. All grades of tumour cells from the most differentiated to the most anaplastic seem to respond similarly. Tumours that respond to endocrine treatment are referred to as "hormone sensitive", but this term can be applied only to the cells that respond, not to the tumour as a whole. Even in tumours that show severe degenerative changes, a few cells showing no signs of damage can usually be found. Often, both primary and secondary tumours respond similarly, but in some cases after prolonged treatment, the primary tumour may still be retarded, although metastatic deposits grow actively. In others, the primary and soft tissue deposits may be inactive while the bone deposits are growing and ultimately kill the patient. Hormone sensitivity is therefore not a property of the tumour as a whole but may vary from part to part of the same tumour. This underlines another general principle in tumour therapy. Most therapeutic agents, such as drugs, hormones or radiation, do not destroy all the cells in a tumour, and the result of treatment may be to leave behind resistant cells that give rise to recurrences. Whether these resistant cells were present in the tumour from the beginning or are produced by treatment is not known. All the tumour cells can be killed as a rule by increasing the dose, but the higher dosage may well kill normal tissues too. Although endocrine treatment will cause regression in about 80% of cases, most relapse eventually even after removal or inhibition of the sources of all the known sex hormones. These tumours have become hormone independent.

Nearly 40 years ago, I drew some conclusions about the effects of treatment, based on figures reported by McDonald (1957) and on others of my own (Franks, 1960). It would seem from these figures that patients with clinical prostatic cancer can be divided into three groups. The first group—about 70–75% of treated patients and 85% of controls—die within 3 years. This includes an estimated 20% of all patients whose disease does not respond to endocrine treatment at all and who die within the first year. After 3 years, the difference in survival between the treated and untreated patients becomes more marked. By 5 years, 25–30% of the treated patients but only 5–6% of the controls survive. This last group is of particular interest since there must be some natural mechanism in these cases that retards tumour growth. I suggested that in the great majority of patients—those dying within the first 3 years—the effect of treatment on survival time may be an indirect effect resulting from the relief of urinary obstruction, control of infection and so on without any direct alteration on the neoplastic process. This would explain the remarkable similarity of results whatever form of treatment is used.

SUMMARY AND CONCLUSIONS

There are inner and outer gland groups in the human prostate. Benign nodular hyperplasia develops from the inner group of glands. Carcinomas arise in the outer glands and spread beyond the prostate at an early stage in the disease. The biological malignancy of prostatic cancer varies from patient to patient and from part to part of the same tumour. Some tumours remain biologically inactive or latent so that there must be some naturally occurring mechanism that controls tumour growth in some cases. This phenomenon is not confined to the prostate but can be found in many other organs, although not so frequently. It may represent a stage in tumour progression or reflect the balance between growth stimulating and inhibiting factors (Franks, 1956b). Our new knowledge of these factors suggests that this may be an area well worth looking at again.

Prostatic cancer patients may be divided into groups that differ in their response to endocrine treatment. These differences may be due to changes in the tumour cells or in the host. A temporary state of tumour retardation or latency follows endocrine treatment in about 70–80% of all cases, but whatever form of treatment is used, about 75% of all patients die within 3 years. Even in tumours that show a marked response, endocrine treatment does not destroy all the tumour cells. Hormone sensitivity is not a property of the tumour as a whole but may vary from part to part of the same tumour.

Almost all the observations that I have outlined here have been described by me and by many others both before and since I first began to work in this field. The fact that benign prostatic enlargement arises in the inner glands was first recorded by Morgagni in 1769. Each subsequent generation has rediscovered the basic facts. We know a little more about the endocrine system and we have better methods for the detection of metastases—in itself a confession of failure—but the main questions remain unanswered.

We need an explanation for the remarkable differences in the sites of origin of benign hyperplasia and carcinoma and for the surprising frequency, age and race distribution of carcinoma as well as methods for assessing the biological malignancy of prostatic—and other—cancers. We need to ask whether screening has any relevance while we have no rational and effective method of treatment. We need to be able to decide both when to treat and how to treat. For the moment, the only reliable indicator of biological malignancy is the behaviour of the tumour in the patient. We need to know whether treatment before there are clinical symptoms influences the course of the disease. Finally, we need to take a new look at experimental approaches. We now have the technology we did not have 50 years ago that may allow us to answer some of these questions.

References

Clifton JA, Philipp RJ, Ludovic E and Fowler WM (1952) Bone marrow and carcinoma of prostate. *American Journal of Medical Sciences* **224** 121–130

Dearnaley DP (1944) Cancer of the prostate. *British Medical Journal* **308** 780–784

Franks LM (1954a) Benign nodular hyperplasia of the prostate:a review. *Annals of the Royal College of Surgeons* **14** 92–106

Franks LM (1954b) Latent carcinoma. *Annals of the Royal College of Surgeons* **15** 236–249

Franks LM (1956a) The spread of prostatic cancer. *Journal of Pathology and Bacteriology* **72** 603–611

Franks LM (1956b) Latency and progression in tumours: the natural history of prostatic cancer. *Lancet* **ii** 1037–9

Franks LM (1960) Estrogen-treated prostatic cancer: the varation in responsiveness of tumour cells. *Cancer* **13** 490–501

Franks LM, Fergusson JD and Murnaghan GF (1958) An assessment of factors influencing survival in prostatic cancer: the absence of reliable prognostic features. *British Journal of Cancer* **12** 321–326

Jewett HJ (1949) Radical perineal prostatectomy for cancer of the prostate: analysis of 190 cases. *Journal of Urology* **61** 277–280

Kirk D (1985) Prostatic carcinoma. *British Medical Journal* **290** 875–876

McDonald E (1957) Natural history of prostatic cancer, In *Proceedings of the 3rd National Cancer Conference,* p 185 Lippincott, Philadelphia

Morgagni G (1769) *The Seats and Causes of Disease Investigated by Anatomy,* pp 460–462, Johnson and Payne, London

The author is responsible for the accuracy of the references.

A Physician's Perspective

R T D OLIVER
London Hospital Medical College, Turner Street, London E1 1BB

Prostate cancer is becoming an increasingly fascinating and economically important disease, with the number of years of life lost among men in 1992 in the UK (72 000) being intermediate between that for breast cancer (226 000) and cervical cancer (35 000) in women. Prostate intraepithelial neoplasia occurs on average 20–30 years before clinically life threatening disease, and we would have an enormous window of opportunity for interfering with the progression of the disease if a simple low cost approach without major morbidity could be developed to eliminate the early stages. The critical issue in justifying the development of this concept is whether all cancers, even the most malignant, start with the differentiated occult type of disease that progresses by clonal evolution with loss of suppressor genes and mutation of oncogenes or whether the more malignant cases are a product of "skip" tumours that mutate so drastically in one step that they bypass the "latent" phase—something that the emerging cytogenetic data on the number of steps of significant loss of heterozygosity may ultimately answer.

Two hypotheses relevant to the development of new approaches to prevent deaths from prostate cancer have arisen from observations on the pathology of the early stages of the disease and other work reported in this volume. The first relates to the protective benefit of genital hygiene and nutrition. The epidemiology studies have demonstrated that past exposure to a venereally acquired disease is the most important risk factor associated with development of prostate cancer. The possibility that diminished use of barrier contraception is the cause of the increased incidence of prostate cancer seen in vasectomized men is another factor supporting the venereal disease hypothesis, whereas consumption of diets low in red meat and high in carrots has been shown to be associated with reduced risk. The observation on the venereal factor is supported by epidemiological evidence that cancer of the prostate follows cancer of cervix and cancer of penis, as well as AIDS, in being high in areas of Africa and South America with a low incidence of circumcision and low in the Middle East, where circumcision is common, and Japan, which is a population with a high level of genital hygiene rituals. The fact that the specific venereal diseases syphilis and gonorrhoea are less important risk factors than a non-specific venereal infection, taken with a failure of any study of human papillomavirus, raises interest in the possibility that there may be low grade pathogenic organism in prostate cancer patients having a role similar to that in *Helico-*

bacter in carcinoma of the stomach. If this were so, the current twin track approach of condoms and an aggressive approach to the treatment of non-specific venereal infection, which is already beginning to show benefits in reducing spread of AIDS in Africa, may also make a major impact on cancers of the prostate, cervix and penis in the course of the next 10–20 years. To investigate this hypothesis further, there need to be more studies focusing on early sexual behaviour and subsequent development of prostate cancer and more detailed age incidence curves for prostate and cervical cancer incidence in Africa and South America.

The second hypothesis to emerge from the presentations reviewed in this volume relate to the possibility that intermittent hormone therapy as opposed to continuous total androgen blockade might slow the rate of progression to androgen independent tumour growth. The longstanding knowledge that chronic continuous exposure to antibiotics is the best way to induce bacterial antibiotic resistance provides adequate justification for pursuit of such studies. This idea was also supported by the results from two small clinical studies in prostate cancer patients reviewed by ??, the most interesting being that involving three patients with early tumours that had gone for more than 18 months without evidence of recurrence after only 3 months' endocrine treatment. The possibility that hormone therapy, by its indirect effect on immune function, might have durable anti-tumour cytotoxic effects instead of the previously presumed cytostatic effects is a secondary reason for more detailed studies of intermittent hormone therapy on early stage tumours, particularly those in the older patients not fit for radical prostatectomy. The new observation that androgen withdrawal could induce regeneration of thymic lymphocytes justifies renewed interest in the possibility that immunotherapy might have a greater role in the treatment of this disease, particularly in the more endocrine responsive tumours. The possibility of using genetic engineering to reconstitute tumours to increase their susceptibility to immunotherapy is a particularly interesting new direction, which is opening up because of the possibility of using the prostate specific antigen promoter as part of the gene therapy construct to improve the specificity of targeting the gene to prostate cancer cells.

Surgery from a UK Perspective

JOHN BLANDY

Emeritus Professor of Urology, The Royal London Hospital, London E1 1BB

There are two opposing ideas of cancer: most surgeons see it as dry rot in timber, calling only for an enthusiastic carpenter, but a minority have come to see it more like woodworm in a valuable antique, requiring emphasis on restoration and preservation of everything that can possibly be saved—that is, Rentokil, rather than ruthless eradication.

With the dry rot school, it is an article of faith that one must cut out the rot before it spreads, and there is much talk of "early" cancer. All of this is understandable because surgeons are better at cutting things out than rebuilding them, and we all love operating.

What a boon it was therefore when Walsh modified Millin's old and rather discredited operation of total retropubic prostatectomy by showing how to stop the bleeding and preserve the nerves and vessels of the penis (Walsh, 1986). The response can only be compared with an evangelical revival. In the USA, the numbers of radical prostatectomies increased sixfold in the 6 years from 1984 (Lu-Yao *et al,* 1993) and a mass search began for cases suitable for the operation.

Within a decade, the indications for the operation had also widened. At first, it was done only for tumours confined to the prostate; next, hormones were given to shrink large tumours until they were operable; finally, in some centres even invasion of the lymph nodes was no longer regarded as a contraindication (Winkler *et al,* 1988) so long as there were not too many secondary tumours, and always supposing someone would pay for the operation.

Patients are easily persuaded by the argument that all cancers start small, so it must be good to get rid of them before they have started to spread. It is difficult to believe that at least 25% of cancers in 70 year olds have been present for at least 20 years (Gleason, 1988) or that cancers do not necessarily progress tamely from A to B to C to D but may stay put or take a short cut (Whitmore, 1988).

Along with the campaign for total prostatectomy usually comes a doom ridden warning of the increase in the incidence of prostatic cancer (Fig. 1). Seldom is it pointed out that this increase in a disease of elderly men is easily explained by the increase in the numbers of men who live to be old (Fig. 2), and by the introduction of prostate specific antigen testing and transrectal ultrasound. In fact, cancer of the prostate causes death in fewer than 0.5% of

Cancer Surveys Volume 23: *Preventing Prostate Cancer: Screening versus Chemoprevention*

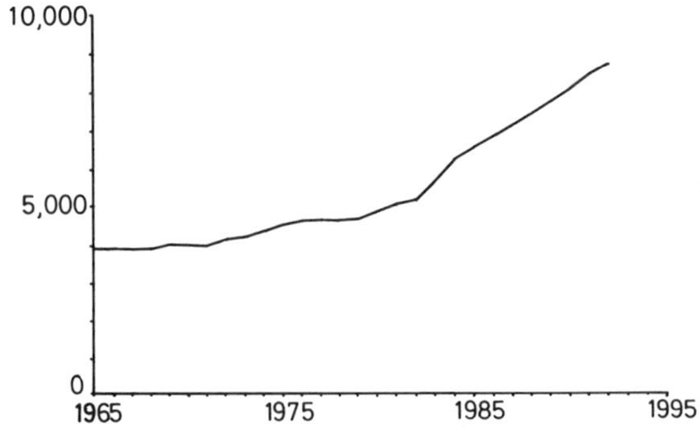

Fig. 1. Cancer of prostate, deaths per annum, England and Wales. Data from Office of Population Census and Surveys

these old men, although more than 30% have cancer (Table 1) (Chodak *et al,* 1994). Indeed, the real question we should be asking is why the other 29.5% do not die.

It is customary to show survival curves of men after radical prostatectomy which are as good as, or even better than, those expected in the same age group, even (in diploid cases) when lymph nodes are involved (Winkler *et al,* 1988). It is rare to point out that these patients are very carefully selected: they are both fit enough to go through a radical prostatectomy and rich enough to have it done in one of the famous centres from which such statistics emanate. It is a different story for US Medicare patients, in whom mortality and morbility are by no means negligible (Lu-Yao *et al,* 1993).

The current enthusiasm for screening for "early" cancer is based on the assumption that radical prostatectomy will save lives. But does it? Wennberg's group have calculated, from a meta-analysis of published studies, that the

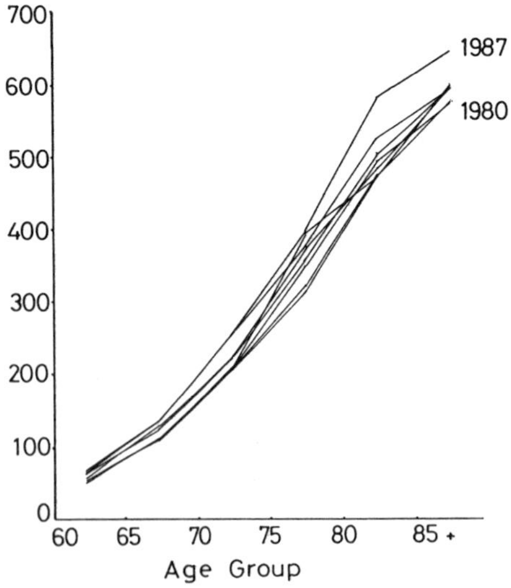

Fig. 2. Cancer of prostate, new registrations per 100 000 population. Data from Office of Population Census and Surveys

TABLE 1. Cancer of prostate[a]

Age group	No of males alive	Deaths from Ca prostate (%)
65–70	1215 000	1325 (0.11)
71–75	784 900	2116 (0.27)
75–80	648 300	2365 (0.41)
81–85	365 700	1545 (0.42)
85+	183 900	873 (0.47)

[a]Office of Population Censuses and Surveys, 1985–1989

results of watchful waiting are better than either total prostatectomy or radiotherapy (Chodak *et al,* 1994), except possibly in the small group of younger patients with undifferentiated cancer:

> In the most optimistic scenario favoring treatment, assuming the highest observed metastatic rate and 100% efficacious treatment, the marginal benefit of treatment for patients with well-differentiated tumors compared with watchful waiting exceeds six months improvement in quality-adjusted life expectancy only for the youngest patients. In all other scenarios treatment for patients with well differentiated tumors results in less than 6 quality-adjusted months and may actually diminish quality-adjusted life expectancy for some patients. (Fleming *et al,* 1993.)

Only a proper prospective randomized trial can adequately compare radical prostatectomy with watchful waiting. In fact, there has been just such a trial, but it has been virtually ignored—I refer to the US Veterans Administration study, whose first report was delayed until 1981 (Byar *et al,* 1981). Paul Madsen, one of the original participants in this VA study, has recently reported the 20 year outcome of this trial. There is still no difference in survival between the treated and untreated groups (Madsen P, personal communication). This is just as one might expect, since radical prostatectomy has not lessened the population based cancer mortality (Lu-Yao *et al,* 1993).

And yet, as a surgeon who has watchfully waited upon all too many patients only to see the cancer spread, I reproach myself with the thought that if only I had cut it out I might have prevented an agonizing death at least in some of my patients. Statistics offer no comfort to the surgeon faced with the individual patient.

We urgently need a way of identifying the small proportion of early confined cancers that are going to spread: "amongst all these kittens, which will become the pussy cats and which will turn into tigers". I hope that the time is not far off when we shall be able to detect the tigers by a marker in blood or urine (Martin *et al,* 1992). In this hope I have been enormously encouraged by what I have learned here in Cambridge at this meeting. And I look forward to the day when there will no longer be any need for the carpenter: instead there will be a kind of genetic Rentokil to reprogram the tiger's genome, and turn it back into a pussy cat.

Is this a pipe dream? It need not be, if only a fraction of the money and effort now spent on screening and radical prostatectomy for localized cancer were diverted to this area of research.

References

Byar DP, Costa DK and Veterans Administration Cooperative Group (1981) VACURG randomised trial of radical prostatectomy for stages I and II prostate cancer. *Urology* **17 (Supplement 4)** 7–11

Chodak GW, Thisted RA, Gerger GS *et al* (1994) Results of conservative management of clinically localised prostate cancer. *New England Journal of Medicine* **330** 242--248

Fleming C, Wasson JH, Albertsen PC, Barry MJ and Wennberg JE for the Prostate Patient Outcomes Research Team (1993) A decision analysis of alternative treatment strategies for clinically localised prostate cancer. *Journal of the American Medical Association* **269** 2650–2658

Fowler FJ, Roman A, Barry MJ, Wasson J, Grace L-Y and Wennberg JE (1993) Patient reported complications and follow up treatment after radical prostatectomy. *Urology* **42** 622–629.

Gleason DF (1988) Histologic grade, clinical stage, and patient age in prostate cancer. *National Cancer Institute Monograph* **7** 15–18

Lu-Yao G, McLennan D, Wasson J and Wennberg JE (1993) An assessment of radical prostatectomy: time trends, geographic variation, and outcome. *Journal of the American Medical Association* **269** 2633–2636

Martin JE, Jenkins BJ, Baithun SI and Blandy JP (1992) The expression of b-HCG and survival in prostatic adenocarcinoma. *Journal of Pathology* **68 (Supplement)**

Walsh PC (1986) Radical retropubic prostatectomy, In: Walsh PC, Gittes RF, Perlmutter AD *et al* (eds). *Campbell's Textbook of Urology*, vol 3, pp 2754–2775, Saunders, Philadelphia

Whitmore WF (1988) Overview: historical and contemporary. *National Cancer Institute Monograph* **7** 7–11

Winkler HZ, Rainwater LM, Myers RP *et al* (1988). Stage D1 prostatic adenocarcinoma: significance of nuclear DNA ploidy patterns studied by flow cytometry. *Mayo Clinic Proceedings* **63** 103–112

The author is responsible for the accuracy of the references.

Surgery from a US Perspective

JEAN B DEKERNION • JOHN R FRANKLIN
ARIE BELLDEGRUN • ROBERT B SMITH
UCLA Division of Urology, Department of Surgery, UCLA School of Medicine, Los Angeles, CA

INTRODUCTION

The incidence of prostate cancer is increasing in the USA, undoubtedly owing partly to increased awareness and the increased use of serum prostate specific antigen (PSA) testing. Simultaneously, the need for any form of definitive therapy is being questioned. The slow progression of many prostate cancers, the primary occurrence in older men and the recognized disparity between the autopsy and the clinical incidence all raise the question of the place of aggressive therapy.

Screening studies by Catalona *et al* (1993) show that tumours can be discovered in early stages, before other clinical suspicion, and that many of these tumours are being detected in young men with greater than a 20 year life expectancy. Although the degree of threat of the tumour to these patients is still unquantified, reason would suggest that removal of the cancer bearing prostate gland in this population would have clinical benefit.

Radical prostatectomy has been the primary method of management of clinically localized prostate cancer in the USA for many years. However, the morbidity of the procedure has dissuaded some from advocating this surgery on a large scale. Anatomical dissection (radical retropubic prostatectomy with dissection of the apex of the prostate and preservation of the neurovascular bundles) (Walsh *et al,* 1987) and further refinements in recent years have greatly reduced the morbidity of the operation, and a better selection of appropriate patients has improved results.

An analysis of the results of radical retropubic prostatectomy at our institution has been reported (Trapasso *et al,* 1994). These results, including a discussion of the value of the serum PSA as an indicator of success or failure of therapy, are discussed below.

Cancer Surveys Volume 23: *Preventing Prostate Cancer: Screening Versus Chemoprevention*

METHODS

The analysis concerns 601 patients who underwent radical retropubic prostatectomy and retroperitoneal lymph node dissection for clinical stages T_1, T_2, N_0 and M_0 treated between 1972 and 1992. Patients who received adjuvant radiotherapy or neoadjuvant hormonal therapy were not included in the analysis. Since the introduction of the Hybritech monoclonal PSA assay, patients have had PSA tested every 6 months as part of their follow-up, in addition to digital rectal examination. Peripheral and central sections of prostatectomy specimens were obtained. In recent years, whole mount sections have been routinely obtained. This has provided accurate pathological staging.

Patients were separated into three groups according to their histopathological findings: group 1—tumour confined to the prostate with no extension into the capsule; group 2—penetration into or through the capsule with or without positive urethral or bladder neck margin; group 3—extension into the seminal vesicles. Tumours were graded according to Gleason's system. Patients whose serum PSA became detectable (above 0.4 ng/ml) were evaluated for clinical metastases, and many underwent ultrasound guided biopsy of the bladder neck and prostatic bed. Patients with a PSA above 0.4 ng/ml were designated chemical failures and presumed to have tumour recurrence.

The time to progression was estimated with the Kaplan-Meier analysis. One standard deviation was used in the Kaplan-Meier estimates. The Cox proportional hazard model was used for group comparisons, with covariate adjustments. The significance of comparisons in groups was measured with the log rank test or the Cox model. The variables examined were interval to any death, interval to death from disease, interval to clinically detectable progression and interval to progression manifested by detectable PSA. Four patients died of unknown causes and were presumed to have died of prostate cancer. Data were analysed for all 601 patients and for a subset of 425 patients operated on since the introduction of anatomical retropubic prostatectomy ("contemporary" series).

RESULTS

The distribution of the clinical staging preoperatively is shown in Table 1. The age of the patients averaged 64.3 years (range 44–80). Follow-up was from 12 to 237 months (median 34 months): 224 patients were followed for more than 5 years and 68 for more than 10 years. For the entire population, the 5 and 10 year all cause (crude) survival rates were 96 ± 1.1(SD)% and 86 ± 3.1(SD)%, respectively. Comparable cause specific survival rates were 98 ± 0.6(SD)% and 94 ± 2.0(SD)%, respectively. Patients were analysed in these groups according to pathological stage (see Methods and Table 2). The respective 5 and 10 year cause specific survival rates were 99 ± 0.7(SD)% and 99 ± 0.7(SD)% for group 1; 100% and 91 ± 0.8(SD)% for group 2; and 93 ± 3.1(SD)% and 89 ± 4.6(SD)% for group 3. Clinical progression occurred in 75 patients, includ-

TABLE 1. Preoperative clinical staging

Stage	No of patients	
T_{1a}	15	(2)
T_{1b}	33	(3)
T_{1c}	114	(19)
T_{2a}	171	(28)
T_{2b}	268	(48)
Total	601	(100)

TABLE 2. Patient characteristics according to degree of tumour extension

	Group 1[a]	Group 2[b]	Group 3[c]
Number of patients	293	215	93
Mean age (years)	62	63	64
Median follow-up (months)	35	34	34

[a]Organ confined tumour
[b]Capsule involved ± positive margin
[c]Positive seminal vesicles

TABLE 3. Probability of survival after radical retropubic prostatectomy according to pathological stage

	Organ confined (%)	Capsule involved (%)	Seminal vesicle extension (%)
Cause specific			
5 years	99	100	93
10 years	99	91	89
Clinical disease free			
5 years	96	89	68
10 years	89	76	60

TABLE 4. Clinical disease free survival (±SD) after radical retropubic prostatectomy

Time of treatment	3 year survival (%)	5 year survival[a] (%)
Before 1987 (n = 176)	86 ± 2.7	79 ± 3.2
1987 onwards (n = 425)	95 + 1.0	94 ± 1.7

[a]Difference in survival 1987 onwards v. pre-1987, $p<0.001$

ing 12 who have died from prostate cancer metastases. Biopsy proven local recurrence was found in 43 patients (7%), 37 of whom underwent external beam radiotherapy. For the entire series, the 5 and 10 year clinical disease free survival rates were 86 ± 2(SD)% and 78 ± 3(SD)%, respectively. The 5 and 10 year clinical disease free survival rates differed among the various pathological groups (Table 3).

The 3 year and 5 year clinical disease free survival for patients treated before 1987 and those treated from 1987 onwards is shown in Table 4. The difference in 5 year survival between the two groups was statistically significant (79 ± 3.2(SD)% v. 94 ± 1.7(SD)%; p=0.001).

A total of 123 patients of the entire group of 601 patients failed by a detectable PSA or by a detectable PSA together with other clinical evidence of tumour recurrence or metastases. The 5 and 10 year non-detectable PSA disease free survivals for the 601 patients were 69 ± 2(SD)% and 47 ± 3(SD)%, respectively. The differences among the three groups were significant: group 1 87% ± 2.6(SD)%; group 2 64 ± 3.2(SD)%; group 3 40 ± 4.8(SD)%. However, in the contemporary series, the 5 year survival of patients with non-detectable PSA levels and no evidence of clinical recurrence was 80 ± 3(SD)%. When the contemporary series was separated into groups, the survival rates were 92 ± 2(SD)% for group 1; 74 ± 3(SD)% for group 2; and 56 ± 3.4(SD)% for group 3.

These data, even in the absence of long term follow-up, show that most patients with organ confined prostate cancer can be cured by radical prostatectomy. The probability of survival is directly influenced by the extent of local tumour extension and is especially adversely affected by invasion of the seminal vesicles. In this study, patients with tumour bearing lymph nodes were excluded from the analysis. It is important to note that a recent study, at our institution and others, has shown that among patients currently being detected with prostate cancer and selected for surgery, the probability of finding a positive lymph node is about 3% (Danella *et al,* 1993). This further supports the value of total prostatectomy.

This study and earlier ones from this institution (Stein *et al,* 1992; Trapasso *et al,* 1994) demonstrate significant differences between non-detectable PSA disease free and clinical disease free survival. The results of recent studies at other centres support this finding (Paulson 1994; Walsh *et al,* 1994; Sincke *et al,* 1994). Furthermore, since the adoption of the anatomical dissection, the disease free survival rates, even considering PSA as an indicator of recurrence, have significantly improved (Trapasso *et al,* 1994). This is also due to better patient selection, possibly as a consequence of tumours being detected in the early stages by serum PSA analysis.

The complications of the operation have gradually decreased in incidence, probably as a result of a better understanding of the apical anatomy and the mechanisms of continence (Andriole *et al,* 1994, Walsh *et al,* 1994). Severe incontinence occurs in fewer than 2% of patients, and stress incontinence has been reported in fewer than 20% (Catalona and Basler, 1993). In selected patients, sparing the corporal nerves results in preservation of potency (Walsh,

1987). The mortality rate at our institution and in other large series varies from 0% to 0.5%. The economic burden of the operation has also remarkably reduced. Combined with a decreased surgical time, reduction in blood loss and blood replacement with autologous blood and use of the non-narcotic analgesic ketorolac, the mean hospital stay at our institution has been reduced to 3 days. Further refinements in the apical dissection have also reduced the time to control of urinary continence after removal of the catheter.

DISCUSSION

The detection of localized prostate cancer will continue to increase as PSA becomes more widely used and as patient awareness improves. A major issue for the future is to define those patients who need treatment and those who will benefit from definitive therapy.

In broad terms, this will probably represent patients with a long life expectancy who have more than 1 cm tumour volume but without very well differentiated malignant potential. In the meantime, further refinement in the technique of radical prostatectomy, with the attendant decreased morbidity, provides a strong argument for this method of intervention. The PIVOT studies sponsored by the US Veteran Administration hospitals will soon begin recruiting patients. This trial will randomize patients of all ages to receive either prostatectomy or observation only and perhaps will better define the impact of treatment. While these results are awaited, many patients will present with prostate cancer, in whom the tumour will threaten their longevity. While we better define this population, we believe that radical prostatectomy remains an effective and worthwhile treatment for many patients with prostate cancer.

SUMMARY

Prostate screening has made it possible to detect organ confined prostate carcinoma in men with a life expectancy of 20 years and longer. These clinically significant malignancies may be successfully eradicated by means of anatomical dissection of the prostate, which minimizes both morbidity and mortality. In a retrospective series of patients with clinically localized prostate cancer who were treated with a radical retropubic prostatectomy and lymph node dissection, 5 and 10 year crude survival rates were 96% and 86%. Survival was compromised by penetration of tumour through the prostatic capsule, and even more significantly by involvement of the seminal vesicles. The use of prostate specific antigen (PSA) concentrations to monitor disease progression before any clinical manifestation revealed that disease free survival was less than previously reported. Patients diagnosed and treated more recently had longer disease free survival than the overall group mainly because of earlier detection with PSA, with consequent lower tumour volumes and stage. In addition, 92 ± 3(SD)% patients with pathologically organ confined tumours, without capsular or seminal vesicle invasion, are clinically disease free with non-detectable PSA at 5 years. Our data therefore show that radical prostatectomy can cure patients with organ confined prostate cancer, with acceptable morbidity. Although the need for cure may be questioned in many patients, young patients with prostate cancer almost certainly benefit from eradication of the malignancy.

References

Andriole GL, Smith DS, Rao G, Goodnough L and Catalona WJ (1994) Early complications of contemporary anatomical radical retropubic prostatectomy. *Journal of Urology* **152** 1858–1860

Catalona WJ and Basler JW (1993) Return of erections and urinary continence following nerve sparing radical retropubic prostatectomy. *Journal of Urology* **150** 905–907

Catalona WJ, Smith DS, Ratcliff TL and Basler JW (1993) Detection of organ confined prostate cancer is increased through prostate-specific antigen-based screening. *Journal of the American Medical Association* **270** 948–954

Danella JF, deKernion JB, Smith RB and Steckel J (1993) The contemporary incidence of lymph node metastases in prostate cancer: implications for laparoscopic lymph node dissection. *Journal of Urology* **149** 1488–1491

Paulson DF (1994) Impact of radical prostatectomy in the management of clinically localized disease. *Journal of Urology* **152** 1826–1830

Stein A, deKernion JB, Smith RB, Dorey F and Patel H (1992) Prostate specific antigen levels and radical prostatectomy in patients with organ confined and locally extensive prostate cancer. *Journal of Urology* **147** 942–946

Trapasso JG, deKernion JB, Smith RB and Dorey F (1994) The incidence and significance of detectable levels of serum prostate specific antigen after radical prostatectomy. *Journal of Urology* **152** 1821–1825

Walsh PC (1987) Radical prostatectomy, preservation of sexual function, cancer control. *Urological Clinics of North America* **14** 663–673

Walsh PC, Partin AW and Epstein JI (1994) Cancer control and quality of life following anatomical radical retropubic prostatectomy: results at 10 years. *Journal of Urology* **152** 1831–1836

Zincke H, Oesterling JE, Blute ML, Bergstralh EJ, Myers RP and Barrett DM (1994) Long-term (15 years) results after radical prostatectomy for clinically localized (stage T2c or lower) prostate cancer. *Journal of Urology* **152** 1850–1857

The authors are responsible for the accuracy of the references.

A Patient's Perspective

CLIVE BOURNE
Prostate Cancer Trust, Purlieu House, 11 Station Road, Epping, Essex CM16 4HA

To be told that one has cancer is devastating; to be diagnosed as having prostate cancer is even worse because it has the spectres of cancer in general coupled with taboos that are whispered in dark corners—incontinence, impotence and, possibly, castration. How can this information be absorbed, much worse passed onto one's family and colleagues? In my own case, I took nearly 6 months to tell my children the facts of what I had been confronted with. It is obviously a matter for the most delicate and sensitive counselling. Having, at the time of my initial diagnosis, been given only 5–8 months to live, I reappraised my blessings—a beautiful wife and four wonderful daughters—promptly sought a second opinion and lived to tell the tale.

Having spent a busy and satisfying working life that involved immersing myself in each new phase of work and developing new skills and activities as a contributor to each success, I was determined to apply the same principles to my own situation as soon as initial fears and shock had been confronted. I quickly realized the magnitude of this problem and the sheer ignorance surrounding it, particularly among the general public but also among doctors.

The problem of prostate cancer is compounded by our social habits and taboos, as men find it difficult to discuss their sexual organs and genital problems, unlike women, whose education has been much expanded by the breast and cervical cancer screening programmes. A cost effective, comprehensive and early screening and prevention programme with consequent widespread publicity would be a vital start to improving a disastrous record of the disease. At the moment, most men know little about it, try to ignore it, or hear it as an aside, often in the men's room, with an emphasis on the disastrous side effects of surgical treatment.

The benefit of eating carrots as a way to reduce the risk of prostate cancer now seems fairly clear from a paper included in this volume. Equally better health education for males from the time of puberty would not go amiss. Although I understand that screening is not universally accepted because of its limited diagnostic precision, I think it needs to be a target, an emphasis on the search for better ways of identifying those with a higher risk. As for new treatment, it seems that, although there are no promises of miracle cures, progress is being made, particularly in reducing the barbarity of the treatment. From the viewpoint of the patient, this has to be progress.

Cancer Surveys Volume 23: *Preventing Prostate Cancer: Screening versus Chemoprevention*

Biographical Notes

Jan Adolfsson, MD, PhD, is associate professor in urology at the Karolinska Institute, Stockholm, and on the staff of the department of urology at Karolinska Hospital.

PRF Bell is professor of surgery at the University of Leicester. His major research interests are vascular surgery and transplantation. Professor Bell has been head of the department of surgery since its inception in 1974.

Arie S Belldegrun, MD, graduated from the Harvard University programme in urology in 1985. From 1985 to 1988 he served as a surgical oncology fellow in the surgery branch at the National Cancer Institute/National Institutes of Health under Dr Steven Rosenberg. In 1988 he joined the faculty at the UCLA School of Medicine. His research focuses on the development of novel immunotherapeutic approaches to kidney and prostate cancers, including gene and vaccine therapy. His main interest is urological oncology, including cancers of the kidney, prostate, bladder and testes. He is a professor of surgery/urology, chief of urology at Olive View/UCLA Medical Center, co-director of the oncology programme at the Jonsson Comprehensive Cancer Center, director of the UCLA Kidney Cancer Program and clinical director of the UCLA Prostate Disease Research Program.

John P Blandy graduated from Oxford University after clinical training at The Royal London and St Peter's Hospitals in London. He was appointed professor of urology at The Royal London Hospital in 1968 and retired in 1992. He is vice-president of the Royal College of Surgeons and past president of the British Association of Urological Surgeons and the European Association of Urology.

Sir Walter Bodmer, director-general of the Imperial Cancer Research Fund, read mathemetatics at Cambridge University and went on to do a PhD in population genetics. He spent nine years at Stanford University, California, working with Joshua Lederberg, before taking up an appointment as professor of genetics at Oxford University in 1970. In 1979 he became director of research at the Imperial Cancer Research Fund and was appointed director-general in 1991. He is also chairman of the Committee on the Public Understanding of Science and president of the International Human Genome Organization. His research interests centre on the expression of HLA determinants in cancer and the genetics and biology of the epithelial cells in the colon from which the majority of colorectal adenocarcinomas are derived.

David G Bostwick, MD, is a diagnostic surgical pathologist whose main interest is in early detection of prostate cancer. He graduated from the University of Maryland in 1979 and completed his training at Stanford University, California. He has held faculty positions at the Universities of Chicago and Maryland, including chairman of pathology at Mercy Medical Center, Baltimore (1986–1991). He has published two books and more than 100 articles, including recent reports on the prognostic significance of tumour volume in prostate cancer. Dr Bostwick is editor-in-chief of the *Journal of Urologic Pathology* and treasurer of the international society of urologic pathology.

Clive J Bourne, unlike the other contributors to this volume, has no qualifications except from the University of Life. He left school at age 14 and founded his own freight forwarding company at 17, having learned the business the hard way in London's docklands. His courier, airports and commercial property group, Seabourne, has won two Queen's awards for export and is now established throughout Europe and the Far East. He is also a lay magistrate and a trustee of the proposed Docklands Museum. He was diagnosed with prostate cancer three years ago and given 9–12 months to live. He immersed himself in the subject, sought other opinions and with treatment has confounded his initial prognosis. He recognized the need for more information and exchanges, hence his efforts in promoting the Cambridge forum.

G Steven Bova received his MD degree in 1984 from Cornell University Medical College, New York, and carried out his urology training at the University of Virginia. He is an assistant professor in the department of urology at the Johns Hopkins School of Medicine, Baltimore.

Harold J Brenner, MB, ChB, FRCR, is chief of oncology at Sheba Medical Center and associate professor of oncology and chairman of the section of oncology at Tel-Aviv University.

James D Brooks received his MD degree from Stanford University in 1988 and is finishing the urology residency programme at Johns Hopkins, Baltimore.

MJG Bussemakers received her PhD degree from the department of biochemistry, University of Nijmegen, The Netherlands, in 1992. She is director of molecular biology in the urology research laboratory in Nijmegen.

Bernard Candas received his biomedical engineering degree in 1981 from Université de Compiègne (France) and received a PhD in physiology from Laval University (Canada) in 1989. With his experience in data analysis and statistics he became systems manager and consultant in biostatistics at the clinical investigation unit of Ottawa Civic Hospital while in postdoctoral training at the Loeb Medical Research Institute from 1989 to 1992. He then joined the CHUL Research Center (Québec City, Canada), where he has been studying the pharmacokinetics of conversion of C19 steroids in peripheral tissues and their modulation by pituitary hormones using techniques of mathematical modelling.

Leland WK Chung obtained his PhD at the University of Oregon Medical School and trained at Johns Hopkins University School of Medicine and the James Buchanan Brady Urological Institute, Johns Hopkins Hospital, under Professor Donald S Coffey. He is professor of urology, biochemistry and molecular biology, and director of the urology research laboratory at the University of Texas MD Anderson Cancer Center. His major research interests include the mechanisms of mesenchymal-epithelial interaction in genitourinary cancers, the role of bone and prostate stroma in prostate cancer metastasis and gene regulation and therapy of urological tumours.

Pejman Cohan received his bachelor's degree in biochemistry from the University of California, Los Angeles. He is currently a fourth year medical student at UCLA. His research interests in oncology have led to work with Dr Owen Witte on the mechanism of transformation of the *BCR-ABL* oncogene and Dr Arie Belldegrun on the target specific gene therapy of prostate cancer.

Lionel Cusan graduated in medicine at Laval University in Québec City after obtaining a PhD in physiology. His major interests are clinical endocrinology and hormone dependent cancers. In 1987 he joined the laboratory of molecular endocrinology at Laval University Medical Center (CHUL), working on the development of the concept of total androgen blockade for the treatment of advanced prostate cancer and the establishment of a prostate cancer screening programme. He currently lectures in endocrinology at Laval University and is head of the hormonal treatment clinic at CHUL.

Jack Cuzick is head of the department of mathematics, statistics and epidemiology at the Imperial Cancer Research Fund in London. He holds a PhD in mathematics and statistics, and previously worked at Columbia University in New York and at Oxford University. His current interests are cancer epidemiology and clinical trials, with special interest in prevention and screening. He is currently chairman of the Tamoxifen Breast Cancer Trial Working Party and is involved in studies on the use of smear based human papillomavirus assays for cervical screening and flexible sigmoidoscopy for colorectal cancer screening. He has a longstanding interest in multiple myeloma and has conducted case-control studies, international mortality studies and prognostic factor studies for this disease.

Edward DeAntoni received MA and PhD degrees from Cornell University. After teaching appointments at Cornell and Boston College, he entered government service in public health. Most recently, he initiated and directed the cancer control programme at the Colorado Department of Health. He was research director for the Cancer Center of Porter Memorial Hospital in Denver before being appointed to the division of urology at the University of Colorado Health Sciences Center.

Jean B deKernion, MD, graduated from Louisiana State University School of Medicine and trained in surgery and urology at the National Cancer Institute, Bethesda, and the University Hospitals of Cleveland, Case Western Reserve University. He moved to the University of California at Los Angeles in 1973 and to Tulane University in 1978, developing urological oncology programmes in each. He returned to UCLA as head of urological oncology in 1982 and became professor and chief of urology in 1985. He is also head of the urological oncology section and director of the genitourinary oncology programme of the Jonsson Comprehensive Cancer Center at UCLA. He is a member of the American Association of Genitourinary Surgeons, the Clinical Society of Genitourinary Surgeons and the American Board of Urology and past president of the Society for Urologic Oncology and the Los Angeles Urologic Society.

Pierre Diamond completed his MD and PhD at Laval University (Québec City) in 1990. His major research interests during his graduate studies in physiology have been hormonal control and on the role of the autonomic nervous system in thermogenesis and in diabetes and metabolism. He joined the laboratory of molecular endocrinology in 1992, where he works in the field of hormone dependent cancer and clinical endocrinology. Since 1993 he has been associate professor of physiology at the school of medicine, Laval University.

Charles Ewing received his BS degree from the University of Maryland in 1992 and is in the masters of science programme at Johns Hopkins University, Baltimore.

Mark R Feneley, MA, FRCS, is a urological research registrar in the department of urology, St Bartholomew's Hospital, London.

Yves Fradet, MD, FRCSC, graduated from Laval University (Québec, Canada) in 1981. After specializing in urology, he spent two and a half years at the Memorial Sloan-Kettering Cancer Center in New York, where he acquired further specialized training in urological oncology and research. Since 1983 he has been head of the research laboratory at Laval University Cancer Research Center at the Hôtel-Dieu de Québec Hospital, where he is also director of the urological oncology section.

John Franklin is a clinical urology oncology fellow at the University of Californa, Los Angeles (UCLA), School of Medicine. He received his medical degree from Columbia University in 1988 and completed his general urology training, also at Columbia University, in 1994. He will continue his studies at UCLA as a research fellow to explore the feasibility of gene therapy in the management of prostate cancer.

LM Franks graduated in medicine at the University of Durham in 1942. After service as a medical officer to an armoured division, he trained in pathology at the Prince of Wales and London Hospitals. In 1951 he joined the new clinical pathological laboratories of ICRF. After working at the Strangeways Research Laboratories in Cambridge and at the Johns Hopkins Hospital, Baltimore, he headed the new department of cellular pathology at ICRF and is now senior consultant scientist and consulting editor of *Cancer Surveys*. His research interests have been in prostate and bladder cancer, ageing and tumour metastasis.

CJ Gallagher, MD, PhD, graduated from the University of Auckland School of Medicine, New Zealand, in 1974 and undertook postgraduate research with Dr Mike Crumpton at the ICRF, receiving his PhD in 1986. He trained in oncology at St Bartholomew's and the Royal Marsden

Hospitals and was appointed senior lecturer and honorary consultant in medical oncology at The Royal London Hospital in 1990. His research interests are in gynaecological tumours and endocrine therapy of cancer.

José-Luis Gomez is a graduate of Cuyo National University, Argentina. His major research interests have been in the field of prognostic factors of prostate cancer and its favourable modification by the use of combined anti-androgen treatments. After graduating in medicine, as a holder of an NCI Terry Fox scholarship, he spent 1982 to 1985 at the Manitoba Cancer Foundation, Winnipeg. His early work was on tumour immunology and on the chemotactic and killing properties of natural killer cells. He joined Laval University Hospital Research Center in 1989, where he carries out clinical trials of hormone dependent neoplasms.

Terry Horsburgh graduated from London University in 1969 and obtained his PhD at the Institute of Urology, London, in 1974 on the effect of ischaemia on kidney function in transplantation. After working at the University of Florida, he joined Professor Brent at St Mary's Hospital Medical School, London, to investigate the induction of transplant unresponsiveness. He joined the department of surgery at Leicester University and is currently senior clinical scientist and lecturer in transplant immunology, with responsibility for clinical laboratory support for the renal and islet transplant programme. His research interest is the immunological basis of transplantation and cancer, especially prostate and gastrointestinal cancers, and its therapeutic manipulation.

William B Isaacs received his PhD from the department of pharmacology and experimental therapeutics of the Johns Hopkins University School of Medicine in 1984 under the guidance of Dr Donald Coffey. From then until 1988 he was a postdoctoral fellow with Dr Alice Fulton of the department of biochemistry at the University of Iowa. He is an associate professor of urology and oncology in the Johns Hopkins University School of Medicine. His primary interest is the molecular biology of tumours of the genitourinary tract.

Elijah O Kehinde, FRCS, graduated from the Medical School, University of Ibadan, Nigeria. He has had clinical training in urology and renal transplantation at University College Hospital of Ibadan, the Institute of Urology, London, and Leicester General Hospital. In 1986–1987 he was awarded the European development fellowship. He is a fellow of the Royal College of Surgeons of England, fellow of the College of Surgeons of Nigeria and a diplomate of the Institute of Urology, London. Currently he is research fellow and registrar in the university departments of surgery and urology at Leicester. His research interests have been in urological and postrenal transplant cancers. Since 1991 he has been carrying out in vitro and in vivo experiments on growth factor inhibitors involved in the progression of hormone resistant prostate cancer.

Timothy Key studied veterinary medicine at Edinburgh University. After working in a small animal practice he obtained an MSc in nutrition and a DPhil in cancer epidemiology. He has worked for the ICRF since 1985 and his main interests are the roles of diet and sex hormones in the aetiology of cancers of the breast and prostate.

Michael G Kirby, MB, BS, MRCS, MRCP, is a general practitioner in Letchworth, Hertfordshire.

Roger S Kirby, MA, MD, FRCS(Urol), is consultant urological surgeon in the department of urology, St Bartholomew's Hospital, London.

David Kirk is a consultant urologist at the Western Infirmary in Glasgow and honorary clinical senior lecturer at Glasgow University. He graduated in medicine from Oxford University. He is a member of the Prostate Cancer Working Party of the Medical Research Council, for whom he is co-ordinating a study comparing immediate versus deferred hormonal treatment for prostatic cancer. He is also chairman of the Prostate Forum and has been particularly active in the promotion of shared care between urologist and general practitioner in managing prostate disease. His main interest is urological oncology.

Fernand Labrie is director of research at the Laval University Medical Center in Québec City. After graduating in medicine and doing internship and residency in internal medicine at Laval University, he received his PhD in endocrinology under the direction of late Professor Claude Fortier at Laval University in 1966. He then pursued postdoctoral training in the department of biochemistry at the University of Cambridge in the laboratory of the late Professor Asher Korner and was visiting fellow at Churchill College. He then trained under Professor Frederick Sanger in the laboratory of molecular biology in Cambridge, where he purified the first mammalian messenger RNA, namely rabbit haemoglobin messenger RNA. In 1969 he founded the laboratory of molecular endocrinology in Québec City and has been its director since. His research interests have been centred on the mechanisms of regulation of the pituitary–gonadal axis, LHRH agonists, prostate cancer, breast cancer and the formation and regulation of sex steroids in peripheral intracrine tissues.

Martin Lemay, FRCPSC, is a graduate of Laval University. He is head of the laboratory of anatomo-pathology at Laval University Medical Center and his research interests are centred on prostate cancer.

Tom McNicholas, MB, BS, FRCS, is consultant urological surgeon, department of urology, Lister Hospital, Stevenage, UK.

Alison McLean, MRCP, DMRD, FRCR, is consultant radiologist, department of diagnostic radiology, St Bartholomew's Hospital, London.

Natu Mistry graduated in biochemistry and pharmacology in 1974 and received the MPhil at the University of Leicester in 1982, investigating immune responses to heart allograft rejection. He is currently involved in developing a tissue culture programme and drug monitoring assays in the department of surgery, Leicester General Hospital.

Ronald A Morton received his MD degree from Johns Hopkins in 1986 then trained in the urology residency programme at Johns Hopkins. He is an assistant professor in the department of urology at Baylor College of Medicine in Houston, Texas.

DWW Newling is head of the department of urology, Free University Hospital, Amsterdam. He is also a member of the board and council of the European Organization for Research on Treatment of Cancer (EORTC) and former chairman of the EORTC genitourinary group.

Benedict Nussbaum, MD, is senior oncologist at Sheba Medical Center with a main interest in urological oncology.

Kenji Oishi, a graduate of Kyoto University, worked for three years with Professor FH Schroeder in Rotterdam, where his major interest was the epithelial-stromal interaction in prostate tissue. After returning to Kyoto University he joined the case-control study on prostate cancer carried out in both Japan and the Netherlands. He is now an associate professor, his research interest being growth factors in prostate tissue.

RTD Oliver, MD, graduated from the University of Cambridge and The London Hospital in 1966. He undertook postgraduate research on HLA and transplantation immunology with Hilliard Festenstein and received an MD in 1974. He trained in oncology with Gordon Hamilton-Fairley at St Bartholomew's Hospital and in urology with John Blandy at St Peter's Hospital and the Institute of Urology. He is currently on the staff of The Royal Hospitals Trust and is professor in medical oncology at The Royal London Hospital Medical College. He runs a clinical research unit carrying out research in urological tumours with a special interest in germ cell tumours and the immunology of cancer.

Hardev Pandha, MRCP, is a senior registrar in in medical oncology at the Hammersmith Hospital, London. He is currently working on a PhD thesis in molecular biology.

Shen Pang received his PhD in molecular biology from Albert Einstein College of Medicine, Yeshiva University, New York, in 1987. He then joined the laboratory of Dr Irvin Chen, UCLA

School of Medicine, Los Angeles, as a postdoctural fellow. In 1992, he was appointed assistant professor in the division of urology, UCLA School of Medicine, Los Angeles.

Carol Parkes graduated in medicine at St Bartholomew's Hospital in 1985. She has been working in epidemiology and public health medicine since 1989, both at the City and Hackney Health Authority and at the Wolfson Institute of Preventive Medicine, part of St Bartholomew's Hospital Medical School. Her research interests have mainly been in cancer screening.

Peter Rath, MD, is senior oncologist at Sheba Medical Center with a main interest in urological oncology.

Peter Rosen is director of the solid oncology program at the University of California at Los Angeles and runs the lymphoma clinic and lymphoma conferences. He is also co-director of the prostate clinic with Dr Belldegrun.

Davinder P Sandhu, MD, graduated from the Royal Free Hospital, London University, in 1980 and received his surgical training in Leicester. He obtained the fellowships of the Royal College of Surgeons of Edinburgh and of Glasgow. He completed his urological training in Manchester and Nottingham. His current post is consultant urological surgeon at the Leicester General Hospital Trust, with research interests in prostate cancer.

Fritz H Schroeder is a chairman and professor at Erasmus University, Rotterdam. He trained in urology at the University of California, Los Angeles. His early work on cell culture of prostate cancer contributed to the establishment of a cell line and a tumour line of prostate cancer. He now also holds an appointment in urology within the European Community.

Hans-Peter Schmid received an MD degree from the University of Zurich Medical School in 1984. Since 1989 he has been resident in urology in the division of urology, University of Basel, Switzerland. In 1990–1991 he was research fellow in urology at the department of urology, Stanford University, California.

Freddy Sitas graduated from the University of the Witwatersrand in 1980, joined the department of sociology at the University of the Witwatersrand as a research officer on health and safety in the foundry industry in 1982 and moved to the epidemiology unit of the South African National Centre for Occupational Health in 1983. In 1987 he joined the ICRF Cancer Epidemiology Unit as a DPhil research student, working on the association between *Helicobacter pylori* and stomach cancer. Since 1990 he has been head of the South African National Cancer Registry. His research interests include the associations between HIV, other infections and cancer, adult health in developing countries and disease surveillance.

Philip Smith is head of the department of urology at St James's Hospital, Leeds. His major research interests have included malignant disease of the urinary tract over the past 20 years. He was co-founder and first chairman of the Urology Group of the European Organization of Research on Treatment of Cancer (EORTC) and chairman of the MRC Urological Working Party for several years.

Robert B Smith, MD, is a professor of surgery/urology at the University of California at Los Angeles and a past chief of staff of the UCLA Medical Center. He graduated from the UCLA School of Medicine in 1963 and took residency training in urology and general surgery at UCLA, completing this in 1969. He is also chief of urology at the Wadsworth Veterans' Administration Hospital. His interests are urological oncology and reconstructive urology.

E Raul Suburu is visiting professor at Laval University. He is a graduate of El Salvador University, Argentina. He trained in diagnostic radiology and since 1988 has focused on early detection of cancer using innovative modalities of imaging and tumour markers. He trained with Dr Fred Lee at St Joseph Mercy Hospital, Ann Arbor, Michigan, in transrectal ultrasound of the prostate and needle biopsy. He carries out a screening programme for prostate cancer.

Samir S Taneja, MD, is a senior resident in urology at the University of California, Los Angeles. He received both undergraduate and medical degrees from Northwestern University,

Chicago, Illinois. His research efforts have focused on the molecular biology of prostate cancer, with a current interest in gene therapy for cancer.

Timothy R Terry, MD, FRCS, graduated from St George's Hospital, London University and completed his surgical and urological training in London and Leeds. His present post is consultant urological surgeon at the Leicester General Hospital Trust. His main interests are urological oncology and reconstructive surgery.

Bernard Têtu graduated in medicine in 1979 and in pathology in 1984 at Laval University. He trained in electron microscopy in Bonn, Germany, in 1983 and in 1986 completed a two year fellowship in oncological pathology at the University of Texas MD Anderson Cancer Center, Houston. He is associate professor of pathology at Laval University and holds a research clinical scholarship from le Fonds de la Recherche en Santé du Québec. His main fields of research are urological pathology and breast cancer.

Thomas Tichler, MD, is deputy chief of oncology and chief of the oncology section at Sheba Medical Center.

Jonathan Waxman, FRCP, is reader in oncology at the Hammersmith Hospital, London. His research interests are hormones and cancer, and urological malignancy.

Judy A W Webb, BSc, MD, FRCP, FRCR, is a consultant radiologist in the department of diagnostic radiology at St Bartholomew's Hospital, London.

George Wilding, MD, is associate professor of human oncology at the University of Wisconsin Comprehensive Cancer Center. He received an MD from the University of Massachusetts in 1980, performing his internship and residency in internal medicine at the University of Massachusetts Medical Center. His medical oncology training was at the National Cancer Institute in the breast cancer section under Marc Lippman until 1988, when he moved to the University of Wisconsin. His clinical research is in the field of experimental therapeutics, and his laboratory focuses on the growth control of human prostate cancer and prostate carcinogenesis.

Peter Wrigley qualified in medicine at Oxford in 1964 and then worked at St Batholomew's Hospital with the late Sir Ronald Bodley-Scott. He obtained his PhD there before returning to clinical work with Professor Paul Beeson in Oxford. He returned to St Bartholomew's Hospital in 1971 and was appointed to the staff in 1974. The development of the Solid Tumour Cancer Service in the 1970s and 1980s was under his direction. He was a founder member, secretary and chairman of the British Stomach Cancer Group. He has been a member of several Medical Research Council cancer committees.

Osamu Yoshida, a graduate of Kyoto University, majored in chemical carcinogenesis of the urinary bladder. He is chairman and professor of the department of urology, Kyoto University. One of his major research interests is the molecular biology of urogenital cancers.

Index

LIST OF PREVIOUS ISSUES

VOLUME 1 1982

No. 1: Inheritance of Susceptibility to Cancer in Man
Guest Editor: W F Bodmer

No. 2: Maturation and Differentiation in Leukaemias
Guest Editor: M F Greaves

No. 3: Experimental Approaches to Drug Targeting
Guest Editors: A J S Davies and M J Crumpton

No. 4: Cancers Induced by Therapy
Guest Editor: I Penn

VOLUME 2 1983

No. 1: Embryonic & Germ Cell Tumours in Man and Animals
Guest Editor: R L Gardner

No. 2: Retinoids and Cancer
Guest Editor: M B Sporn

No. 3: Precancer
Guest Editor: J J DeCosse

No. 4: Tumour Promotion and Human Cancer
Guest Editors: T J Slaga and R Montesano

VOLUME 3 1984

No. 1: Viruses in Human and Animal Cancers
Guest Editors: J Wyke and R Weiss

No. 2: Gene Regulation in the Expression of Malignancy
Guest Editor: L Sachs

No. 3: Consistent Chromosomal Aberrations and Oncogenes in Human Tumours
Guest Editor: J D Rowley

No. 4: Clinical Management of Solid Tumours in Childhood
Guest Editor: T J McElwain

VOLUME 4 1985

No. 1: Tumour Antigens in Experimental and Human Systems
Guest Editor: L W Law

No. 2: Recent Advances in the Treatment and Research in Lymphoma and Hodgkin's Disease
Guest Editor: R Hoppe

No. 3: Carcinogenesis and DNA Repair
Guest Editor: T Lindahl

No. 4: Growth Factors and Malignancy
Guest Editors: A B Roberts and M B Sporn

VOLUME 5 1986

No. 1: Drug Resistance
Guest Editors: G Stark and H Calvert

No. 2: Biochemical Mechanisms of Oncogene Activity: Proteins Encoded by Oncogenes
Guest Editors: H E Varmus and J M Bishop

No. 3: Hormones and Cancer: 90 Years after Beatson
Guest Editor: R D Bulbrook

No. 4: Experimental, Epidemiological and Clinical Aspects of Liver Carcinogenesis
Guest Editor: E Farber

VOLUME 6 1987

No. 1: Naturally Occurring Tumours in Animals as a Model for Human Disease
Guest Editors: D Onions and W Jarrett

No. 2: New Approaches to Tumour Localization
Guest Editor: K Britton

No. 3: Psychological Aspects of Cancer
Guest Editor: S Greer

No. 4: Diet and Cancer
Guest Editors: C Campbell and L Kinlen

VOLUME 7 1988

No. 1: Pain and Cancer
Guest Editor: G W Hanks

No. 2: Somatic Cell Genetics and Cancer
Guest Editor: L M Franks

No. 3: Prospects for Primary and Secondary Prevention of Cervix Cancer
Guest Editors: G Knox and C Woodman

No. 4: Tumour Progression and Metastasis
Guest Editor: I Hart

VOLUME 8 1989

No. 1: Colorectal Cancer
Guest Editor: J Northover

No. 2: Nitrate, Nitrite and Nitroso Compounds in Human Cancer
Guest Editors: D Forman and D E G Shuker

No. 3: A Critical Assessment of Cancer Chemotherapy
Guest Editor: A H Calvert

No. 4: Biological Response Modifiers
Guest Editors: F R Balkwill and W Fiers

VOLUME 9 1990

No. 1: Haemopoietic Growth Factors: Their Role in the Treatment of Cancer
Guest Editor: M Dexter

No. 2: Germ Cell Tumours of the Testis: A Clinico-Pathological Perspective
Guest Editors: P Andrews and T Oliver

No. 3: Genetics and Cancer— Part I
Guest Editors: W Cavenee, B Ponder and E Solomon

No. 4: Genetics and Cancer— Part II
Guest Editors: W Cavenee, B Ponder and E Solomon

VOLUME 10 1991

Cancer, HIV and AIDS
Guest Editors: V Beral, H W Jaffe and R A Weiss

VOLUME 11 1991

Prostate Cancer: Cell and Molecular Mechanisms in Diagnosis and Treatment
Guest Editor: J T Isaacs

VOLUME 12 1992

Tumour Suppressor Genes, the Cell Cycle and Cancer
Guest Editor: A J Levine

VOLUME 13 1992

A New Look at Tumour Immunology
Guest Editors: A J McMichael and W F Bodmer

VOLUME 14 1992

Growth Regulation by Nuclear Hormone Receptors
Guest Editor: M G Parker

VOLUME 15 1992

Oncogenes in the Development of Leukaemia
Guest Editor: O N Witte

VOLUME 16 1993

The Molecular Pathology of Cancer
Guest Editors: N R Lemoine and N A Wright

VOLUME 17 1993

Pharmacokinetics and Cancer Chemotherapy
Guest Editors: P Workman and M A Graham

VOLUME 18 1993

Breast Cancer
Guest Editors: I S Fentiman and J Taylor-Papadimitriou

VOLUME 19/20 1994

Trends in Cancer Incidence and Mortality
Guest Editors: R Doll, J F Fraumeni Jr and C S Muir

VOLUME 21 1994

Palliative Medicine: Problem Areas in Pain and Symptom Management
Guest Editor: G W Hanks

VOLUME 22 1995

Molecular Mechanisms of the Immune Response
Guest Editors: W F Bodmer and M J Owen